H. Yasuda · H. Kawaguchi (Eds.)

New Aspects in the Treatment of Failing Heart

With 100 Figures Including 1 in Color

Springer-Verlag
Tokyo Berlin Heidelberg New York London
Paris Hong Kong Barcelona Budapest

Dr. Hisakazu Yasuda, Emeritus Professor
Dr. Hideaki Kawaguchi

Department of Cardiovascular Medicine
Hokkaido University School of Medicine
N-15, W-7 Sapporo 060 Japan

ISBN-13:978-4-431-68221-9 e-ISBN-13:978-4-431-68219-6
DOI: 10.1007/978-4-431-68219-6

Printed on acid-free paper

Softcover reprint of the hardcover 1st edition 1992

Preface

I am delighted to welcome all of the participants to the satellite symposium of the 14th International Society of Heart Research (ISHR) in Sapporo. I would like to thank all participants for their interest and effort in helping us make this symposium possible, especially those who have travelled long distances to be here with us. It is a real honor and privilege for us to host this meeting and invite our colleagues to Sapporo. Since the ISHR in Japan approved the decision to hold this symposium in Sapporo 2 years ago, our members have exerted their utmost efforts in planning and organizing a substantial program to look into the pathogenesis and treatment of heart failure from new viewpoints. Here, I would like to list the names of these members and express my sincere appreciation for their cooperation: Drs. S. Onodera and T. Abiko from Asahikawa; Drs. H. Saito, A. Kitabatake, M. Kanno, M. Minami, H. Kawaguchi, T. Kohya, and H. Okamoto from Sapporo; and all members of ISHR in Sapporo and the Japan Heart Foundation.

With regards to the purpose of this symposium, "New Aspects in the Treatment of Failing Heart", I would like to mention our thoughts very briefly. Heart failure is a syndrome that occurs because of myocardial failure following work overload such as hypertension, valvular diseases, myocardial ischemia, and inflammation, as well as unknown etiologies such as cardiomyopathy. With the development of heart failure, various mechanisms compensating for the reduction in cardiac performance may be mobilized to maintain the cardiovascular homeostasis. Well-known compensatory mechanisms in heart failure include cardiac enlargement in Frank-Starling mechanisms, cardiac hypertrophy, increased heart rate, and increased activity of a series of neurohormonal factors, such as sympathetic nerve activity catecholamines, the renin-angiotensin-aldosterone system, the vasopressin system, atrium natriuretic peptide, and prostaglandins. These factors serve to optimize preload and afterload in heart failure, to increase myocardial contractility, to maintain arterial blood pressure and organ blood flow, and to improve the heart failure syndrome. However, as heart failure progresses, the degree of neurohormonal activation tends to increase, and this overactivation can lead to exaggerated congestive symptoms and cause cardiac arrhythmia and other inappropriate feedback responses. In short, this inadequate adaptation often leads to a deterioration of heart failure rather than to its amelioration. Recently, it has been found that drugs such as vasodilators and ACE inhibitors, which lessen the over-activated compensatory mechanism, are very useful. It has also been discovered that some cardiotonic drugs, which improve cardiac contractility, are rather unfavorable as they disturb the quality of life and are not suitable for the prolongation of life. The frontiers of research in heart failure have advanced from cardiac physiology to the biochemistry of heart muscle and more recently to new areas, such as cardiac molecular and genetic biology and technology.

The proceedings of this symposium will present (1) the process of ischemic myocardial damage in heart failure, (2) biochemical abnormalities in cardiomyopathy, (3) signal transduction in diseased myocardial cells, (4) electrophysiological abnormalities of the failing heart, and (5) recent concepts in drug therapy for failing heart. We think these basic mechanisms may change the ideas behind heart failure, and this may also contribute to the development of a new therapy for heart failure.

I am sure you will find the topics interesting and informative. We hope that you will all contribute to further clarification of the problems we are faced with now. Finally, on behalf of all the members of the organizing committee of the satellite symposium, we would like to thank all participants in this symposium.

HISAKAZU YASUDA
HIDEAKI KAWAGUCHI

Contents

IX: Left Ventricular Hypertrophy and Myopathy

List of Contributors

I: Ischemic Myocardial Damage

Postischemic Myocardial Dysfunction (Myocardial "Stunning"): Role of Oxidative Stress

Xiao-Ying Li, Marcel E. Zughaib, Mohamed O. Jeroudi, Craig Hartley, Jian-Zhong Sun, Selim Sekili, and Roberto Bolli

Section of Cardiology, Department of Medicine, Baylor College of Medicine, Houston, TX 77030, USA

KEYWORDS: Oxygen Free Radicals; Myocardial Reperfusion; Postischemic Myocardial Dysfunction; Myocardial Stunning; Spin Trapping

INTRODUCTION

It is now recognized that spontaneous reperfusion after coronary spasm or thrombosis is a common occurrence in patients with coronary artery disease. In addition, coronary reperfusion by means of thrombolytic therapy, percutaneous transluminal angioplasty or bypass surgery is rapidly emerging as the fundamental strategy in the management of acute ischemic syndromes. The recent appreciation of the role of reperfusion in the natural history of coronary artery disease, coupled with the explosive growth of interventional recanalization, has provided the impetus to investigate the consequences of restoring blood flow to the ischemic myocardium. Experimental studies have demonstrated that, although early reperfusion limits or even prevents necrosis, this beneficial effect does not lead to immediate functional improvement; rather, the return of contractility in tissue salvaged by reperfusion is delayed for hours, days or even weeks [1-9], a phenomenon that has been termed "stunned myocardium" [10].

The stunned myocardium has recently become the focus of considerable interest because of its potential role in negating the benefits of reperfusion. A critical but still unresolved issue relates to the mechanism responsible for this contractile abnormality. Clearly, if effective clinical therapies aimed at preventing postischemic dysfunction are to be developed, its pathogenesis must be elucidated. In the past 8 years several experiments have been reported that suggest that myocardial stunning may be mediated in part by the generation of cytotoxic oxygen-derived free radicals. The purpose of this article is to critically review the evidence supporting this hypothesis and to discuss its pathophysiologic clinical implications.

Definition

Postischemic dysfunction, or myocardial stunning, is the mechanical dysfunction that persists in myocardium reperfused after reversible ischemia. Thus, postichemic dysfunction must be distinguished from the contractile abnormalities occurring *during* ischemia and from those associate with infarction. Implicit in this definition is that postischemic dysfunction, no matter how prolonged, is a reversible phenomenon, provided that sufficient time is allowed for the myocardium to recover.

Effect of Antioxidants on Myocardial Stunning After a Brief Coronary Occlusion

In the early 80s, a number of investigators, including ourselves, postulated that reactive oxygen metabolites (e.g., superoxide anion ($\cdot O_2^-$), hydrogen peroxide (H_2O_2), and hydroxyl radical ($\cdot OH$)) contribute to myocardial stunning. To test this hypothesis, we employed an open-chest dog preparation in which the left anterior descending coronary artery is occluded for 15 min and then reperfused [1]. We found that administration of superoxide dismutase (SOD) and catalase significantly enhanced recovery of function after reperfusion [2]. In a subsequent study [3], we found that neither enzyme alone significantly improved recovery of function in the stunned myocardium; however, when they were combined, contractile recovery was significantly greater than that observed in controls or in dogs receiving either agent alone. These results suggest that *both* $\cdot O_2^-$ and H_2O_2 contribute to the cellular damage responsible for myocardial stunning. To determine whether $\cdot O_2^-$ and H_2O_2 contribute to stunning by direct cytotoxicity or via formation of other species like the highly reactive ·OH radical, we used dimethylthiourea, (an ·OH scavenger that is more effective than traditional ·OH scavengers [4] and that does not react with $\cdot O_2^-$ or H_2O_2 *in vitro* [5]). We observed that dimethylthiourea produced a significant and sustained improvement in the function of the stunned myocardium [5]. These results were further corroborated by studies using *N*-2-mercaptopropionyl glycine (MPG). MPG is a powerful scavenger of ·OH with no effect on $\cdot O_2^-$ or H_2O_2 *in vitro* [6], readily enters the intracellular space, is active orally, and effectively attenuates myocardial stunning *in vivo* [5,6]. In addition, the iron chelator, desferrioxamine, was found to attenuate postischemic dysfunction [7,8], presumably through prevention of the iron-catalyzed formation of ·OH (through the Haber-Weiss or Fenton mechanisms) and of the propagation of ·OH-initiated lipid peroxidation [9]. Taken together, these results suggest that the ·OH radical (or one of its reactive products) is a mediator of postischemic dysfunction and that the beneficial effects of SOD and catalase previously demonstrated [2,3,10-12] are due in part to prevention of ·OH generation.

The studies discussed above [2,3,5-8,10-12] consistently support the oxyradical hypothesis, but their significance is limited by the fact that they were all performed in open-chest animals. Thus, artifacts due to the combined effects of anesthesia, hypothermia, surgical trauma, volume and ionic imbalances, unphysiologic conditions and attending neuro-humoral perturbations, as well as other potentially confounding variables, cannot be excluded. Indeed, we [13] have recently demonstrated that the severity of myocardial stunning induced by a 15-min coronary occlusion is greatly exaggerated in open-chest as compared with conscious dogs, even when differences in collateral flow are taken into account and fundamental physiological variables in the open-chest preparation are carefully kept within normal limits. The striking differences between the two models indicate the presence of artifacts in the open-chest dog and raise the possibility that results obtained in this model may not be applicable to more physiological conditions. It was therefore essential that the oxyradical hypothesis be tested in conscious animal preparations. Recently, we [13] observed that the combined administration of SOD and catalase in conscious, unsedated dogs subjected to a 15-min coronary occlusion produced a significant enhancement of the recovery of function that was sustained for at least 6 h after reflow. No subsequent deterioration occurred, indicating that postischemic depression of contractility is not a useful "protective" response to injury. Similar findings were obtained with desferrioxamine and MPG [14]. These results [13,14] indicate that the oxyradical hypothesis developed in open-chest models is applicable to conscious models.

In summary, numerous investigations from several independent laboratories [2,3,5-8,10-13] uniformly suggest that oxygen metabolites play a significant role in the genesis of myocardial stunning after a 15-min period of ischemia, both in open-chest and in conscious animals. It seems clear that a portion of the damage is mediated by ·OH. However, the available evidence suggests that myocardial stunning cannot be simplistically ascribed to a single oxygen species, and that *all of the three* initial metabolites of oxygen ($\cdot O_2^-$, H_2O_2 and ·OH) contribute to the cellular injury responsible for postischemic dysfunction. Iron also appears to play a role in stunning, presumably by catalyzing the formation of ·OH. The relative contributions of the various oxygen metabolites remain to be definitively established.

Direct Evidence for the Oxyradical Hypothesis

The studies reviewed heretofore [2,3,5-8,10-13] are limited by the fact that the evidence for a causative role of oxygen metabolites in postischemic dysfunction was indirect and, therefore, inconclusive. In order to definitively validate the oxyradical hypothesis of stunning, it was necessary to directly demonstrate and quantitate free radical generation in the presence and absence of antioxidant interventions.

We used the spin trap, α-phenyl *N-tert*-butyl nitrone (PBN), and electron paramagnetic resonance (EPR) spectroscopy to detect and measure production of free radicals in our *in vivo* model of postischemic dysfunction (15-min coronary occlusion in open-chest dogs) [15].

Following infusion of PBN, EPR signals characteristic of PBN radical adducts were detected in the venous blood draining from the ischemic-reperfused vascular bed [16]. The EPR signals were consistent with a mixture of different secondary lipid radicals, such as alkyl and alkoxyl radicals. The myocardial production of radicals began during coronary occlusion but increased dramatically after reperfusion, peaking at 2 to 4 min. After this initial burst, production of radicals abated but did not cease, persisting up to 3 h after reflow [16]. There was a linear, positive relation between the magnitude of adduct production and the magnitude of ischemic flow reduction, indicating that the intensity of free radical generation after reflow is proportional to the severity of the antecedent ischemia [16]: the greater the degree of hypoperfusion, the greater the subsequent production of free radicals and, by inference, the severity of reperfusion injury. In a subsequent study [17], we found that SOD plus catalase suppressed the production of free radicals in the stunned myocardium, indicating that these radicals result from univalent reduction of oxygen. Importantly, the inhibition of free radical production was associated with improvement of myocardial stunning [17]. More recently, we observed that MPG [6] or desferrioxamine [18], administered just before reperfusion, markedly attenuated myocardial stunning and the associated production of PBN adducts; however, the same agents given 1 min *after* reperfusion did not attenuate myocardial stunning or initial PBN adduct production. Thus, three different antioxidant interventions (SOD plus catalase, MPG, and desferrioxamine) reduced postischemic dysfunction at the same doses and under the same experimental conditions in which they reduced formation of PBN adducts. These circumstances strongly suggest that there is a cause-and-effect relationship between the production of free radicals in the stunned myocardium and the depression of contractility.

More recently, we have demonstrated, using PBN, that free radicals are also produced in the stunned myocardium in the *conscious* dog after a 15-min occlusion [19], with a time-course similar to that observed in the open-chest dog. These results [19] provide important evidence that the generation of free radicals observed in open-chest animals [6,15-18,20] is not an artifact due to the unphysiologic conditions associated with this preparation. In another recently reported study [21], we have used aromatic hydroyxylation of phenylalanine to investigate whether the hydroxyl radical is generated in the stunned myocardium. We have found that hydroxylated derivatives of phenylalanine (*ortho*-, *meta*-, and *para*-tyrosine) are released in the local coronary venous blood during the first few minutes of reperfusion after a 15-min occlusion, both in open-chest and in conscious dogs [21], indicating that ·OH is produced in the stunned myocardium upon reperfusion. *The similarity of the results obtained in our canine model of stunning with two completely different techniques (spin trapping [6,15-20] and aromatic hydroxylation [21]) further corroborates the concept that reactive oxygen species play a significant role in the pathogenesis of postischemic ventricular dysfunction.*

In summary, measurements of free radicals in experimental models of stunned myocardium [6,15-21] provide direct evidence supporting a pathogenetic role of oxygen metabolites. Specifically, these studies indicate that 1) free radicals are produced in the stunned myocardium in both open-chest and conscious dogs after reversible regional ischemia; 2) the univalent pathway of reduction of oxygen is the source of the radicals; and 3) inhibition of free radical reactions results in enhanced recovery of contractility (i.e., the radical reactions are *necessary* for postischemic dysfunction to occur).

Time Course of Free Radical-Induced Damage in the Stunned Myocardium

We have observed that infusion of the antioxidant MPG attenuated postischemic dysfunction to a similar extent whether the infusion was started before ischemia or 1 min before reperfusion; however, infusion started 1 min *after* reflow was ineffective [6], suggesting that the critical radical-mediated injury occurs in the first few moments of reperfusion. We have subsequently obtained similar results with desferrioxamine [18]. Furthermore, the spin trap, PBN, enhances contractile recovery in open-chest animals even when the infusion is commenced 20 s before reflow; the magnitude of the protective effect is similar to that observed when the infusion is started before ischemia [16]. That a substantial portion of the cellular damage responsible for stunning occurs immediately after reflow is further corroborated by direct measurements of free radicals [6,16,17] and lipid peroxidation products [22] in the stunned myocardium, both of which have shown a burst in the initial moments after reperfusion. Free radical inhibition *during* this initial burst, but not *after* the first 5 min of reperfusion (i.e., *after* the initial burst), will result in functional improvement [6]. *These observations suggest that the free radicals important in causing myocardial stunning are those produced immediately after reflow.*

In summary, myocardial stunning appears to be, in part, a form of oxyradical-mediated "reperfusion injury." *This concept may have significant therapeutic implications, because it suggests that antioxidant therapies begun after the onset of ischemia could still be effective in preventing postischemic dysfunction; however, a delay in the implementation of such therapies until after reperfusion would result in loss of efficacy.*

CONCLUSIONS

In conclusion, the studies summarized in this review provide strong evidence to support the hypothesis that oxygen-derived free radicals play an important role in the pathogenesis of postischemic myocardial dysfunction. It must be stressed, however, that myocardial stunning is a *multifactorial* phenomenon and other derangements, such as impaired calcium homeostasis, also play an important role in its pathogenesis [23]. With the increasing use of therapeutic recanalization and the recognition that spontaneous reperfusion occurs commonly, there is a growing need to elucidate the mechanisms that are responsible for the adverse sequelae of reperfusion. The hypothesis that oxyradicals contribute to postischemic dysfunction provides not only a conceptual framework for developing investigative strategies aimed at elucidating the pathophysiology of ischemic injury, but also a rationale for testing clinically applicable interventions designed to prevent this undesirable sequela of reperfusion.

ACKNOWLEDGEMENTS

The excellent secretarial assistance of Valerie R. Price is gratefully acknowledged. The work reported here was supported in part by NIH Grants HL-43151 and by NIH SCOR Grant HL-42267.

REFERENCES

1. Zhu WX, Myers ML, Hartley CJ, Roberts R, Bolli R (1986) Validation of a single crystal for measurement of transmural and epicardial thickening. Am J Physiol **251**: H1045-H1055
2. Myers ML, Bolli R, Lekich RF, Hartley CJ, Roberts R (1985) Enhancement of recovery of myocardial function by oxygen free-radical scavengers after reversible regional ischemia. Circulation **72**: 915-921
3. Jeroudi MO, Triana FJ, Patel BS, Bolli R (1990) Effect of superoxide dismutase and catalase, given separately, on myocardial "stunning." Am J Physiol **259**: H889-H901
4. Fox RB (1984) Prevention of granulocyte-mediated oxidant lung injury in rats by a hydroxyl radical scavenger, dimethylthiourea. J Clin Invest **74**: 1456
5. Bolli R, Zhu WX, Hartley CJ, *et al.* (1987) Attenuation of dysfunction in the postischemic "stunned" myocardium by dimethylthiorea. Circulation **76**: 458-468
6. Bolli R, Jeroudi MO, Patel BS, *et al.* (1989) Marked reduction of free radical generation and contractile dysfunction by antioxidant therapy begun at the time of reperfusion: evidence that myocardial "stunning" is a manifestation of reperfusion injury. Circ Res **65**: 607-622
7. Bolli R, Patel BS, Zhu WX, O'Neill PG, Charlat ML, Roberts R (1987) The iron chelator desferrioxamine attenuates postischemic ventricular dysfunction. Am J Physiol **253**: H1372-H1380
8. Farber NE, Vercellotti GM, Jacob HS, Pieper GM, Gross GJ (1988) Evidence for a role of iron-catalyzed oxidants in functional and metabolic stunning in the canine heart. Circ Res **63**: 351-360
9. Halliwell B, Gutteridge JMC (1984) Oxygen toxicity, oxygen radicals, transition metals and disease. Biochem J **219**: 1-14
10. Przyklenk K, Kloner RA (1986) Superoxide dismutase plus catalase improve contractile function in the canine model of the "stunned" myocardium. Circ Res **58**: 148-156

11. Gross GJ, Farber NE, Hardman HF, Warltier DC (1986) Beneficial actions of superoxide dismutase and catalase in stunned myocardium of dogs. Am J Physiol **250**: H372-H377
12. Murry, CE, Richard VJ, Jennings RB, Reimer KA (1989) Free radicals do not cause myocardial stunning after four 5 minute coronary occlusions. Circulation **80**(Suppl II): II-296 (*abstr.*)
13. Triana JF, Unisa A, Bolli R (1990) Antioxidant enzymes attenuate myocardial "stunning" in the conscious dog. FASEB J **4**: A622 (*abstr.*)
14. Sekili S, Li XY, Zughaib M, Sun JZ, Bolli R (1991) Evidence for a major pathogenetic role of hydroxyl radical in myocardial "stunning" in the conscious dog. Circulation **84**(Suppl II): II-656
15. Bolli R, McCay PB (1990) Use of spin traps in intact animals undergoing myocardial ischemia/reperfusion: A new approach to assessing the role of oxygen radicals in myocardial "stunning." Free Rad Res Comms **9**: 169-180
16. Bolli R, Patel BS, Jeroudi MO, Lai EK, McCay PB (1988) Demonstration of free radical generation in "stunned" myocardium of intact dogs with the use of the spin trap α-phenyl *N-tert*-butyl nitrone. J Clin Invest **82**: 476-485
17. Bolli R, Jeroudi MO, Patel BS, *et al.* (1989) Direct evidence that oxygen-derived free radicals contribute to postischemic myocardial dysfunction in the intact dog. Proc Natl Acad Sci USA **86**: 4695-4699
18. Bolli R, Patel BS, Jeroudi MO, *et al.* (1990) Iron-mediated radical reactions upon reperfusion contribute to myocardial "stunning." Am J Physiol **259**: H1901-H1911
19. Zughayb M, Sekili S, Li XY, Triana JF, McCay PB, Bolli R (1991) Detection of free radical generation in the "stunned" myocardium in the conscious dog using spin trapping techniques. FASEB J **5**: A704
20. Leiboff RL, Arroyo CM, Schaer GL, *et al.* (1988) Free radical generation in an *in vivo* model of regional myocardial stunning. FASEB J **2**: A818 *(abstr.)*
21. Bolli R, Kaur H, Li XY, Triana JF, Halliwell B (1991) Demonstration of hydroxyl radical generation in "stunned" myocardium of intact dogs using aromatic hydroxylation of phenylalanine. FASEB J **5**: A704
22. Romaschin AD, Rebeyka I, Wilson GJ, Mickle DAG (1987) Conjugated dienes in ischemic and reperfused myocardium: an *in vivo* chemical signature of oxygen free radical mediated injury. J Mol Cell Cardiol **19**: 289-302
23. Bolli R (1990) Mechanism of myocardial "stunning." Circulation **82**:723-738

Degradation of Membrane Phospholipids in the Ischemic and Reperfused Heart

GER J. VAN DER VUSSE and ROBERT S. RENEMAN

Department of Physiology, Cardiovascular Research Institute Maastricht, University of Limburg, 6200 MD Maastricht, The Netherlands

Key words: phospholipids, heart, injury, ischemia, reperfusion.

INTRODUCTION

Under normal circumstances cardiac cells provide sufficient amounts of energy by oxidative degradation of substrates such as fatty acids, glucose and lactate to fulfil their energy requirements. Contraction and relaxation of the myofibrils consume over 70% of ATP produced by mitochondrial activity, the remaining part is used for transport of ions across membranes, and maintenance of cellular integrity. The plasmalemma, the membrane enclosing the content of living cells, plays a crucial role in the complex process of maintenance of integrity. As soon as the plasmalemma is no longer capable of maintaining a barrier between the extracellular and intracellular compartments, the cell will die (1). Loss of semi-permeable properties of the plasmalemma results in release of metabolites and cytoplasmic proteins, required for enzymatic or transport processes, and influx of extracellular macromolecules and calcium ions into the interior of the injured cell (1). This condition, usually designated as cell death, will be followed by degenerative changes such as lysis of the cellular remnants by lysosomal enzymes and by macrofages invading the damaged area of the heart. A variety of pathophysiological derangements may lead to death of cardiac cells. The most common cause of cellular injury and cell death is ischemia (insufficient blood supply to the heart). Restoration of flow to previously ischemic areas may inflict additional damage upon the injured cells.

It is generally recognized that the mechanism underlying ischemia and reperfusion-induced damage is a multifactorial process involving alterations in cellular ion homeostasis, contractile behaviour of myofibrils, mitochondrial energy conversion, chemical composition of membranes, structure of the cytoskeleton and its attachment to the plasmalemma, permeability of lysosomal membranes and capacity to scavenge oxygen free radicals.

Despite several decades of scrutinous investigations, the precise nature of the chain of events leading from reversible changes in cellular functioning to cell death has only been partly elucidated. Since disruption of cellular membranes is supposed to be a key event in the onset of cell death, it has been hypothetized that enzymatic degradation of membrane phospholipids is involved in the ultimate step of loss of cellular integrity (2).

In this survey, the potentially detrimental role of impaired phospholipid homeostasis in ischemic and reperfused heart will be discussed. Special attention will be paid to physical changes in the lipid bilayer, the interaction between cytoskeleton and cellular membranes and hydrolytic degradation of phospholipids, being the important building block of biological membranes.

Cardiac membranes

Like other mammalian cells, the plasmalemma of cardiomyocytes is mainly composed of phospholipids, cholesterol and proteins. Phospholipids are present in a variety of species. Phosphatidyl choline, phosphatidyl ethanolamine, phosphatidyl inositol and phosphatidyl serine are the main constituents of the plasmalemma. Sphingomyelin, the backbone of which is sphingosine instead of glycerol, is also present in the plasmalemma (2). The plasmalemma is composed of two leaflets. The hydrophilic head groups of the phospholipids in the outer leaflet of the lipid bilayer point towards the extracellular space. The hydrophilic head groups of phospholipids, aligned in the inner leaflet, face the cytoplasmic compartment. The distribution of the various membrane phospholipids over the two leaflets is asymmetric. The inner leaflet is composed of phosphatidyl ethanolamine, phosphatidyl serine, phosphotidyl inositol and phosphatidyl choline. The outer leaflet is relatively enriched in phosphatidyl choline and sphingomyelin (3). The asymmetrical distribution is maintained by an ATP-dependent aminophospholipid translocase (4). The hydrophobic fatty acyl chains of the membrane phospholipids form the core of the lipid bilayer. To compensate for differences in fluidity, the outer leaflet accomodates more cholesterol than the inner leaflet (2). Proteins are present in the lipid bilayer to regulate specific functions of the plasmalemma, such as transport of ions and hydrophylic compounds, and signal transduction.

The stability of biological membranes is determined by a variety of factors. Chemical composition of the acyl chains of the phospholipids, the amount of cholesterol in the membranes, the distribution of phospholipid species over inner and outer leaflet, and the physical arrangement of phospholipid molecules in the leaflets influence the stability of the plasmalemma. Additional strength to the membrane is provided by structures present in the intra- and extracellular compartment in close proximity of the plasmalemma. Inside the cardiomyocyte parts of the cytoskeleton form a subcortical lattice, which is attached to the sarcolemma through vinculine in the Z-band region. Other cytoskeletal proteins are thought to play also a role in anchoring the plasmalemma to cytoskeletal structures (1). The outer leaflet of the plasmalemma is connected to an outer lamina or basement membrane. The phospholipid moieties inside the membrane are involved in a continuous turnover process. Fatty acyl chains are removed by enzymatic action of phospholipases and replaced by other fatty acyl chains to keep the membrane in an optimal condition.

Ischemia and reperfusion-induced damage of cardiac membranes

Prolonged ischemia results in loss of plasmalemmal integrity and, hence, in cell death. The mechanism leading to plasmalemmal disruption is incompletely understood. Overt destruction of the membrane is most likely preceded by destabilization of the lipid bilayer. Loss of stability of the plasmalemma can be caused by physical and chemical alterations in the lipid bilayer and its immediate surroundings. A shift of cholesterol molecules from the plasmalemma to mitochondrial structures, as has been observed by Rouslin and colleagues (5), will alter plasma membrane fluidity which may add to destabilization of the lipid bilayer. Acidification of the cytoplasmic compartment of ischemic cells may cause solidification of the negatively charged phosphatidyl inositol and phosphatidyl serine. As a result, lateral phase separation of lipids may occur (6). This process has been visualized by electronmicroscopic evaluation of membranes of ischemic cardiac cells. Aggregation of intramembranous particles (=integral proteins) are readily observed, which is attributed to the formation of lipid domains in the membrane. In addition to the clustering of intramembranous particles, extrusion of lipid material from membranes of cells under ischemic conditions has been reported (6,7). Extrusion of lipids might be the consequence of membrane destabilization caused by loss of phospholipid asymmetry. The latter process might occur due to the fact that phosphatidyl ethanolamine prefers to form non-bilayer configurations (the so-called hexagonal II phase). Under normal conditions this tendency is suppressed by proteins and other types of phospholipids present in the membrane. Increased concentrations of Ca^{2+} in the vicinity of the inner leaflet of the plasmalemma are thought to stimulate the formation of non-bilayer structures. When phospholipids in the lipid bilayer are organized in the hexagonal II phase, phospholipid asymmetry cannot be maintained. Under normal circumstances, the amino phospholipid translocator immediately restores the asymmetric composition of the membrane (4). In the ischemic cell the activity of this pump is most likely impaired due to low ATP and high intracellular Ca^{2+} levels. Extrusion of lipids results in the formation of multilamellar vesicles (6, 7). Detachment of the cytoskeleton from the inner leaflet of the phospholipid bilayer may also add to destabilization of the membrane. The formation of blebs, filled with mitochondria and other cytoplasmic material, as has been observed in ischemic cells, is most likely caused by impaired cytoskeleton-sarcolemma interactions. The precise mechanism underlying impaired anchoring of the sarcolemma is incompletely understood. Enhanced calpain activity by high intracellular Ca^{2+} concentrations may give rise to enzymatic degradation of proteins responsible for proper attachment of membrane and cytoskeletal lattice.

A variety of studies indicate that enzymatic degradation of phospholipids also add to destabilization of the membrane of the ischemic cardiac cell. Especially the accumulation of unesterified arachidonic acid in ischemic and ATP depleted cells has lead to this notion (2). Both phospholipase A_2 and phospholipase C (in combination with diacylglycerol hydrolase) are able to remove fatty acyl chains from the parent phospholipid molecule. The activity of these enzymes might be enhanced by alterations in the ionic environment of the enzyme (enhanced Ca^{2+} levels) or physical changes in the lipid bilayer such as solidification of phospholipids (extrusion of lipid material). Moreover, decreased levels of ATP, a substance required for activation of the fatty acids to acylCoA, representing the first step in reacylation of hydrolyzed phospholipids, and increased contents of AMP, a well-known inhibitor of acylCoA synthetase, will also impair proper phospholipid homeostasis (8). In addition to loss of phospholipids from the membrane, accumulation of fatty acids and lysophospholipids in the membrane may add to bilayer destabilization.

Overt disruption of the plasmalemma will take place when physical forces are exerted on the unstable membrane (1). Forces generated by ischemic contracture of the myofibrils and by osmotic loading of the injured cells might exceed the level tolerable by the destabilized membrane. As a consequence, the membrane will lose its semi-permeable properties, metabolites and intracellular proteins wil be released and extracellular material (Ca^{2+}, macromolecules) will invade the damaged cell. This process may occur during ischemia, but also after restoration of flow, when uncontrolled influx of water into the cytoplasmic compartment and resumption of myofibrillar contraction occur. Other events that take place during the initial phase of reperfusion, such as peroxidation of lipid material in the membrane and cytoplasmic Ca^{2+} overloading, may further compromise the unstable condition of the plasmalemma.

Since membrane destabilization and destruction is a multifactorial process, it cannot be excluded that phospholipase A_2 mediated events play a crucial role in ischemia and reperfusion induced damage of cardiac structures. This notion is substantiated by observations that phospholipase inhibitors such as quinacrine and mepacrine are able to attenuate damage inflicted upon ischemic tissue (2). Additional evidence has been provided by studies showing that antibodies against phospholipase A_2 administered to the heart prior to and after a period of ischemia, protected the hearts against the deleterious effects of ischemia and reperfusion (9). Further experiments are required to rate the significance of the latter findings in the pharmacological treatment of patients suffering from ischemic heart disease.

REFERENCES

1. Ganote CE, Van der Heide RS (1990) Importance of mechanical forces in ischemic and reperfusion injury. In: Piper HM (ed) Pathophysiology of severe ischemic myocardial injury. Kluwer Academic Publ. Dordrecht. pp 337-355.
2. Van der Vusse GJ, Van Bilsen M, Sonderkamp T, Reneman RS (1990) Hydrolysis of phospholipids and cellular integrity. In: Piper HM (ed) Pathophysiology of severe ischemic myocardial injury. Kluwer Academic Publ. Dordrecht. pp. 337-355.
3. Post JA, Langer GA, Op den Kamp JAF, Verkley AJ (1988) Phospholipid asymmetry in cardiac sarcolemma. Analysis of intact cells and gas-dissected membranes. Biochim Biophys Acta: 943: 256-266.
4. Zwaal RFA, Bevers EM, Comfurius P, Rosing J, Tilly RHJ, Verhallen PFJ (1989) Loss of membrane phospholipid asymmetry during activation of blood platelets and sickled red cells: mechanisms and physiological significance. Mol Cell Biochem 91: 23-31.
5. Rouslin W, MacGee J, Gupte S, Wesselman A, Epp DE (1982) Mitochondrial cholesterol content and membrane properties in porcine myocardial ischemia. Am J Physiol 242: 11254-11259.
6. Verkley AJ, Post JA (1987) Physico-chemical properties and organization of lipids in membranes: their possible role in myocardial injury. Basic Res Cardiol 82 (Suppl 1): 85-91.
7. Schrijvers AHGJ, De Groot MJM, Heynen VVTh, Van der Vusse GJ, Frederik PM, Reneman RS (1990) Influence of the duration of ischemia and reperfusion on multilamellar vesicles in isolated rabbit hearts: a morphometrical and ultrastructural study using tannic acid based fixation. J Mol Cell Cardiol 22: 653-665.
8. Van Bilsen M, Van der Vusse GJ, Willemsen PHM, Coumans WA, Roemen THM, Reneman RS (1989) Lipid alterations in isolated, working rat hearts during ischemia and reperfusion: Its relation to myocardial damage. Circ Res 64: 304-314.
9. Prasad MR, Popescu LM, Moraru II, Liu X, Maity S, Engelman RM, Das DK (1991) Role of phospholipases-A2 and phospholipase-C in myocardial ischemic reperfusion injury. Am J Physiol 260: H877-H883.

Protective Effects of Antiarrhythmic Agents on Oxygen-Deficiency-Induced Contractile Dysfunction of Isolated Perfused Hearts

SATOSHI TAKEO, KOUICHI TANONAKA, JIAN-XUN LIU, and YASUTAMI OHTSUKA

Department of Pharmacology, Tokyo College of Pharmacy, Hachioji, 192-03 Japan

KEYWORDS: Quinidine, Disopyramide, Lidocaine, Ischemia/reperfusion injury, Hypoxia/reoxygenation injury

INTRODUCTION

Some of antiarrhythmic agents have been shown to reduce ischemia/reperfusion injury (1-3). Although this may be in part attributed to prevention of ventricular arrhythmias (4-7), other unknown mechanisms might also be involved in the effects of particular antiarrhythmic agents. The present study was undertaken to determine whether or not, prevention of oxygen-deficiency/oxygen-replenishment-induced injury is a generalized phenomenon for an antiarrhythmic agent. To test this, we used three antiarrhythmic agents, lidocaine, disopyramide and quinidine, and also used two oxygen-deficiency/oxygen-replenishment models, hypoxic/reoxygenated and ischemic/reperfused hearts.

MATERIALS AND METHODS

In the first set of experiments, isolated rabbit hearts were subjected to hypoxia/reoxygenation. The hearts were perfused at 37°C at a constant flow rate of 16 ml/min with the Krebs-Henseleit solution of the following composition (mM); NaCl 120, KCl 4.8, $MgSO_4$ 1.2, KH_2PO_4 1.2, $CaCl_2$ 1.25, $NaHCO_3$ 25 and glucose 11. The buffer was previously oxygenated with a gas mixture of 95% O_2 + 5% CO_2. Hypoxia was induced by perfusing the heart for 20 min with the buffer previously saturated with a gas mixture of 95% N_2 + 5% CO_2, pH 7.4. In the hypoxic buffer, glucose was replaced with 11 mM mannitol. After hypoxic perfusion, the heart was reoxygenated for 45 min with the oxygenated buffer containing glucose as above. The heart was preloaded with 1.5 g of initial resting tension and isometric tension development was estimated as contractile force. The heart was paced at 180 beats/min throughout the experiment except for the first 15 min reoxygenation. Treatment with either lidocaine or disopyramide was performed from 8 min after the onset of hypoxia to the end of hypoxia at a flow rate of 300 µg/min (69 or 55 µM, respectively). After reoxygenation, myocardial calcium content was determined by an atomic absorption method as described previously (8). The perfusate eluted from hypoxic and reoxygenated heart was collected and sampled for determination of purine and base contents (ATP metabolites) (8), and creatine kinase activity (9).

In the second set of experiments, isolated rat hearts were subjected to ischemia/reoxygenation. The hearts were perfused at a constant flow rate of 8 ml/min with the Krebs-Henseleit solution containing glucose as described above. A latex balloon was inserted into left ventricular cavity and a 5-mmHg of the initial resting pressure was preloaded. Changes in ventricular developed pressure (LVDP), dP/dt and left ventricular end-diastolic pressure (LVEDP) were measured via a pressure-transducer. The heart was first subjected to 35 min-global ischemia and followed by 60 min-reperfusion with the buffer as described above. The heart was paced at 300 beats/min throughout the experiment except for the first 15 min-reperfusion. Treatment of perfused hearts with quinidine was performed for the last 3 min of preischemia at a concentration of 30 μM. Tissue ion content and, creatine kinase activity and ATP metabolites of the perfusate were determined according to the same methods as above.

In the third set of experiments, rat atrial muscles were isolated and suspended in an organ bath filled with the buffer containing glucose as described above except for that a higher concentration of $CaCl_2$ (2.5 mM) was employed. The maximal driving frequency, the stimulus frequency which the atria could not follow, was determined according to the method described previously (10).

RESULTS AND DISCUSSION

1. Effects on hypoxic/reoxygenated hearts

Hypoxia/reoxygenation resulted in very little cardiac contractile recovery (6% of initial), sustained rise in resting tension (420% of initial) and perfusion pressure (135% of initial). When the hearts were treated with either 69 μM lidocaine or 55 μM disopyramide, the posthypoxic contractile activity was greatly improved (Fig. 1). Reoxygenation-induced rise in resting tension and increase in perfusion pressure were also profoundly suppressed by treatment with either lidocaine or disopyramide. The findings indicate that treatment with the antiarrhythmic agents are effective in the improvement of posthypoxic cardiac performance. Tissue calcium was accumulated by hypoxia/reoxygenation under the present experimental conditions (1.6-fold increase), which was virtually abolished by treatment with either lidocaine or disopyramide (Fig. 2). The results suggest that hypoxia/reoxygenation-induced ionic imbalance, particularly calcium accumulation, is prevented by both antiarrhythmic agents. This may be effective in reducing derangements of calcium overload-induced biochemical abnormalities such as activation of phospholipases (11) and neutral proteases (12). A marked release of creatine kinase from the reoxygenated heart was observed, but little from the hypoxic heart. Lidocaine and disopyramide completely inhibited the release of creatine kinase from the perfused heart. The release of creatine

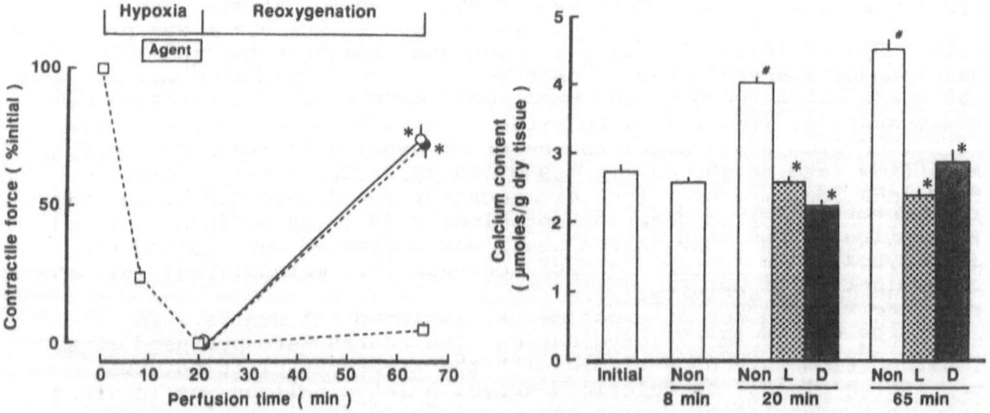

Fig. 1 and 2. Contractile force and calcium content of hypoxic/reoxygenated hearts without (□, Non) and with either lidocaine (○, L) or disopyramide (●, D), respectively.

kinase implies a loss of cytosolic macromolecules across the sarcolemma following myocardial cell death or changes in cell membrane permeability. The findings suggest prevention of hypoxia/reoxygenation-induced loss of membrane integrity by the antiarrhythmic agents. ATP metabolites of the perfusate were appreciably increased during hypoxia, and more markedly during reoxygenation. Release of ATP metabolites was reduced by treatment with both antiarrhythmic agents. Since purine nucleosides and bases are permeable across cardiac cell membrane, the findings suggest protecting effects of these agents on hypoxia/reoxygenation-induced facilitation of metabolite loss across the sarcolemma. No incidence of contractile irregularity was observed in isolated rabbit hearts during hypoxia and reoxygenation under the present experimental conditions regardless of treatment with or without the antiarrhythmic agents.

2. Effects on ischemic/reperfused hearts
To generalize the effects of an antiarrhythmic agent on oxygen-deficient and oxygen-replenished hearts, we attempted the second set of experiments. That is, isolated rat hearts were subjected to 35-min global ischemia and 60 min-reperfusion with and without quinidine-treatment. Ischemia/reperfusion resulted in no generation of LVDP and, increases in LVEDP (15-fold increase) and perfusion pressure (30% increase). Treatment of the heart with quinidine enhanced postischemic contractile recovery (Fig. 3). This was associated with suppression of postischemic rise in perfusion pressure. The results indicate that treatment with quinidine is beneficial for postischemic cardiac performance. Tissue ion content of the reperfused heart was determined in the absence and presence of quinidine treatment (Fig 4). Tissue sodium was increased after ischemia and this increase was further augmented by reperfusion. Tissue calcium was also increased after reperfusion, but not after ischemia. In contrast, tissue potassium was decreased after ischemia and after reperfusion, and tissue magnesium after reperfusion. When the heart was treated with 30 µM quinidine, suppression of both the increase in tissue sodium and calcium and the

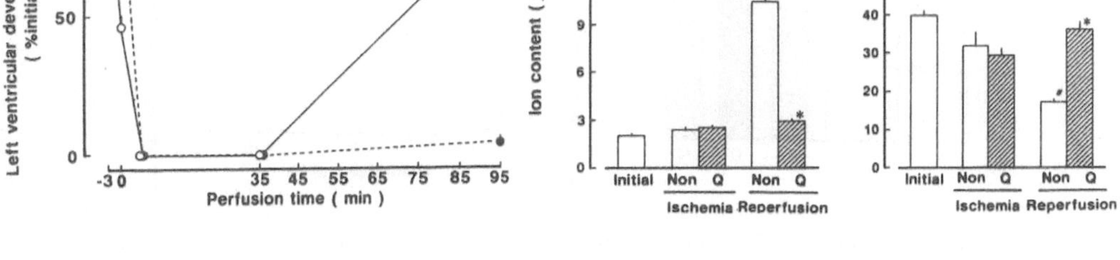

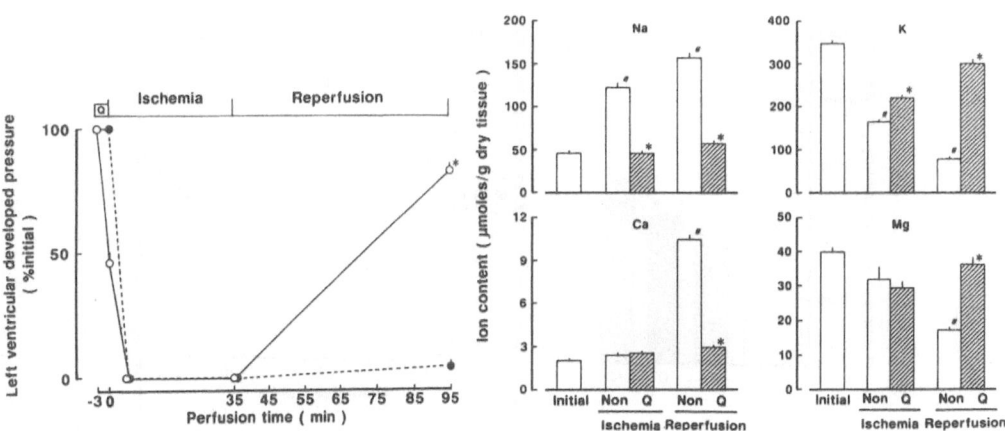

Fig. 3 and 4. Left ventricular developed pressure and ion contents of ischemic/reperfused hearts without (●, Non) and with quinidine (○, Q), respectively.

decrease in tissue potassium and magnesium was seen. The results indicate that ischemia/reperfusion-induced ionic imbalance across the sarcolemma is prevented by quinidine. The release of creatine kinase from hearts was greatly increased upon reperfusion. Treatment with quinidine resulted in a depression of the release of creatine kinase. ATP metabolites were released minimally from the ischemic heart and markedly from the reperfused heart. Both suppressive effects were the same as those in hypoxic/reoxygenated hearts. Contractile irregularities were examined during reperfusion. Incidence of the irregularity of ischemic/reperfused hearts was minimal when they were not treated with quinidine, possibly due to complete contractile failure upon reperfusion. Contractile irregularities were, however, elicited when the heart was treated with 30 µM quinidine. Thus, the benefit of antiarrhythmic agents on ischemic/reperfused hearts are unlikely attributable to their depression of reperfusion-induced arrhythmias.

3. Effects on atrial muscle

In the third set of experiments, the rat left atrial muscle was isolated and its maximal driving frequency was determined. As shown in the left panel of Fig. 5, the maximal driving frequency of the left atria was depressed by 69 µM lidocaine, 55 µM disopyramide and 30 µM quinidine, which were found to be effective in improving posthypoxic or postischemic recovery of cardiac contractile force. The right panel in Fig. 5 shows a relationship between the concentrations of quinidine which revealed significant postischemicc contractile recovery and, the rate of depression of maximal driving frequency or the rate of recovery of postischemic contractile force. The results strongly suggest a close relationship between improvement of postischemic contractile recovery and effects on maximal driving frequency of the atria. These results postulate that antiarrhythmic agents prevent oxygen-deficiency/oxygen-replenishment injury, probably not due to antiarrhythmic effects on the heart but to membrane protecting effects against oxygen-replenishment-induced loss of cardiac cell membrane integrity.

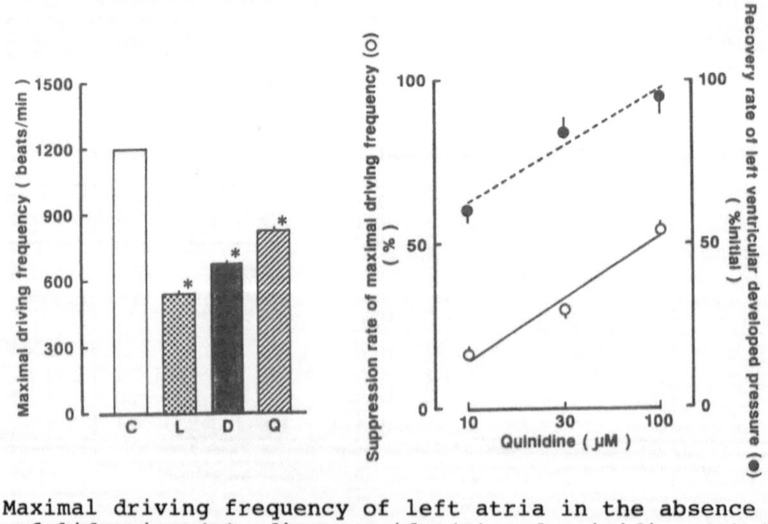

Fig. 5 Maximal driving frequency of left atria in the absence (C) and presence of lidocaine (L), disopyramide (D) and quinidine (Q) (left panel), and the relationship between concentration of quinidine used and, either efficacy on maximal driving frequency (○) or recovery of left ventricular developed pressure (●).

ACKNOWLEDGMENT

This work was in part supported by the grant of Fujisawa Foundation.

REFERENCES

1. Bergey JL, Nocella K, McCallum JD (1982) Acute coronary artery occlusion-reperfusion-induced arrhythmias in rats, dogs and pigs: Antiarrhythmic evaluation of quinidine, procainamide and lidocaine. Eur J Pharmacol 81: 205-216

2. Tosaki A, Balint S, Szekeres L (1988) Protective effect of lidocaine against ischemia and reperfusion-induced arrhythmias and shifts of myocardial sodium, potassium, and calcium content. J Cardiovasc Pharmacol 12: 621-628

3. Hanaki Y, Sugiyama S, Hieda N, Taki K, Hayashi H, Ozawa T (1989) Cardioprotective effects of various class I antiarrhythmic drugs in canine hearts. J Am Coll Cardiol 14: 219-224

4. Mannings S, Crome R, Isted K, Coltari DJ, Hearse DJ (1985) Reperfused ventricular fibrillation. Modification by pharmacological agents. Adv Myocardiol 6: 515-528

5. Polwin W, McDonald FM, Brinkmann C, Hirche Hj, Addicks K (1987) Effects of lidocaine on catecholamine release in the ischemic rat heart. J Cardiovasc Pharmacol 9: 6-11

6. Tzivoni D, Keren A, Granot H, Gottlieb S, Benhorin J, Stern S (1983) Ventricular fibrillation caused by myocardial reperfusion in Prinzmetal's angina. Am Heart J 105: 323-325

7. Goldberg S, Greenspon AJ, Urban PL, Muza B, Berger B, Walinsky P, Maroko PR (1983) Reperfusion arrhythmia; A marker of restoration of antegrade flow during intracoronary thrombolysis for acute myocardial infarction. Am Heart J 105: 26-32

8. Takeo S, Tanonaka K, Matsumoto M, Miyake K, Minematsu R (1988) Cardioprotective action of alpha-blocking agents, phentolamine and bunazosin, on hypoxic and reoxygenated myocardium. J Pharmacol Exp Ther 246: 674-681

9. Bergmeyer HU, Rich W, Butter H, Schmidt E, Hillmann G, Kreuz FH, Stamm D, Lang H, Szasz G, Lane D (1970) Standardization of methods for estimation of enzyme activity in biological fluids. Z Klin Chem Biochem 8: 658-660

10. Tanonaka K, Matsumoto M, Minematsu R, Miyake K, Murai R, Takeo S (1989) Beneficial effect of amosulalol and phentolamine on post-hypoxic recovery of contractile force and energy metabolism in rabbit hearts. Brit J Pharmacol 97: 513-523

11. Chien KR, Pfau RG, Faber JL (1979) Ischemic myocardial cell injury: Prevention of chlorpromazine of an accelerated phospholipid degradation and associated membrane dysfunction. Am J Pathol 97: 505-530

12. Reddy MK, Etlinger JP, Rabinowitz M, Fischman DA, Zak R (1974) Removal of Z-lines and a-actinin from isolated myofibrils by a calcium-activated neutral proteases. J Biol Chem 250: 4278-4284

Ischemic Myocardial Damage

KAZUO ICHIHARA

Department of Pharmacology, Asahikawa Medical College, Asahikawa, 078 Japan

KEYWORDS: isolated perfused rat heart, ischemia, ATP, creatine phosphate

INTRODUCTION

When ischemia occurs in the heart, utilization of fatty acids is inhibited, resulting in accumulation of fatty acyl esters in the heart cells, and then glycolysis is accelerated to produce adenosine triphosphate (ATP) anaerobically. However, the level of ATP decreases during ischemia, because ATP supply to the heart cell is not sufficient. There are two major causes of the myocardial damage induced by ischemia; ATP depletion [1] and accumulation of long chain fatty acyl esters [2]. Therefore we examined the relation between the recovery of mechanical function of the heart during reperfusion after brief ischemia and the levels fatty acyl esters and ATP.

MATERIALS AND METHODS

Hearts were removed from fed male Sprague-Dawley rats weighing 300-400 g and perfused by the working heart technique with Krebs-Henseleit bicarbonate buffer containing 11 mM glucose and 1.2 mM palmitate at 37 °C. Ischemia was induced for 20 min by lowering the afterload pressure from 60 to 0 mmHg [3]. When the heart was reperfused, the afterload pressure was again raised to 60 mmHg. In some experiments, the heart was perfused with some interventions, i.e. the buffer containing 20 mM KCl or 17 µM propranolol, or the buffer precooled at 10 or 20 °C during ischemia.

At the end of the experiments, the hearts were frozen with clamps cooled in liquid nitrogen. The frozen heart sample was pulverized and used for determining the metabolites levels.

RESULTS AND DISCUSSION

Ischemia produced the heart arrest with a marked decrease in the tissue levels of ATP and creatine phosphate. When the heart was perfused without intervention during ischemia, the mechanical function (peak aortic pressure x heart rate) of the arrested heart due to ischemia was not recovered by reperfusion. The myocardial protective interventions preserved the ATP and creatine phosphate stores from being exhausted during ischemia and made the mechanical function of the heart recover almost completely during reperfusion. Figure 1 shows the mechanical function of the reperfused heart as a function of the ATP level in the reperfused heart. This result indicate that recovery of mechanical function of the heart after reperfusion depends upon how much ATP can recover during reperfusion.

Long chain fatty acyl CoA and acyl carnitine esters are known to have membrane detergent properties [2]. In Fig. 2, relation between

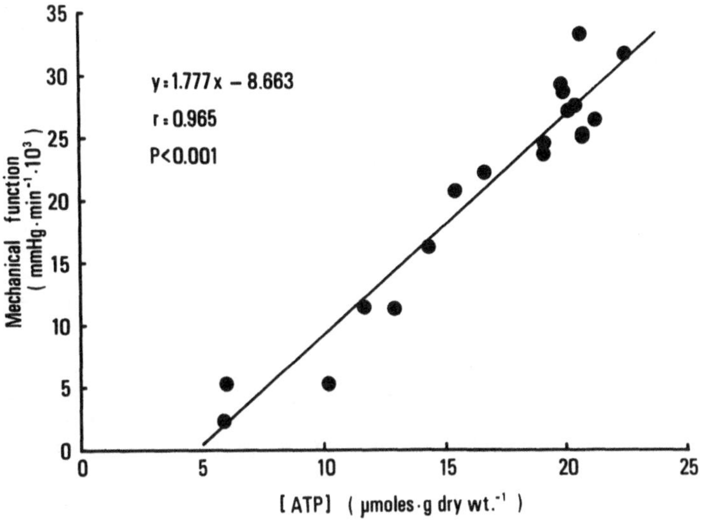

Fig. 1 Relation between the mechanical function and ATP level in the reperfused heart. Perfused hearts were made ischemic for 20 min with or without myocardial protective interventions, and then reperfused for 20 min with the normal perfusate.

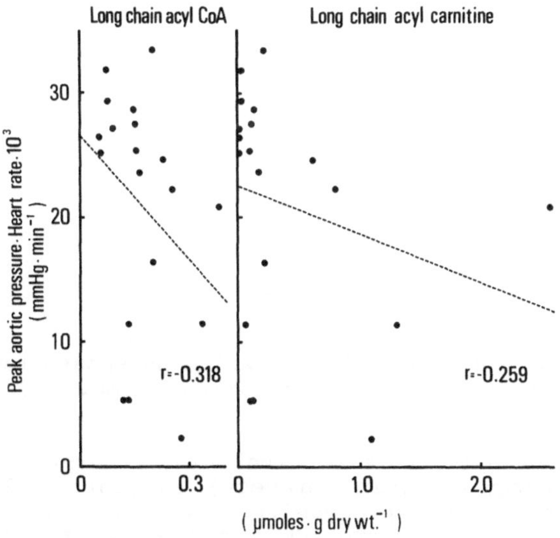

Fig. 2 Relation between the mechanical function and long chain fatty acyl CoA and fatty acyl carnitine levels in the reperfused heart. The heart sample was the same as shown in Fig. 1.

the mechanical function and the levels of long chain fatty acyl CoA and acyl carnitine in the reperfused heart is illustrated. There are no significant correlations between them. This result indicates that recovery of the cardiac mechanical function after reperfusion is not influenced by accumulation of long chain fatty acyl CoA and carnitine. High levels of fatty acyl CoA and carnitine esters may not be a major cause of ischemic myocardial damage [4].

Changes in the creatine phosphate level before and after ischemia and after reperfusion are illustrated in Fig. 3. The creatine phosphate level was decreased by ischemia, and increased to twice the preischemic level by reperfusion following ischemia. As mentioned above, the ATP level was increased to only 60 % of the preischemic level by reperfusion. The creatine phosphate level in the reperfused heart with myocardial protective interventions was less than that in the reperfused heart without interventions, although the mechanical function of the heart with interventions was fully recovered by reperfusion. When the mechanical function of the reperfused heart was plotted as a function of the creatine phosphate level in the reperfused heart, the mechanical function was inversely proportional to the creatine phosphate level [5].

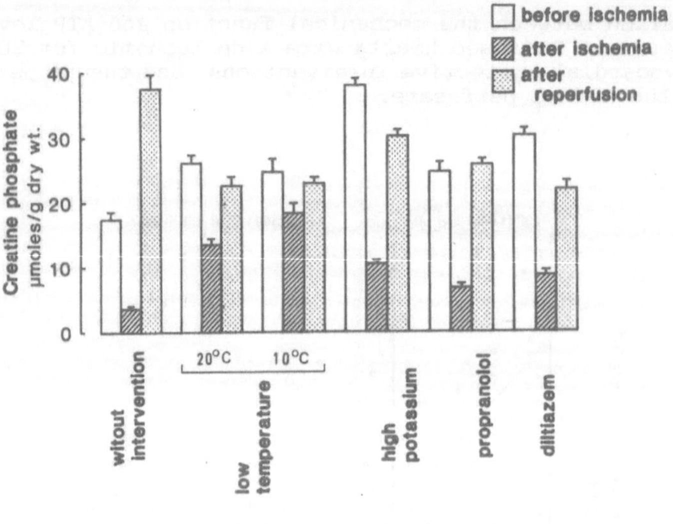

Fig. 3 Changes in the myocardial creatine phosphate level induced by ischemia under several conditions and reperfusion.

Creatine phosphate carries the high energy phosphate from mitochondrion (energy-producing process) to contractile elements in cytoplasm (energy-consuming process)(Fig. 4). Because the heart beats continuously, energy must be provided for the myocardium continuously. A fraction (⁘) of the creatine phosphate pool, which is coupled with the energy-consuming process, always liberates high energy phosphate. Therefore, when the creatine phosphate level is biochemically measured in the myocardium, it will be identical with a residual fraction (□) of the total creatine phosphate pool. If the cardiac work increases, the size of the fraction being measured biochemically decreases, because the turnover rate of ATP and creatine phosphate in the energy-consuming process must increase. These findings suggest that the myocardial cell in the reperfused heart following brief ischemia can produce high energy phosphates, even when its mechanical function and ATP level cannot recover.

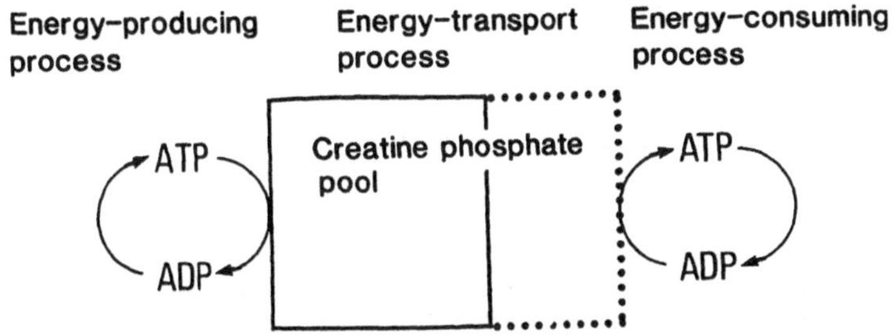

Fig. 4 The speculative role of creatine phosphate pool in the energy cycle of myocardial cells. Creatine phosphate carries the high energy phosphate from mitochondrion to contractile elements in cytoplasm. Because the turnover rate of a fraction (⁞) of creatine phosphate pool at the energy-consuming process is rapid, only the residual fraction (□) can be measure biochemically.

Figure 5 shows the cause of ischemic myocardial damage. In the normal heart, ATP synthesized with mitochondrial respiration transfers its high energy phosphate to creatine in mitochondria. Then the creatine phosphate move to cytosol, and give the high energy phosphate back to

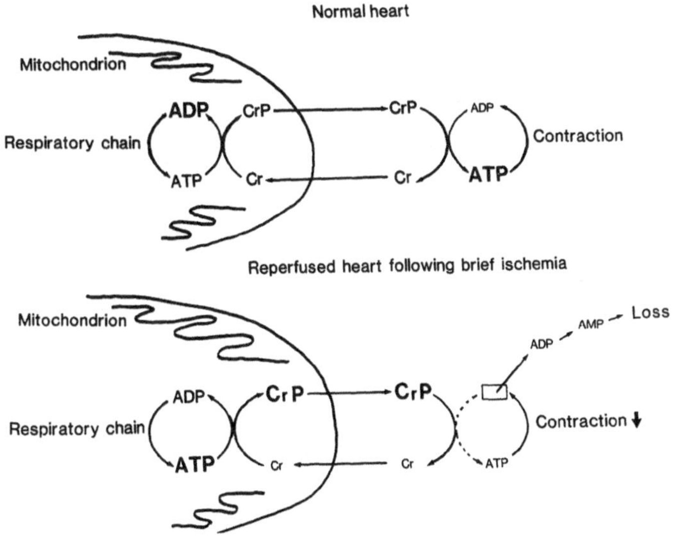

Fig. 5 A cause of myocardial ischemic damage. Creatine phosphate cannot transfer its high energy phosphate to ADP near contractile elements, because of loss of ADP at the energy-consuming process.

adenosine diphosphate (ADP) at the compartment including contractile elements, in order to resynthesize ATP. In the reperfused heart following brief ischemia, mitochondrial respiration can synthesize ATP, and creatine phosphate move to the compartment near the contractile elements. However, creatine phosphate cannot transfer its high energy phosphate to ADP at the energy-consuming process, because the loss of adenine nucleotide induced by ischemia decreases the size of ADP pool near the contractile elements.

It is concluded that the myocardial cell damage induced by brief ischemia may be due to decrease or disappearance of ADP pool in the compartment near the contractile elements.

REFERENCES

1. Ichihara K, Abiko Y (1983) Effects of diltiazem and propranolol on irreversibility of ischemic cardiac function and metabolism in the isolated perfused rat heart. J Cardiovasc Pharmacol 5: 745-751
2. Katz AM, Messineo FC (1981) Lipid-membrane interactions and the pathogenesis of ischemic damage in the myocardium. Circ Res 48: 1-16
3. Ichihara K, Morgan HE (1991) Limitations of the one-way ball valve: a device for making the isolated rat heart ischemic. J Appl. Cardiol 6: 195-198
4. Ichihara K, Neely JR (1985) Recovery of ventricular function in reperfused ischemic rat hearts exposed to fatty acids. Am J Physiol 249: H492-H497
5. Ichihara K, Abiko Y (1984) Rebound recovery of myocardial creatine phosphate with reperfusion after ischemia. Am Heart J 108: 1594-1597

II: Cardiomyopathy

Role of Protein Kinase System in the Signal Transduction of Stretch-mediated Myocyte Growth

YOSHIO YAZAKI and ISSEI KOMURO

Third Department of Internal Medicine, The Faculty of Medicine, University of Tokyo, Tokyo, 113 Japan

ABSTRACT

To examine the molecular mechanisms by which mechanical stimuli induce protooncogene expression, we cultured rat neonatal cardiocytes in deformable dishes and imposed an in vitro mechanical load by stretching the adherent cells. Myocyte stretching increased total cell RNA content and mRNA levels of c-fos and skeletal α-actin followed by activation of protein synthesis. CAT assay indicated that sequences containing a serum response element were required for efficient transcription of c-fos gene by stretching. This accumulation of c-fos mRNA was suppressed by protein kinase C inhibitors at the transcriptional level and inhibited markedly by down-regulation of protein kinase C. Moreover, myocyte stretching increased inositol phosphate levels. These findings suggest that mechanical stimuli might directly induce protooncogene expression possibly via protein kinase C activation. Furthermore, we observed the activation of MAP kinase by myocytes stretching. This result suggest that MAP kinase activation might increase in efficiency of protein synthesis on ribosomes induced by mechanical stimuli.

KEYWORDS: protooncogenes, cardiac hypertrophy, mechanical stimulus, protein kinase C, MAP kinase

INTRODUCTION

During the process of cardiac hypertrophy, the expression of specific genes, such as protooncogenes and fetal-type genes of contractile proteins, was induced as well as an increase in protein synthesis. The "immediate early genes" such as protooncogenes and heat shock protein genes are induced as an early response to pressure overload, and "late responsive genes" such as fetal contractile protein genes and the atrial natriuretic peptide gene are reexpressed as a later event. Recently, many hormones and growth factors have been reported to induce cardiac hypertrophy and specific gene expression in cultured cardiac myocytes. However, whether hemodynamic overload directly stimulates cellular hypertrophy and specific gene expression in cardiac myocytes without the participation of humoral factors remains unknown.

In the present study, to examine whether mechanical stimuli are directly coupled to specific gene expression, we cultured neonatal rat cardiac myocytes in deformable silicone culture dishes with defined serum-free medium, imposed mechanical stimuli by stretching adherent myocytes and examined protooncogene expression. Furthermore, using protooncogene induction by stretching, we studied the signal transduction pathway of mechanical stimuli on cardiacmyocytes. We also observed the activation of MAP kinase which is proposed to activate S6 kinase of rebosomes resulting in increased efficiency of protein synthesis.

RESULTS AND DISCUSSION

Mechanical Load Stimulates Cell Hypertrophy and Specific Gene Expression

We devised deformable culture dishes to impose mechanical stimuli directly on cardiac myocytes. Whole culture dishes were made of silicone. The bottom of the dish is 1-mm-thick, and it is highly transparent because of no inorganic filler in either component. We mechanically expanded the dishes with the plastic frame and increased their length uniaxially. Following expanding the length of the dishes, attached cardiac myocytes were stretched. The resting length of the myocytes was increased parallel to the axis of expansion by the same percent length as the dish[1]. This method allowed us to do more detailed analysis, such as quantitative assessment of mRNA levels, because we could obtain larger scaled samples.

We prepared primary cultures of cardiac myocytes from the ventricles of 1-day-old Wistar rats. A cardiac myocyte-rich fraction was obtained by preplating method. Myocytes not attached to the preplated dishes were plated into laminine-coated silicone dishes at a field density of 1×10^5 cells / cm^2. A nonmuscle cell-rich fraction was obtained by preplating the cells into silicone dishes for the first hour.

The effect of myocyte stretch on amino acid incorporation into cardiac proteins was firstly examined. To avoid the effect of serum, we performed this experiment after 2 days in the serum-free, chemically defined medium. Myocytes were stimulated by 10% increase in the length of the attached dishes. At this point, more than 90% of cells were beating. The incorporation of [^{14}C]phenylalanine was significantly increased 2 hours after stretch and the stimulation was maintained for over 12 hours. This finding suggests that mechanical stress stimulates cardiac cellular hypertrophy.

To ascertain whether mechanical stress induces specific genes, such as protooncogenes and fetal-type isogenes of contractile proteins as observed in the heart in vivo, we examined the expression of c-fos and skeletal α–actin gene. Northern blot analysis revealed that c-fos was rapidly and transiently expressed by stretching myocytes. The level of c-fos mRNA was increased as early as 15 minutes after the passive stretch of myocytes, and reached the maximum level at 30 minutes, followed by a decline to the undetectable level. The kinetics of this c-fos expression by stretching is the same as those when cells are stimulated with serum or growth factors. This protooncogene expression was observed abundantly in cardiac myocyte-rich fraction rather than in nonmuscle cell-rich fraction. This result confirmed that the stimulation of c-fos gene expression by stretching occurred in cardiac myocytes. The induction of c-fos mRNA depended on the extent of expansion of the dishes. The stimulation of c-fos gene expression was recognized by 5% increase in the length of the dishes. The maximum stimulation was obtained by 20% of stretch.

The level of skeletal α–actin mRNA was also accumulated after the passive stretch of myocytes. Skeletal α–actin mRNA was significantly increased 4 hours after stretching, and gradually accumulated up to 2 days during stimulation. Because it has been known that acute pressure overload induces cardiac hypertrophy and the gene expression, such as protooncogenes and fetal-type isogenes of contractile proteins in the heart in vivo, our observations revealing the expression of c-fos and skeletal α–actin gene by myocytes stretching, suggested that stretching cardiac myocytes in vitro could substitute for hemodynamic overload in vivo.

Transcriptional Activation of c-fos Gene by Myocyte Stretching

To examine whether the c-fos gene expression by myocytes stretching was regulated at the transcriptional level or post-transcriptional level, we analyzed its promoter function by CAT assay method[2]. We linked the 5' flanking region of the fos gene including its promoter, to the 5' end of the chloramphenicol acetyltransferase (CAT) encoding sequences in the plasmid and transfected this plasmid into primary cultures of neonatal rat cardiac myocytes and measured CAT activity of the cell extracts. The pSVO CAT construct containing the entire coding sequences of the procaryotic CAT gene minus its promoter showed very little CAT activity in either the absence or presence of stretch stimulation. By contrast when pSVO fos CAT, which contained the 5' c-fos flanking region, was introduced into the system, myocytes stretching for 48h reproducibly caused more than a 7-fold increase in CAT activity but there was little activity without stretching. When the pSV2CAT construct, which contained SV40 enhancer and early promotor sequences, was introduced into myocytes, a large amount of CAT activity was observed. However, additional activity was not obtained after stretching. Furthermore, the run-on study using myocyte nuclei also revealed the accumulation of c-fos mRNA by stretching. These results suggested that the c-fos gene expression by stretching was regulated at the transcriptional level and that the stretch response element was located in the 5' flanking region of the c-fos gene.

These results revealed that mechanical stress markedly induced the expression of c-fos protooncogene without the participation of humoral factors. Therefore, hemodynamic overload itself seems to be one of the main factors to stimulate the expression of the c-fos gene in the heart in vivo. Recently, Fos, the protein which the fos gene encodes, was elucidated to be localized in the nucleus and to bind to the 12-0-tetradecanoylphorbol-13-acetate-responsive elements of some genes, followed by the activation of their gene transcription in cooperation with the transcription factor AP-1. These observations suggest that some early responsive gene products like Fos may stimulate other subsequent gene expressions in the heart under conditions of hemodynamic overload.

To identify the sequences essential for the transcription of the fos gene induced by stretching, we analyzed effects of deletion of the 5' flanking region of the gene on CAT activity.

Mechanism of c-fos Gene Expression by Myocyte Stretching

Deletion mutagenesis of the 5'-flanking region of the c-fos gene indicated that the sequences between -227 and -404 base pairs were required for the efficient transcription of the fos gene by myocyte stretching. Since it has been known that there were serum and cAMP responsive element in this region , we hypothesized that three known factors, cAMP, protein kinase C and tyrosine kinase, are involved in c-fos gene stimulation by stretching.

Thus, we carried out desensitization study to determine which protein kinase system plays a central role in the signal transduction induced by mechanical stress. We pretreated myocytes with either phorbol esters (TPA), epidermal growth factor (EGF) or forskolin for 24h to down-regulate individual protein kinases, C kinase, tyrosine kinase or A kinase, respectively, and then treated again with one of these inducers. Thirty minutes after the treatment, we assessed the mRNA level of c-fos with Northern blot analysis. Our results showed that, after the pretreatment with TPA, c-fos stimulation was not obtained only with TPA. Again, the pretreatment with EGF or forskolin induced desensitization against the stimulation with EGF or forskolin, respectively. The most important observation was that only the pretreatment with TPA desensitized myocytes against stretch. These results suggest that the induction of c-fos gene by myocyte stretching might be caused by the activation of protein kinase C.

To confirm this possibility, we examined the effect of protein kinase C inhibitors on the expression of c-fos by myocyte stretching. H-7 strongly inhibited c-fos mRNA induction by stretching, whereas H-1004 inhibited it weakly, depending on their Ki value for protein kinase C. Staurosporin also strongly inhibited c-fos induction. Furthermore, the treatment of myocytes with TPA induced both c-fos and skeletal α–actin mRNA.

Finally, to examine the mechanism for the activation of protein kinase C by myocyte stretching, we measured phosphatidyl inositol turnover after myocyte stretching. Immediately after stretching, the activation of phosphatidyl inositol turnover was observed in myocytes. One minute after stretching, inositol monophosphate and bisphosphate significantly increased and reached about two-fold levels of control after 5 minutes. We could not detect the elevation of inositol trisphosphate levels at either time point. However, these results suggest that mechanical stress might stimulate protein kinase C activity via phospholipase C activation in cardiac myocytes. Recently, mechanical stress has been reported to induce prostagrandin production in skeletal and endothelial cells via phospholipase C pathway. These reports might support our hypothesis. However, further investigation is necessary to elucidate the precise molecular mechanisms how mechanical load activates phospholipase C or protein kinase C[2].

Activation of MAP Kinase by Myocyte Stretching

Mitogen-activated protein kinase, MAP kinase is a serine / threonine protein kinase, which can be activated by a variety of stimuli such as growth factors and TPA, and is proposed to be a general intracellular signaling molecule to link between events at cell surface and those in the nucleus and ribosome. Recent reports indicated that MAP kinase can phosphorylate and activate S6 kinase of ribosomes resulting in increased efficiency of protein synthesis[3,4]. Thus, in order to further define the intracellular signals by which mechanical stimuli result in increased protein synthesis, we examined whether mechanical stimuli can activate MAP kinase.

We labeled cardiac myocytes with P^{32} orthophosphate and stretched, solubilized and immunoprecipitated with specific autibodies against MAP kinase. Our results showed that stretching myocytes increased phospholyration of the protein of 43 KDa by appriximately 6-fold. Other bands were not increased. This protein was identified to the 43 KDa MAP kinase, MAP II kinase, by western immunoblotting.

To address the question, whether increased phosphorylation of MAP II kinase by stretching is indeed associated with increased kinase activity, we measured kinase activity of cell lysate by the phosphorylation of myelin basic protein, MBP as substrate. The phosphorylation of MBP was stimulated maximally 10-20 minutes after stretching by approximately 1.8 fold.

To directly determine whether the phosphorylation of MBP is induced by MAP kinase itself, cell lysates were electrophoresed on SDS-polyacrylamide gels containing MBP. After renaturation, the gels were incubated with γ-P^{32} ATP and magnesium. We observed an increased phosphorylation of MBP at 43 KDa after stretching. This increased phosphorylation was also observed when myocytes were treated with TPA. These data demonstrate that stretching myocytes increased 43 KDa MAP kinase, MAP II kinase activity. We also observed the phosphorylation of MBP at 70 KDa, but the identity of this kinase activity is unknown at present.

Our results strongly suggested that MAP kinase is stimulated by mechanical stress Via PKC activation, and this activated MAP kinase probably phosphorylates and stimulates S6 kinase of ribosome accompanied by an increased protein synthesis. Recently, MAP kinase has been shown to phosphorylate and activate the protooncogene product, c-jun. Therefore, the induction of c-fos and possibly activation of c-jun Via MAP kinase activation by stretching, can synergrstically activate the function of AP 1 comples.

ACKNOWLEDGMENT

This investigation was supported in part by Grant-in-aid for Scientific Research from the Ministry of Education, Science and Culture of Japan, Grants from the Ministry of Welfare and Uehara Memorial Foundation, and for Basic Research on Cardiac Hypertrophy from Vehicle Racing Commemorative Foundation.

REFERENCES

1) Komuro I, Kaida T, Shibazaki Y, Kurabayashi M, Katoh Y, Hoh E, Takaku F, Yazaki Y (1990) Stretching cardiac myocytes stimulates protooncogene expression. J. Biol. Chem. 265:3595-3598

2) Komuro I, Katoh Y, Kaida T, Shibazaki Y, Kurbayashi M, Hoh E, Takaku F, Yazaki Y (1991) Mechanical loading stimulates cell hypertrophy and specific gene expression in cultured rat cardiac myocytes. J. Biol. Chem. 266:1265-1268

3) Ahn NG, Krebs EG (1990) Evidence for an epidermal growth factor-stimulated protein kinase cascade in swiss 3T3 cells. J. Biol. Chem. 265:11495-11501

4) Ahn NG, Seger R, Bratlien RL, Diltz CD, Tonks NK, Krebs EG (1991) Multiple components in an epidermal growth factor-stimulated protein kinase cascade. J. Biol. Chem. 266:4220-4227

Cellular Mechanisms of Left Ventricular Hypertrophy

CHRISTOPHE LECLERCQ, JEAN-MARIE MOALIC, DANIÉLE CHARLEMAGNE, PASCALE MANSIER, CLAUDE SAINTE-BEUVE, FRANCOISE RANNOU, BRIGITTE CHEVALIER, and BERNARD SWYNGHEDAUW

U 127-INSERM, Hopital Lariboisiére, Paris, France

KEY WORDS: left ventricular hypertrophy, membrane proteins, calcium ATPase, ryanodine channels, (Na^+, K^+) ATPase, adrenergic receptors.

Cardiac hypertrophy is the physiological adaptation of the heart to chronic hemodynamic overload. Hypertrophy produces an adaptational advantage both by multiplying the contractile units and by normalizing wall stress. On the other hand, hypertrophy might be detrimental. For example, the decrease of the maximum unloading velocity, beneficial at the fiber level, is detrimental in terms of diastolic function and cardiac output [reviewed in 1].
Changes due to chronic overload exist both in myocyte and in non-myocyte cells. Every cellular component is modified in cardiac hypertrophy : the cellular membranes, the membrane proteins, the contractile apparatus, and also the extracellular matrix. Most of these changes are species specific and for example, the modifications of the myosin heavy chain which exist in the overloaded rat ventricle do not exist in guinea pigs or humans. Cardiac remodeling is both quantitative and qualitative and is a consequence of several changes in gene expression [1]. The aim of this article is to review the different modifications observed at the cellular level in the hypertrophied myocytes with a particular attention to the membrane structure.

<u>The external cellular membrane of the hypertrophied myocytes</u> (table 1).

The membrane surface of a myocyte from a normal adult rat can be quantitated on sections using morphological techniques [2] or by measuring the membrane capacity of the cells, the differences observed between these two methods are explained by the fact that the electrophysiologic study takes into account all the microvillosities of the external membrane. In the adult heart, it is well-known that cardiac hypertrophy induced by chronic overload results from both a hypertrophy of the myocyte without cell division and a hypertrophy of the non-myocytes cells which is accompanied by cell divisions [1, 3]. The average cellular volume of the myocyte and thus the average cell surface both increase in parallel with the degree of hypertrophy whist the surface/volume ratio remain constant [2]. Nevertheless the three components of the cell membrane do not increase in the same manner during mechanical overload. For example, for a cardiac hypertrophy of 60 %, the actual surface of the sarcolemma increases by 35 %, that of the intercalated discs by 55 % and that of the T-tubule by 100% [2]. The increase in membrane surface, as deduced from membrane capacity is higher than that deduced from morphologic studies. In a same model and with the same percentage of hypertrophy the membrane increases by 50 % with morphometrical measurements and by 103 % with electrophysiologic studies. The proteins of the membrane are unequally distributed on the membrane surface and the new distribution that may be imposed by the adaptational process is unknown.

<u>The membrane proteins of the hypertrophied myocyte</u> (Table 2).

Besides the change of the membrane structure itself, several modifications are observed in the membrane proteins. Three groups of membrane proteins can be distinguished in the normal myocytes of the adult rat. (i) The very abundant membrane proteins: the calcium-activated Adenosine TriPhosphatase (Ca^{2+} ATPase) of the sarcoplasmic reticulum (SR) (around 100 million molecules per myocyte). (ii) Proteins as (Na^+, K^+) ATPase which are abundant (100,000 to 500,000 molecules per cell) and then (iii) the rare proteins, as the calcium channels, the muscarinic and $\beta1$ or $\alpha1$ adrenergic receptors (10,000 to 80,000 molecules per cell).

The density of these different membrane proteins has been calculated by dividing the number of molecules per cell by the total membrane surface, the number of myocytes per left ventricle remaining constant during cardiac hypertrophy.

Calcium channels

The number of calcium channels per left ventricle has been calculated in the rat after specific binding with radioactive DiHydroPyridine, DHP. In the rat but also in the guinea pig [4, 5] the number of DHP receptors is significantly higher in the whole hypertrophied heart than in the control. Nevertheless, since the hearts are bigger the density of DHP receptors remains constant during hypertrophy. The measurements of the number of functional calcium channels has been made by the patch clamp technique on isolated cells. The differences observed between the patch clamp and the binding technique suggest that only 5 % of the total channels are functional. During cardiac hypertrophy, the measurements of the activity of these channel show that the intensity of calcium current per cell is increased, but the density per unit of membrane surface area remains unchanged which means that the quantity of functional calcium channels also increases with the degree of hypertrophy [6, 7].

Ryanodine channels

During the excitation-contraction coupling, the release of calcium from SR as activated by the rapid influx of calcium through the SL calcium channels. This release is mediated by the ryanodine receptors which are the calcium channels of the SR in cardiac hypertrophy, the alterations of these channels might be responsible of the modification of action potential, calcium transient, and contractility. Both in rats and guinea pigs, the density of ryanodine receptors estimated by specific binding with ^{3}H-ryanodine is decreased in cardiac hypertrophy [8] and the diminution is more pronounced in guinea pig than in rats. In contrast the total number of receptors remains unchanged in the hypertrophied rat heart and is slightly diminished after banding aorta in guinea pig. These differences emphasize the species-specificity of the adaptational process. Rat and guinea pig both have a different intra-myocardial calcium metabolism and it is not really surprising that the fundamental basis of their respective adaptational process is not the same [8].

Ca^{2+} ATPase of SR.

After contraction, the Ca^{2+} ATPase of the SR pumps back the intracellular calcium into the SR. The Ca^{2+} ATPase activity, but also the number of Ca^{2+} ATPase molecules and the mRNA content have been measured in cardiac hypertrophy in rats. The number of Ca^{2+} ATPase molecules per myocyte and/or per left ventricle is unmodified in the hypertrophied heart while the density per unit of surface membrane area is decreased. This protein belongs to a family of genes which are not activated by the process of adaptation, consequently both the enzyme and the corresponding messenger RNA are diluted during the commpensatory growth of the heartt. Such a molecular change could explain the diminution of intracellular calcium movements and is responsible for the decrease in calcium uptake by the isolated SR. This depressed density might also explain the decreased velocity of relaxation in the hypertrophied cardiac muscle. Similar results have been reportted in the human failing heart. [9, 10].

Na^{+}, Ca^{2+} exchange.

The activity of the Na^{+} /Ca^{2+}- exchange which is the main mechanism for calcium extrusion out of the cell has been studied in the hypertrophied heart rat. Both influx and efflux of calcium are significantly depressed compared to control heart. [11, 12].

β adrenergic and muscarinic receptors

The inotropic effect of the β adrenergic system is modulated by the G proteins, the adenylate cyclase and the activations of cAMP-dependent protein kinases. The β adrenergic systems increases [Ca]i during systole by the phosphorylation of the calcium channels. This system is also well-known to stimulate the rate of relaxation by activiting the Na^{+}/Ca^{2+} exchange and the Ca^{2+} ATPase of SR. The decreased effect of isoproterenol on contracility [14] and on the amplitude of the calcium current observed in cardiac hypertrophy may result from a modification of the adrenergic systems, e g, adrenergic receptors, G proteins and /or adenylate cyclase [13]. During compensatory cardiac hypertrophy in rat, the density of both the β adrenergic and the muscarinic receptors decreases in parallel. Since the number of these receptors remains constant per myocyte the ratio β adrenergic/muscarinic receptors is unchanged in this model [14]. Nevertheless in this model there are also evidence for a diminished inotropic effect of forskolin, a well-known activator of adenylate cyclase, suggesting that several other alterations are located "down the road". Recent unpublished data from this laboratory have shown that the relative amount of the mRNA coding for the β adrenergic receptor is lower suggesting that this gene does also belongs to the same family than that of the gene of the Ca^{2+} ATPase of SR. By contrast we also found a normal density in the α_s subunit of the G protein suggesting that this peptide belongs to another group of genes whichh respons to hemcdynamic overload as the sarcolemmal calcium channels.

In human hearts, modifications of the β adrenergic system were found with some differences regarding the etiology. The density in β1 adrenergic receptors drops while that of the α_i subunit of the G protein is augmented [15]. Whether or not the differences between human and rat are species-specfic is unknown. They may be related to the fact that experimental models of heart failure are rare and poorly reproducible whilst by contrast most of the biochemisrtry in human heart has been made using failing hearts NYA class III or IV.

(Na^+, K^+) ATPase.

The (Na^+, K^+) ATPase is directly responsible for the intracellular Na^+ and K^+ homeostasis and indirectly for that of the calcium through the Na^+, Ca^{2+} exchange. In the rat, three genes encoding the α catalytic subunit are expressed: α1, α2, α3. These isoforms differ by their affinity for both sodium and ouabain. α1 exhibits a low affinity for ouabain and is present at every step of the development. α2 has a high affinity and is only expressed after birth and in the adult heart, the last one, α3, also has a hight affinity for ouabain but is specific of the neonatal heart. [16].

There are two possibilities to understand the changes in the (Na^+, K^+) ATPase during the hypertrophic process. (i) The biochemical approach consists in studying the caracteristics of the enzyme with regard to ouabain binding or inhibition of the activity by the glycoside. A low and a high affinity site were found in both the control and the hypertrophied rat and guinea pig hearts, they both are modified, but the adaptation of the (Na^+, K^+) ATPase to chronic overload seems to be species-specific. In the hypertrophied rat heart, the total activity of the enzyme is normal but a large increase in the sensitivity to ouabain is observed. This increase is correlated with a 2 fold augmentation in the number of high affinity sites. In the guinea pig the specific activity of the enzyme of the low affinity sites is more importtant that than of the high affinity sites [8]. (ii) The other approach was to investigate the expression of the mRNA encoding the three types of catalytic subunits of the (Na^+, K^+) ATPase. In the hypertrophied rat heart, no changes in the mRNA of the α1 isoform per mg of total RNA was found. Regarding the two others isoforms, α2 and α3, we observed a decrease in the α2 isoform by 40 % and a two-fold increase in α3. Therefore hypertrophy induces an up-regulation of the α3 gene, normally expressed in the neonatal heart [17]. In other models of cardiac hypertrophy induced by hypertension, alterations in the expression of the (Na^+, K^+) ATPase genes were also observed with a repression of the expression of the gene coding for the α2 isoform. This both quantitative and qualitative changes at cellular level must be taken into account for treatment and pharmacological research.

Cardiac hypertrophy due to chronic overload alters the density and the number of membrane proteins in such a way that calcium homeostasis becomes potentially fragile.

REFERENCES

1. Swynghedauw B (1990) Cardiac hypertrophy and failure. Paris, London INSERM J. Libbey Pub, 740 pp.

2. Anversa P, Loud A, Giacomelli F et al (1978) Absolute morphometric study of myocardial hypertrophy in experimental hypertension. Lab Invest 38 : 597-609

3. Korecky B, Rakusan K (1978) Normal and hypertrophic growth of the rat heart : changes in cell dimensions and number. Am J Physiol 234 : H123-H128.

4. Mayoux E, Callens F, Swynghedauw B, Charlemagne D (1988) Adaptational process of the cardiac Ca^{2+} channels to pressure overload : Biochemical and physiological properties of the DHP receptors in normal and hypertrophied rat hearts. J Cardiovasc Pharmacol 12 : 390-396

5. Primot I, Mayoux E, Oliviero P, Charlemagne D (1991) Effect of pressure overload on cardiac Ca^{2+} antagonist binding sites of guinea pig. Comparison with adaptational response of the hypertrophied rat heart. Cardiovasc Res 25 : 875-880.

6. Reuter H (1983) Calcium channel modulation by neurotransmitters, enzymes and drugs. Nature 301: 569-572.

7. Schwartz LM, Mc Clerley EW, Almers W (1985) DHP receptors in muscle and voltage-dependant but most are functionnal calcium channels. Nature 314 : 747-51.

8. Sainte Beuve C, Leclerq C, Rannou F, Oliviero P, Mansier P, Chevalier B, Swynghedauw B, Charlemagne D (1992) Remodeling of the hypertensive heart. Kidney International 41: suppl. 37 in press.

9. De la Bastie D, Levitsky D, Rappaport L, Mercadier JJ, Schwartz K, Lompré AM (1990) Function of the sarcoplasmic reticulum and expression of its Ca^{2+} ATPase gene in pressure overload-induced cardiac hypertrophy in the rat. Circ Res 66: 554-564

10. Nagai R, Zarain-Herzberg A, Alpert N, Periasamy M (1989) Regulation of myocardial Ca^{2+} ATPase and phospholamban mRNA expression in response to pressure overload and thyroid hormone. Proc Natl Acad Sci USA 86 : 2966-2970

11. Hanf R, Drubaix I, Lelievre LG (1988) Rat cardiac hypertrophy : altered sodium calcium exchange activity in sarcolemmal vesicles. FEBS Letters 236 : 145-149

12. Andrawis NJ, Kuoth, Giacomelli F, Wiener J (1988) Altered calcium regulation in the cardiac plasma membrane in experimental renal hypertension. J Mol Cell Cardiol 20 : 625-634

13. Swynghedauw B (1990) Changes in membrane proteins in chronic mechanical overload of the heart. Am J Cardiol 65 : 30 G - 33 G

14. Mansier P, Chevalier B, Mayoux E, Swynghedauw B (1990) Membrane proteins of the myocytes in cardiac overload. Br J Clin Pharmac 30: 43S-48S

15. Bristow MR, Anderson FL, Port DJ, Feldman A (1991) Differences in adrenergic neuroeffector mechanism in ischemic versus idiopathic dilated cardiomyopathy. Circulation 84: 1024-1039.

16. Orlowski, Lingrel JB (1990) Thyroid and glucocorticoid hormones regulate the expression of multiple Na, K-ATPase genes in culture neonatal rat cardiac myocytes. J Biol Chem 265 : 3462-3470.

17. Charlemagne D, Maixent JM, Preteseille J, Lelièvre LG (1986) Ouabain binding sites and Na^{+}/K^{+} ATPase activity in rat cardiac hypertrophy. Expression of the neonatal form. J Biol Chem 261: 185-189.

Table I

External membrane and sarcoplasmic reticulum of hypertrophied cardiac myocyte in adult rat.

	Normal	Hypertrophied
Cell length (μm)	100	117
Cell width (μm)	20	23*
Cell volume (μm^3)	11,500	18,300*
Cell surface (μm^2)	7,000	11,800*
T Tubules (μm^2)	2,300	4,800*
non tubular sarcolemma	4.500	6,100*
Cell surface (pF capacitance)	13,300	27,100*
Surface / volume (pm-1)	0.60	0.68
Sarcoplasmic reticulum surface	10,000	18,000*
Myocytes number per ventricle x 10^6	46	46

* $p < 0.01$ Data from [13]

Table II

Changes in membrane proteins in rat cardiac hypertrophy.

	Number per cell	Density per surface
β1 adrenergic receptors	Normal	Decreased
Muscarinic receptors	Normal	Decreased
Calcium channels	Increased	Normal
(Na^+, K^+) ATPase high affinity site	Increased	Increased
(Na^+, K^+) ATPase low affinity site	Normal	Decreased
Ca^{2+} ATPase SR	Normal	Decreased
Ryanodine channels	Normal	Decreased

PI Response and Calcium Overload in Cardiomyopathic Hamster Heart Cell

HIDEAKI KAWAGUCHI, MIKAKO SHOKI, HITOSHI SANO, TOSHIYUKI KUDO, HIROFUMI SAWA, HIROSHI OKAMOTO, NAOKI MOCHIZUKI, YUKA ENDO, HISAKAZU YASUDA, and AKIRA KITABATAKE

Department of Cardiovascular Medicine, Hokkaido University School of Medicine, Sapporo, 060 Japan

KEYWORDS:phosphatidylinositide-specific phospholipase C, Inositol-1,4,5 trisphosphate, cardiomyopathy

INTRODUCTION

Plasma membrane inositol phospholipids were breakdown by hormones and neurotransmitters through the mediation of the specific receptors (1-4). This phosphatidylinositol (PI) turnover pathway generates two second messengers, inositol-(1,4,5)-trisphosphate (IP_3) and sn-1,2-diacylglycerol (DAG) (5,6). DAG stimulates membrane-bound phospholipid-dependent, Ca^{2+}-dependent protein kinase C (7), while IP_3 releases Ca^{2+} from stores in the sarcoplasmic reticulum (8,9). The physiological significance of this PI-turnover pathway is not still clear in any mammalian cell system. It is controversial whether IP_3 stimulates Ca^{2+} release from SR in cardiac myocytes.

Syrian cardiomyopathic hamsters (BIO 14.6 and BIO 53.58) display hereditary abnormalities of the cardiac and skeletal muscles which are inherited as an autosomal recessive trait (10). BIO 14.6 cardiac involvement results in initial myocardial hypertrophy that is followed by cardiac dilatation and death from congestive heart failure (11). It is thought the cardiomyopathic hamster provides a useful model of human cardiac diseases such as hypertrophic cardiomyopathy (12,13).

In this report, we determined the role of PI-response in inducing myocardial cell damage and cardiac myocyte hypertrophy in dilated and hypertrophic cardiomyopathic hamster heart cells.

MATERIALS and METHODS

Experimental Protocol

Experiments were carried out using male hypertrophic cardiomyopathic (BIO 14.6) and dilated (BIO 53.58) cardiomyopathic hamsters aged 5, 10, 20 and 30 weeks (Bio Breeders, Fitchburg, Massachusetts)(13). F1b hamsters were used as control. Six experiments in triplicate were analyzed in all the studies, and results were expressed as the mean ± SEM. Statistical significance was determined using ANOVA.

Cell preparation

Cardiac myocytes from BIO 14.6, BIO 53.58 and F1b hamsters were prepared in phosphate buffer (PB) according to a previously reported method (14), and then cultured in Ham's F-10 medium with 10% fetal calf serum (FCS) until use. Freshly prepared cells were maintained at 37° C in a humidified 5% CO_2/95% air atmospher. Cells were then subcultured for assay in 35-mm dishes at 3 x 10^5/dish in 1 ml of PB containing 1 mM $CaCl_2$ and used within 2 hours.

Phospholipase C activity

For the determination of the cellular phospholipase C activity, cells (1x10^5) were first labeled with 5 μCi of [^{3}H]myoinositol. Labeling was performed for 24 hr in PB with 0.3%

FCS, after which cells were washed three times with PB. Cells were then incubated with the indicated concentrations of NE, 5 mM 2,3-diphosphoglyceric acid (2,3-DPG; this concentration inhibited the dephosphorylation of IP_3 and IP_4 by 98%), and 10 mM LiCl for the indicated periods in the presence of 1 μM metoprolol. and then terminated with chloroform/methanol (2:1, v/v). Phospholipids were fractionated by TLC using a chloroform/methanol/acetic acid/water solvent system (50:30:8:4, v/v). For the separation of polyinositol-phosphatides, the aqueous phase was applied to an AG1 x8 column in format form (100-200 mesh; Bio-Rad), and inositol phosphates were separated by an ammonium gradient system (0.2-1.2 M) plus 0.1 M formic acid (15). For a more detailed analysis, including the separation of inositol phosphate isomers, samples were filtered and separated by high-performance liquid chromatography (Whatman Partisil 10 SAX anion-exchange column with a guard column) using a gradient of ammonium formate and phosphate (16). The release of IP_3 was also determined by using an IP_3-binding protein system (myoinositol-(1,4,5)-trisphosphate assay system, Amersham, UK).

Calcium release from sarcoplasmic reticulum

Left ventricles were minced and homogenized for 60 seconds by a polytron homogenizer (PT-19, Kinematica, Switzerland) in 5 volumes (vol/wt) of 0.1 M Tris-HCl (pH 7.4). The homogenate was centrifuged at 1,000g for 10 minutes, and the resultant supernatant was centrifuged at 14,000g for 20 minutes to remove mitochondria. The supernatant was centrifuged at 45,000g for 30 minutes according to previously published methods (16). The pellet was washed twice with the same buffer and suspended in 0.6 M KCl and 10 mM tris(hydroxymethyl)methyl-2-aminomethane-sulfonic acid (TES) pH 7.4. The suspension was centrifuged at 45,000g for 30 min. The resultant pellet was suspended in 150 mM KCl and 1 mM TES pH 7.1 and used for each assay as sarcoplasmic reticulum.

$^{45}Ca^{2+}$ (4 μCi) was loaded into freshly prepared sarcoplasmic reticulum by incubating 400 μg of sarcoplasmic reticulum in a final reaction mixture of 400 μl in cytosolic buffer (KCl 120 mM, NaCl 10 mM, KH_2PO_4 1 mM, $NaHCO_3$ 5 mM, HEPES 10mM, pH 7.1), $MgCl_2$ 5mM, and ATP 5 μM for 10 min. The final free Ca^{2+} concentration was calculated according to the method of Fabiato and Fabiato (18) and adjusted to 1 μM. In Ca^{2+} release experiments, IP_3 was added to the 100 μl-aliquot of $^{45}Ca^{2+}$-loaded sarcoplasmic reticulum in the presence of 1 mM EGTA, 10 mM LiCl and 5 mM 2,3-diphosphoglycerate (2,3-DPG; this concentration of 2,3-DPG inhibited the dephosphorylation of IP_3), and immediately mixed with the reaction medium. Ca^{2+} release started from this time. The experiments were carried out at 37° C. After the indicated incubation periods, the incubation mixture was filtered through a 0.45 Millipore filter, washed three times with 3 ml of cytosolic buffer, and counted in 5 ml of Ready Gel. The zero-time Ca^{2+} content of the sarcoplasmic reticulum was obtained by diluting the original incubate and immediately filtering it through a Millipore filter. The total sarcoplasmic reticulum calcium content was 388 2 nmol/mg protein. There was no differences between two groups in calcium content of sarcoplasmic reticulum.

RESULTS

The heart weight/body weight was higher in 5-20 weeks of ages of BIO 14.6 hamsters than in F1b hamsters. There is no difference in it at 30 weeks of age between both hamsters. On the other hand, it was lower in all age groups of BIO 53.58 hamsters than in F1b hamsters.

Polyphosphoinositide-specific phospholipase C activity was studied. Myocardial cells isolated from 10-week-old BIO 14.6, BIO 53.58, and F1b hamsters were incubated with the indicated concentrations of NE and 1 μM metoprolol in the presence of 10 mM LiCl and 5 mM 2,3-DPG for 90 sec. NE induced the hydrolysis of PI, but lysoPI accumulation was not observed. This indicates that phospholipase has substrate specificity towards PI, and suggests that phospholipase C was activated but not phospholipase A_2. There was no significant difference between the BIO 14.6 and BIO 53.58 hamsters. The PIP_2-PLC activity of isolated cells was markedly enhanced by NE stimulation in both types of cardiomyopathic hamster. IP_3 release was enhanced by NE from the age of 5 weeks to 30 weeks. At this stage, the release of IP_3 in response to NE was significantly activated in both BIO 14.6 and BIO 53.38 hamsters (Fig.2). This acceleration of PI-turnover may affect Ca^{2+} flux into cells. As previously reported, the basal intracellular calcium concentration without NE stimulation was higher in BIO 53.58 hamsters than in BIO 14.6 and F1b hamsters (19).

Intracellular calcium levels in BIO 53.58 hamsters aged 5–20 weeks were significantly higher than those of age-matched BIO 14.6 hamsters, but there was no significant differences between two types of cardiomyopathic hamsters at 30 weeks of age. The sarcoplasmic reticulum (SR) function of cardiomyopathic hamster hearts were investigated. As shown in figure 3, calcium uptake into SR increase in BIO14.6, but it decreased in BIO 53.58. The addition of IP_3 to $^{45}Ca^{2+}$-preloaded sarcoplasmic reticulum from F1b, BIO 14.6 and BIO 53.58 in a medium containing 1 μM free Ca^{2+} induced a transient release of Ca^{2+} and achieved a maximum effect at 10 μM IP_3 for 1 min-incubation at 37° C. The Ca^{2+} release from sarcoplasmic reticulum in BIO 14.6 was significantly higher than in F1b. On the other hand, calcium release from SR decreased in BIO 53.58 (Fig.4).

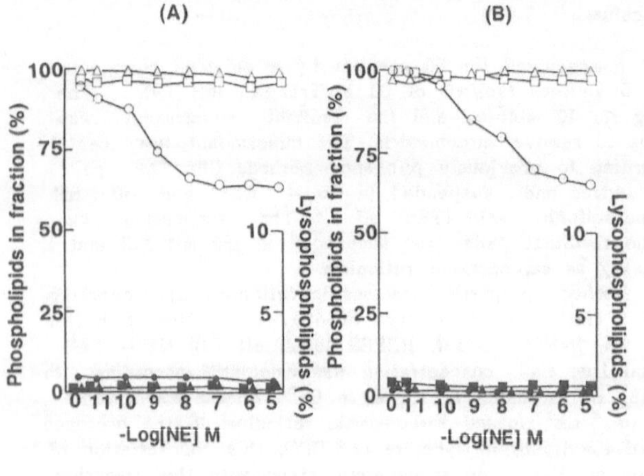

Fig.1 Phospholipid hydrolysis stimulated by NE. Phospholipid hydrolysis was determined as described in Materials and Methods. BIO 14.6 (A), BIO 53.58 (B) △:phosphatidylcholine, ○;phosphatidylinositol,□;phosphatidylethanolamine, ▲;lysophosphatidylcholine, ●;lysophosphatidylinositol, ■;lysophosphatidylethanolamine (from ref 21)

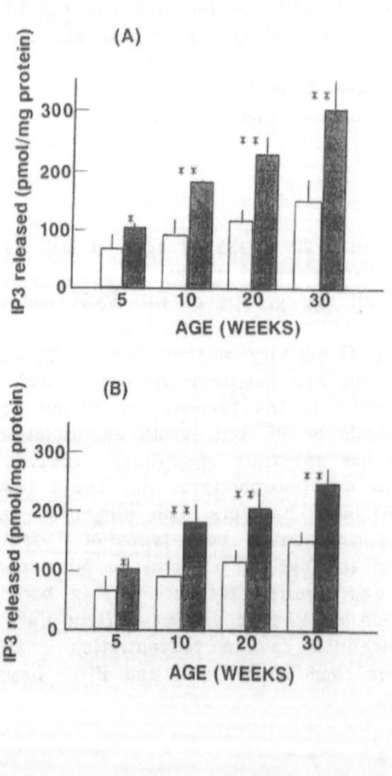

Fig.2. Effects of norepinephrine stimulation on IP_3 release (A)BIO 14.6 8 (hatched bar), (B) BIO 53.58 aged 5–30 weeks (hatched bar) and F1b (open bar). *$p<0.05$ compared with age-matched F1b, **$p<0.001$ compared with age-matched F1b. (from ref 21)

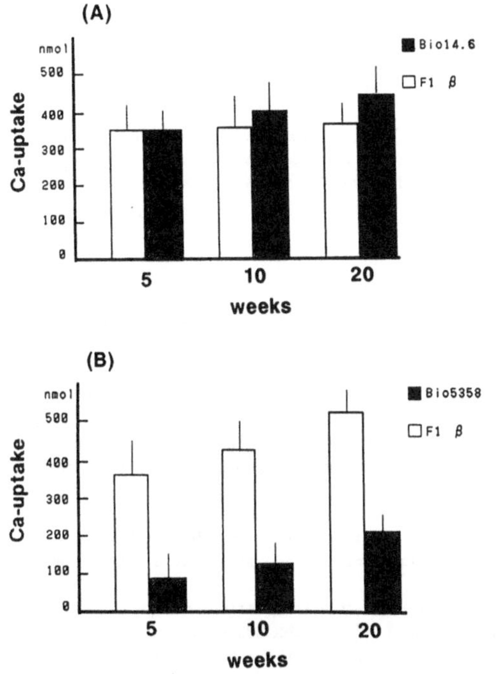

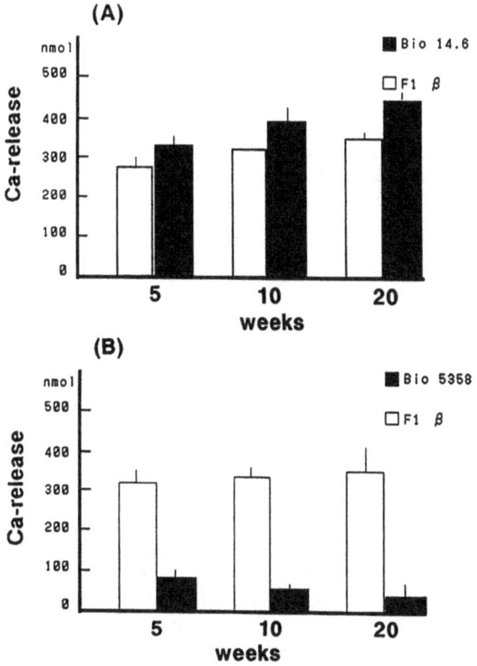

Fig.3. Ca^{2+}-uptake into Sarcoplasmic reticulum Ca^{2+} uptake was determined as described in Materials and methods. (from ref 21)
Fig.4. Ca^{2+}-release from Sarcoplasmic reticulum stimulated by IP_3. Ca^{2+}-release was determined as described in Materials and methods. (from ref 21)

DISCUSSION

In our experiment, the accumulations of polyphosphoinositides after stimulation with NE were significantly enhanced in cardiac myocytes of cardiomyopathic hamster. These results suggest the possibility that the enhanced phosphatidylinositol-4,5-bisphosphate-IP_3-Ca^{2+} pathways and the DAG-PKC pathway may increase protein synthesis in the BIO 14.6 heart. However, this hypothesis does not explain how myocardial cell damage occurs in BIO 53.58 hamsters. In both animals, the phosphatidylinositol metabolism and the polyphosphoinositide metabolism are enhanced, but one develops cardiac hypertrophy and the other develops cardiac dilatation. This difference may be partly explained by the cytosolic Ca^{2+} concentration as reported elsewhere (25). The cytosolic Ca^{2+} concentration was quite high in BIO 53.58 hamsters aged 4-30 weeks, but in BIO 14.6 hamsters, it increased at 30 weeks of age. As mentioned above, an increase in the PI-response may raise the cytosolic Ca^{2+} level, but in BIO 14.6 hamsters aged 4-20 weeks it was still low than in BIO 53.58 hamsters. These results suggest that the intracellular calcium handling is seriously disturbed from a very young age in BIO 53.58 hamsters. On the other hand, it appears to be well-preserved in the early stages of hypertrophic cardiomyopathy in BIO 14.6 hamsters. Our results supported this hypothesis. Calcium uptake into sarcoplasmic reticulum decreased in Bio53.58 hamsters compared to BIO 14.6 and F1b hamsters (26). These results show that α_1-adrenergic receptor stimulation may cause intracellular calcium overload because of deterioration of sarcoplasmic reticulum function in BIO 53.58 hamsters.

CONCLUSION

These results suggest that PI response may produce high intracellular calcium levels in both BIO 14.6 and BIO 53.58 myocytes. In addition, in BIO 53.58 hamster the sarcoplasmic reticulum deteriorate in function. It was concluded from these results that a prolonged high intracellular calcium level may lead to the death of BIO 53.58 myocytes.

ACKNOWLEDGMENT

This research was supported in part by a Research Grant for Cardiomyopathy from the Ministry of Health and Welfare of Japan and Grants-in-Aid for Scientific Research from the Ministry of Education, Science and Culture of Japan, 01870041, 02404042, and 02454250.

REFERENCES

1.Brown JH, Buxton IL, Brunton LL(1985) α_1-adrenergic and muscarinic cholinergic stimulation of phosphoinositide hydrolysis in adult rat cardiomyocytes. Circ Res 57:532-537
2.Fasolato C, Pandiella A, Meldolesi J, Pozzan T (1988) Generation of inositol phosphate, cytosolic Ca^{2+}, and ionic Fluxes in PC12 Cells treated with bradykinin. J Biol Chem 263:17350-17359
3.Baker KM, Singer HA (1988) Identification and characterization of guinea pig angiotensin II ventricular and atrial receptors: coupling to inositol phosphate production. Circ Res 62:896-904
4.Dubyak GR, Cowen DS, Meuller LM(1988)Activation of inositol phospholipid breakdown in HL60 cells by P2-purinergic receptors for extracellular ATP.J Biol Chem 263:18108-18117
5.Berridge MJ (1984) Inositol trisphosphate and diacylglycerol as second messengers. Biochem J 220:345-360
6.Williamson JR, Cooper RH, Joseph NE, Thomas AP (1985) Inositol trisphosphate and diacylglycerol as intracellular second messengers in liver. Am J Phys 248:C203-C216
7.Nisizuka Y (1983) Phospholipid degradation and signal translation for protein phosphoryla tion. Trend Biochem Sci 8:13-16
8.Putney JW (1987) Formation and actions of calcium-mobilizing messenger, inositol 1,4,5-trisphosphate. Am J Physiol 252:G149-G157
9.Ehrlich BE,Watras J (1988) Inositol 1,4,5-trisphosphate activates a channel from smooth muscle sarcoplasmic reticulum. Nature 336:583-586
10.Bajusz E (1969) Hereditary cardiomyopathy:a new disease model. Amer Heart J 77:686
11.Strobeck JE, Factor SM, Bhan A, Sole M, Liew CC, Fein F, Sonnenblick EH (1979) Hereditary and acquired cardiomyopathies in experimental animals:mechanical,biochemical, and structual features. Ann NY Acad Sci 317:59-88
12.Homburger F, Baker JR, Nixon CW Whitney R (1962) Primary generalized polymyophaty and cardiac necrosis in an inbred line of Syrian hamsters. Med Exp 6:339-345
13.Bajuz E, Baker JR, Nixon CW, Homburger F (1969) Spontaneous hereditary myocardial degeneration and congestive heart failure in a strain of Syrian hamsters. Ann NY Acad Sci 156:105-129
14.Glick MR, Burns AH, Reddy WJ (1974) Dispersion and isolation of beating cells from adult rat Heart. Anal Biochem 61:32-42
15.Merritt JE, Taylor CW, Rubin RP, Putney JW (1986) Isomers of inositol trisphosphate in exocrine pancreas. Biochem J 238:825-829
16.Batty IR, Nahorski SR, Irvine RF (1985) Rapid formation of inositol 1,3,4,5-tetrakisphosphate following muscarinic receptor stimulation of rat cerebral cortical slices. Bio chem J 232:211-215
17.Nakanishi T, Jarmakini JM (1988) Developmental changes in myocardial mechanical function and subcellular organelles. Am J Physiol 246:H615-H625
18.Fabiato A, Fabiato F (1975) Contractions induced by a calcium-triggered release of calcium from the sarcoplasmic reticulum of single skinned cardiac cells. J Physiol (London) 249:469-495
19.Kawaguchi H, Shoki M, Sano H, Kudo T, Sawa H, Okamoto H, Sakata Y, Yasuda H (1991) Phospholipid metabolism in cardiomyophatic hamster heart cells. Circ Res 69:1015-1021
20.Whitmer JT, Kumar P, Solaro RJ(1988) Calcium transport proper ties of cardiac sarcoplasmic reticulum from cardiomyopathic syrian hamster (BIO 53.58 and 14.6):Evidence for a quantitative defect in dilated myopathic hearts not eividence in hypertrophic hearts. Circ Res 62:81-85
21.Kawaguchi H, Shoki M, Sano H, Kudo T, Sawa H, Okamoto H, Sakata Y, Yasuda H (1992) The studies of cell damaging and cell growth factor which induce cardiomyopathy. Jpn Cic J in press

Mitochondrial DNA Mutations in Cardiomyopathy

Takayuki Ito[1], Kazuki Hattori[1], Toshihiro Obayashi[1], Masashi Tanaka[2], Satoru Sugiyama[2], and Takayuki Ozawa[2]

Department of Internal Medicine II[1], and Biomedical Chemistry, Faculty of Medicine[2], University of Nagoya, Nagoya, 466 Japan

KEY WORDS: cardiomyopathy, mitochondrial DNA, MELAS, mutation

INTRODUCTION

Mitochondria have their own DNA, 16,569 base pairs, which encodes mRNA genes for 13 subunits of four complexes of the oxidative phosphorylation system, 22 tRNAs required for translation of their mRNA, and two rRNA [1]. The mutation rate in mitochondrial DNA (mtDNA) is more than 10 times higher than that of nuclear DNA [2]. This is due to absence of introns, lack of DNA-binding proteins such as histones, simple DNA repair mechanism, and constant exposure to active oxygen. Mitochondria occupy a pivotal position in cellular energy metabolism, and deterioration of various enzymes linked with energy metabolism in mitochondria due to mtDNA mutations has been shown to be involved in the case of mitochondrial cytopathy or mitochondrial myopathy [3,4,5]. Using advanced gene technology, we have developed rapid and accurate methods for the detection of mutations of mtDNA and total sequences of mtDNA. We review: (1) mtDNA mutations in cardiomyocytes of patients with dilated or hypertrophic cardiomyopathy, (2) a patient with hypertrophic cardiomyopathy associated with left ventricular dilatation, (3) a patient with mitochondrial myopathy, encephalopathy, lactic acidosis, and stroke-like episodes (MELAS) showing hypertrophic cardiomyopathy, and (4) a patient with fatal infantile cardiomyopathy.

MATERIALS AND METHODS

Patients

Study (1): Cardiac tissue specimens were obtained from 16 patients with hypertrophic or dilated cardiomyopathy of unknown etiology and from a person who died from an accident as a normal control. Patient-13 was familial dilated cardiomyopathy. Autopsied frozen myocardiums of patient-5, 9, and 11 reported by Ozawa et al. [6] were used.

Study (2): A 43-year-old man with a twenty year history of cardiomegaly was admitted to hospital because of general malaise and dyspnea on exertion. The chest X ray showed cardiac enlargement with a 68% cardio-thoracic ratio and evidence of pulmonary congestion and bilateral effusion. The echocardiogram showed left ventricular enlargement, diffuse hypokinesis in wall motion. The ejection fraction was 20%. The cardiac index was 2.5 $l/min/m^2$. The endomyocardial biopsy samples showed myofiber hypertrophy and marked disarray, which are characteristic of hypertrophic cardiomyopathy, although the hemodynamic features resembled dilated cardiomyopathy. Family history showed that his younger sister also had hypertrophic cardiomyopathy. Two years after the first admission, he died of heart and renal failure. Autopsied frozen heart muscle, skeletal muscle and liver of this patient reported by Hattori et al. [7] and Ozawa et al. [8] were used.

Study (3): A 37-year-old man was admitted to a hospital because of abdominal pain, vomiting, and fainting. He had lactic acidosis, hypertrophic cardiomyopathy, and stroke-like episodes, and died of heart failure. Ragged-red fibers were observed on skeletal muscle biopsy.

Study (4): A 1-year-old boy was admitted to a hospital because of general weakness. He was an only child of non-consanguineous healthy parents. A chest roentgenogram revealed severe cardiomegaly with a cardiothoracic ratio of 71%. Cyanosis and stiffness of neck were found. Blood analysis indicated anemia, metabolic acidosis, and increased levels of muscle enzymes. The patient developed bradycardia and convulsions, and died of heart failure on the 7th hospital day. Frozen autopsied myocardium of this patient reported by Tanaka et al. [9,10] was used.

Preparation of DNA and Analysis of mtDNA deletions

Total DNA was extracted from 5mg of biopsied or autopsied heart muscles as previously reported [11]. Southern blot analysis [4] and the PCR [11] for detection of mtDNA deletions were performed as described. The total mtDNAs from the patients were sequenced by using a fluorescence-based automated direct sequencing technique [10] using an Applied Biosystems Model 373A DNA Sequencer. The base sequences of the oligonucleotide primers are shown in Table I.

Table I. SYNTHESIZED PRIMERS USED FOR PCR

Primers	Sequences 5' → 3'	Complementary site**		
L116	AACTCAAAGGACCTGGCGGT	1,161	to	1,180
L853	ACGAAAATCTGTTCGCTTCA	8,531	to	8,550
H38	AAATTTGAAATCTGGTTAGG	400	to	381
H617	CGGGGAAACGCCATATCGGG	6,190	to	6,171

* The first letter of the primer, L or H, specifies its priming strand.
** Numbering of the mtDNA is done according to Anderson and colleagues.

RESULTS AND DISCUSSION

Study (1): Fig. 1-A shows the PCR amplification of mtDNA from the heart muscle using primers L853 and H38. Multiple abnormal bands including a 1.0-kb fragment, which means a 7.4 kb-deletion of mtDNA, could be detected in patients 5, 6, 7, 8, 9, 10, 11, 12, 13, 14, and 16. Deleted mtDNA was detected in 5 of 6 patients with dilated cardiomyopathy. We further performed PCR using another pair of primers, L116 and H617, the distance between them was 5.0 kb (Fig. 1-B). We verified that the amounts of the 5.0-kb fragment were almost the same in all patients. Accordingly, the amount of mtDNA as template might be similar among these patients. The deletion was confirmed by the primer shift PCR method [11] and PCR Southern method [11]. These results indicate that the PCR products observed here are not artifacts but are amplified from the deleted mtDNA. Sequence of the region surrounding the deletion is shown in Fig. 2. The crossover sequence was demonstrated to be a 12-bp directly repeated sequence of 5'-CATCAACAACCG-3', which was located at the boundaries of the deletion between the ATPase6 gene and the D-loop region. The deletion spanned 7,436 bp from position 8,649 to position 16,084. mtDNA with a 7.4 kb deletion frequently existed among specimens from patients with dilated cardiomyopathy with or without family history. These result suggest that heart mtDNA deletions may contribute to accelerate pump failure in patients with dilated cardiomyopathy.

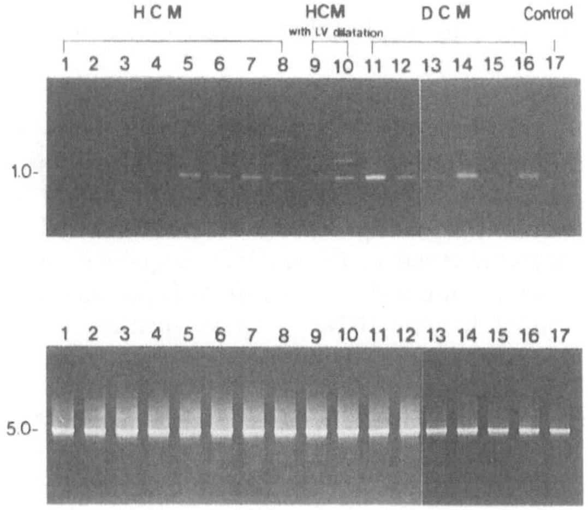

Fig. 1

A: Detection of the deleted mtDNA in hearts of patients with cardiomyopathy using the PCR method. The mtDNA fragments were amplified using primers L853 and H38, separated on a 1% agarose gel, and stained with ethidium bromide. Sizes of amplified fragments are indicated in kb.
B: PCR amplification using primers L116 and H617, the distance between them is 5.0 kb.

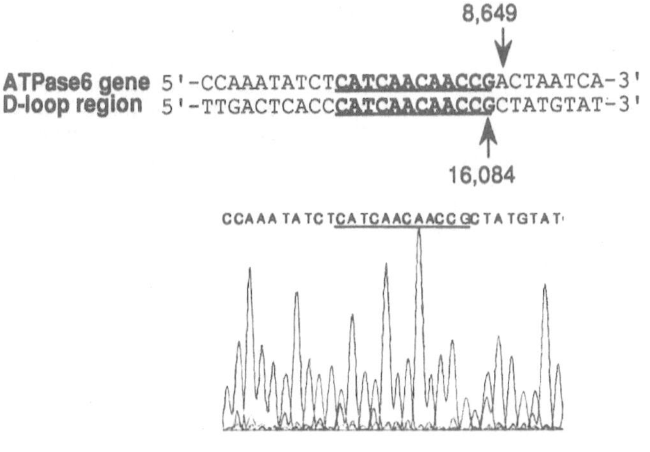

Fig. 2

Fluorescence-based automated sequencing of the deleted mtDNA from the heart muscle in patient-11 with cardiomyopathy. The single 12-bp direct repeat (5'-CATCAACAACCG-3') in the 7.4 kb-deleted mtDNA exists downstream of the 5' portion of the ATPase6 gene and upstream of the 3' portion of the D loop.

Study (2): In the primary PCR amplification of mtDNAs from the heart muscle, skeletal muscle, and liver of patient using primer L853 and H38, multiple abnormal fragments (3.1 kb, 2.4 kb, 2.3 kb, 2.0 kb, 1.7 kb, 1.4 kb, and 1.0 kb), which mean 5.3 kb, 6.0 kb, 6.1 kb, 6.4 kb, 6.7 kb, 7.0 kb and 7.4 kb-deletions of mtDNA respectively, were detected. The sizes and the amounts of deletions were different among these organs. The crossover sequence of one mutant mtDNA was demonstrated to be a 12-bp directly repeated sequence of 5'-CATCAACAACCG-3', which was the same as that in Study 1. Another mutant mtDNA was demonstrated to have no directly repeated sequence, and was revealed to jump from position 8,992 to position 16,072 of mtDNA resulting in a 7,079 bp deletion. This patient had two unique point mutations in the tRNA genes. A G-to-A transition at nucleotide position 5821 in the tRNA^{Cys} gene and an A-to-G transition at position 15,951 in the tRNA^{Thr} gene were found. Both transitions would decrease the stability of the aminoacyl acceptor stem. In the presence of these deleted and mutant mtDNAs, the integrity of electron transport chain would be destroyed, resulting in significant impairment of adenosine triphosphate production and consequent heart failure.

Study (3): We identified an A-to-G transition at 3,243 in the tRNA$^{Leu\ (UUR)}$ gene in a patient with MELAS. This mutation located at the 5' end of the dihydrouridine (DHU) loop of this tRNA molecule (Fig. 3). This mutation was observed in another MELAS patient [12] and was absent in controls. The A at position 3243 in the dihydrouridine loop of the tRNA molecule is strictly conserved in the mtDNA sequences in bovine, mouse, rat, chicken, *Xenopus laevis*, sea urchin, and *Drosophila yakuba*, and an A-to-G transition would disturb the function of leucine tRNA. These results indicate that mtDNA mutations especially the A-to-G transition in the tRNA^{Leu} gene are related to MELAS. This A-to-G transition creates an *Apa*I restriction site, because this enzyme cleaves the mutant sequence (GGGCCC) but not the wild-type sequence (GAGCCC). This convenient method is useful for genetic diagnosis of MELAS. In patients with hypertrophic cardiomyopathy accompanied by lactic acidosis, genetic analysis of mtDNA is recommended.

Mitochondrial tRNA^{Leu} (UUR)

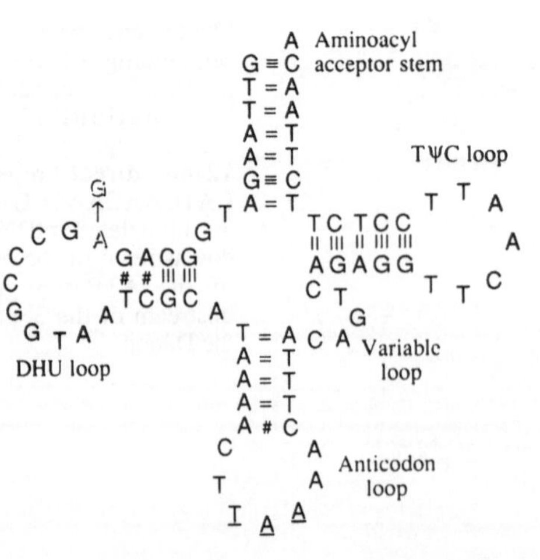

Fig. 3

A-to-G transition in tRNA^{Leu}. Bars indicate hydrogen bonds; # indicates non-standard base pairs found in tRNA. Nucleotides A (normal) and G (mutation) at position 3,243 are highlighted.

Study (4): The respiratory enzyme activity of isolated heart mitochondria were analyzed. The activities of Complex I and Complex IV were decreased to 31% and 33% of control values, respectively. The activity of Complex II was 309% of control, indicating selective defects in Complex I and IV. We sequenced the mtDNA from the patient's heart. We found several nucleotide substitutions which would cause the replacement of amino acids that are conserved among species. One point mutation at nucleotide position 7,673 in the CO2 gene alters conserved isoleucine to valine. We also found an A-to-G base transition at nucleotide position 4,317 in the $tRNA^{Ile}$ gene (the TψC loop). We also found a C-to-T transition at nucleotide position 3,254 in the $tRNA^{Leu}$ gene (the D stem), and a C-to-T transition at nucleotide position 5,554 in the $tRNA^{Trp}$ gene (the variable loop region). It is suggested point mutations in the tRNA genes in mtDNA might cause severe dysfunction of the respiratory chain and might cause early development of heart failure.

In conclusion, it is suggested that mtDNA deletions and point mutations which induce base substitutions in the protein coding genes and the tRNA genes, are important contributory factors to the genesis of some forms of cardiomyopathy.

REFERENCES

1. Anderson S, Bankier AT, Barrell BG, De Bruijin MHL, Coulson AR, Drouin J, Eperon IC, Nierlich DP, Roe BA, Sanger F, Screier PH, Smith AJH, Staden R, Young IG (1981) *Nature* 290: 457
2. Brown WM, George M, Wilson AC (1979) *Proc Natl Acad Sci USA* 76: 1967
3. Dimaouro S, Bonilla E, Zeviani M, Nakagawa M, Devivo DC (1985) *Neurol Prog* 17: 521
4. Ozawa T, Yoneda M, Tanaka M, Ohno K, Sato W, Suzuki H, Nishikimi M, Yamamoto M, Nonaka I, Horai S (1988) *Biochem Biophys Res Commun* 154: 1240
5. Ito T, Hattori K, Tanaka M, Sugiyama S, Ozawa T (1990) *Jpn Circ J* 54: 1214
6. Ozawa T, Tanaka M, Sugiyama S, Hattori K, Ito T, Ohno K, Takahashi A, Sato W, Takada G, Mayumi B, Yamamoto K, Adachi K, Koga Y, Toshima H (1990) *Biochem Biophys Res Commun* 170: 830
7. Hattori K, Ogawa T, Kondo T, Mochizuki M, Tanaka M, Sugiyama S, Ito T, Satake T, Ozawa T (1991) *Am Heart J* 122: 866
8. Ozawa T, Tanaka M, Sugiyama S, Ino H, Ohno K, Hattori K, Ohbayashi T, Ito T, Deguchi H, Kawamura K, Nakane Y, Hashiba K (1991) *Biochem Biophys Res Commun* 177: 518
9. Tanaka M, Ino H, Ohno K, Hattori K, Sato W, Ozawa T (1990) *Lancet* i: 1452
10. Tanaka M, Ino H, Ohno K, Ohbayashi T, Ikebe S, Sano T, Ichiki T, Kobayashi M, Wada Y, Ozawa T (1991) *Biochem Biophys Res Commun* 174: 861
11. Hattori K, Tanaka M, Sugiyama S, Ohbayashi T, Ito T, Satake T, Hanaki Y, Asai J, Nagano M, Ozawa T (1991) *Am Heart J* 121: 1735
12. Tanaka M, Nishikimi M, Suzuki H, Ozawa T, Nishizawa M, Tanaka K, Miyatake T (1986) *Biochem Biophys Res Commun* 140: 88

Disrupted Microtubule Structure in the Ischemic and Failing Myocardium — The Role of Calcium Overload

Masatsugu Hori[1], Hiroshi Sato[1], Kunimitsu Iwai[1], Seiji Takashima[1], Noritake Hoki[3], Masatake Fukunami[3], Masashi Naka[4], Hidetake Kurihara[5], Akira Kitabatake[6], Michitoshi Inoue[2], and Takenobu Kamada[1]

The First Department of Medicine[1] and the Medical Information Science[2], Osaka University School of Medicine, Osaka, 553 Japan and Osaka Prefectural Hospital, Osaka, 558 Japan [3] and Osaka Minami National Hospital, Osaka, 558 Japan[4] and Shionogi Research Laboratory, Osaka, 553 Japan[5] and The Department of Cardiovascular Medicine, Hokkaido University School of Medicine, Sapporo, 060 Japan[6]

KEYWORDS: microtubule, cytoskeleton, Ca overload, ischemia, failing myocardium

Introduction

The architecture of eukaryotic cells is finely organized and the cytoplasm of the cells contains an elaborate and dynamic network of three types of cytoskeletal filaments, i.e., the microtubules, intermediate filaments, and microfilaments. Microtubules are difined as the proteinacous organellas, composed of subunits of tubulin molecules assembled into long tubular structures, with an average exterior diameter of 24 nm, capable of changes in the length by assembly and disassembly of their subunits [1]. Although much information has accumulated regarding the *in vitro* or *in vivo* nature of microtubules since 1961 when the word "microtubule" was proposed, our understanding as to the roles of this oligometric structure in vivo cardiomyocytes remained limited, because previous electronmicroscopic studies which depict only the cross-sectional view of microtubules in an ultrathin section could not provide us three dimentional structures of the microtubules. Recently, we developed the immunofluorescense technique that enables us to stain the microtubules in the tissue section [2]. Since the structural integrity of the microtubules which supports the cytoskeletal framework of the cell are regulated by intracellular Ca^{2+} [3], Ca overload in the ischemic and failing myocardium [4] could affect the microtubule structure.

Microtubule Assembly and Disassembly

The *in vitro* polymerization of tubulin dimers into microtubule-like structure is carried out in many laboratories since the original observation of Weisenberg [5], and several conditions which regulate the microtubule assembly have been elucidated; the concentration of tubulin solution, guanosine nucleotides, Ca^{2+}, Mg^{2+} ions and temperature. Several proteins e.g., MAPs, tau factor, are closely linked to the microtubules and attatched to tubulin polymers. They are involved in assembly, stabilizing the microtubules. A microtubule filament has a difinit polarity; GTP mainly links to the (+) end, and liberation of tubulin dimers and GDP occur at the (-) end. In *in vitro* steady-state conditions, a continuous treadmilling of tubulin molecules along the microtubules takes place. Dynamic instability, switching the steady state between polymerization (growth) and depolymerization (shrinkage), is perturbated by an increase in Ca^{2+} concentration in solution and by phosphorylation of tubulin or MAPs, leading to disassembly of mictorubules. These observations may suggest a possibility that Ca overload disrupts the microtubule structure. In fact, it is known that in the cultured cells, intracellular injections of Ca^{2+} and the treatment with calcium ionophore disrupt the microtubule structure [3, 6]. If the Ca overload disturbes dynamic instability of microtubule of the *in vivo* heart, disruption of microtubule structure may be observed in the injured myocytes such as ischemic injury, catecholamine injury, and myocardial failure.

Microtubule Structure in Cardiomyocyte

The technique for staining of the microtubule structure is described elsewhere [2]. In the normal canine hearts, immunohistochemical staining of microtubule using anti-ß-tubulin monoclonal antibody demonstrates a fine structure of microtubules as the tortuous filaments loosely organized throughout the cytoplasma, which mainly composed of longitudinal and transverse filaments (Fig. 1). These filaments form a lattice-like network; some of them are localized at the perinuclear space and encircle the nucleus. In the cross section of the cells, microtubules are stained as a number of small dots irregularly distributed throughout the cytoplasm. These filamentous stains are specific for the microtubule since the characteristic structures disappear when the anti-tubulin antibody was deleted in the staining precedure. Moreover, treatment with colchicine, which inhibits polymerization of tubulin, markedly diminished the immunoreactivity of microtubules; the microtubule filaments are finely fragmented into regular and short debris of depolymerized microtubules.

Fig. 1. Microtubule staining of ventricular myocardium (nonischemic) with mouse monoclonal antibody against ß-tubulin.

Disruption of Microtubule Structure in Ischemic Injury

Twenty minutes of ischemia is a critical period that renders the cell irreversible. In the previous study, we tested the serial changes of microtubule structure in the canine ischemic myocardium. Fifteen minutes after occlusion of the left anterior descending coronary artery, minimal changes were observed in the microtubule staining. After 20 minutes of ischemia, however, small patchy lesions composed of several myocytes appeared where the immunoreactivities of microtubule were completely lost. Thirty minutes after coronary occlusion, patchy lesions with complete loss of microtubule staining were distributed transmurally, whereas the cross striations of actin filaments were almost intact. The size of the lesions ranged 100 to 240 μm in length in longitudinal sections and 15 to 60 μm in diameter in cross sections, which are similar to those after 20 minutes of ischemia. After 60 minutes of ischemia, the lesions were increased in both size and number. The lesions in the subendocardial layer are composed of more than 100 myocytes and are larger than those in the epicardial layer (Fig. 2). The microtubules located in the peripheral area of the cells tended to disrupt earlier than the perinuclear microtubules. The cross striation of the actin filaments were sporadically disrupted in the cells in which microtubules stainigs were completely lost. In a large number of cells patterns of cross striation of myofibrils were almost normal or minimally affected, indicating that microtubule may disrupt earlier than actin filaments of sarcomeres in the process of ischemic injury.

One may raise a question whether the microtubule disruption indicates irreversible injury. Semi-quanitication of area with microtubule disruption and area with necrosis estimated by TTC staining technique revealed that these areas were comparable, indicating that disruption of microtubule structure reflects severe cellular injury destined to be irreversible change. In contrast, the myocyte with intact microtubule structure were not irreversibly injured, supported by the results that percent areas of myocytes with intact actin filaments and microtubules were not different between before and after reperfusion, and that the ultrastructural signs of irreversible injury were not observed in the myocytes that had intact actin filaments and microtubules. Therefore, these results indicate that disruptions of microtubules occur before the irreversible change and may be an early sign of irreversible injury.

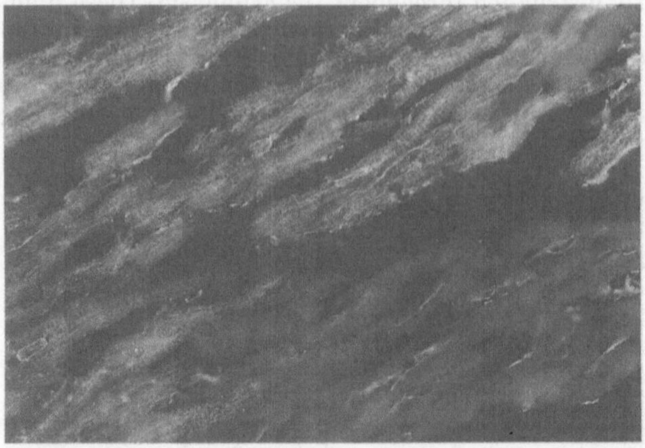

Fig. 2. Microtubule staining of 60-minute ischemic myocardium with mouse monoclonal antibodies against ß-tubulin. A lesion that decreased or lost the immunoreactivities of microtubules is shown.

The patterns of microtubule disruption during ischemia were distinct from those of microtubule disassembly by colchicine treatment, i.e., a complete loss of microtubule staining is observed in the ischemic myocardium. This suggests that mechanism of microtubule disappearance during ischemia may be different from depolymerization of tubulin. It shoud be noted that reperfusion after ischemia has been reported to induce Ca overload [7,8] which may depolymerize the microtubule assembly. Our preliminary results support this possibility since reperfusion after 15 minutes of ischemia induced disruption of microtubule structure mainly around the nucleus without any evidence of irreversivle injury [9]. Thus, this indicates that microtubule structures in the cardiomyocytes are injured during reperfusion prior to the irreversible injury.

Disruption of Microtubule Structure in Catecholamine Injury

A large body of evidence suggests that excessive sympathetic activity in patients with chronic heart failure deteriorates the function of the failing myocardium, and catecholamine may also induce cellular injury and dysfunction of the myocardium. Although a number of possible mechanisms of cellular injury have been raised, intracellular Ca overload may play a key role in the progression of cardiac muscle dysfunction [10-13]. Disruption of microtubule structure may also occur in catecholamine injury through Ca overload. To test the hypothesis that norepinephrine which is often elevated in patients with heart failure disrupts microtubule structures, continuous subcutaneous infusion of norepinephrine was performed with male Wister-Kyoto rat weighing 200g [14]. A small incision was made and an Alzet Osmotic Minipump (Model 1003D) was implanted. The osmotic pump allows the administration of drugs at a constant rate of 1.0μl/h for more than 3 days, and 2, 20, 200μg/kg/h of norepinephrine were administrated for 6 or 24 hours. A low dose of norepinephrine infusion for 6 hours resulted in a minimal change in microtubule structure. However, infusion for 24 hours of a low dose of norepinephrine and a modest dose of norepinephrine infusion for 6 hours caused disruption of microtubules. A modest dose of norepinephrine infusion for 24 hours increased systolic blood pressure from 116±6 to 152±4 mmHg and increased plasma norepinephrine concentration from 430±40 to 17100±3700 pg/ml and further disrupted the network of microtubule in 40±6% of the total area. A large dose of norepinephrine infusion caused more marked changes of microtubules. These dose- and duration-dependent disruptions indicate that microtubule disruption could be induced with even a small dose of norepinephrine, which is often administered clinically and further imply a possibility that microtubule structure is disrupted in uncompensated heart failure.

Disruption of Microtubule Structure in a Human Failing Heart

The presence of Ca overload has been postulated in the myocyte obtained from patients with severe heart failure due to cardiomyopathy (4). Since Ca overload and catecholamine stimulation disrupt microtubule structure in experimental model [3,14,15], abnormal microtubule structure may be observed in biopsied samples obtained from a patient with heart failure. To test this possibility, we fixed the biopsied samples obtained from the patients with heart failure by immersion fixation with PLP fixation [16]. Figure 3 shows the microtubule stains of specimens obtained from the left ventriclar wall of a patient with dilated cardiomyopathy. The patients has been followed for more than 4 years due to mild heart failure. Cardiac function was depressed and ejection fraction assessed by echocardiography was 21% and left ventricular end-diastolic pressure was 16 mmHg. The specimen was composed of the myocytes in which immunoreactivities varied from cell to cell; immunoreactivities were completely lost in many cells, although several cells show a fine reticular network of microtubule.

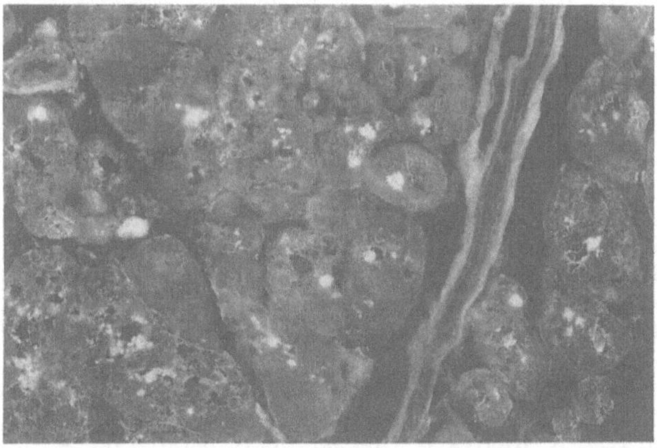

Fig. 3. Microtubule staining of left ventricular myocardium in patients with dilated cardiomyopathy. The specimen was composed of the myocytes in which immunoreactivities varied from cell to cell; immunoreactivities were completely lost in many cells, although several cells show a fine reticular network of microtubule.

It is conceivable that microtubule structure supports and maintains the architecure of the cell in addition to transporting vesicles such as mitochondria, endoplasmic reticulum, sarcoplasmic reticulum, and other membranous organellas [17]. Thus, microtubule disruption may contribute to maldistribution of cellular component, which in turn may affect the myocardial function.

Conclusion

We uncovered the changes of microtubule structure in the various types of failing myocardium both in experimental models and a human specimen. Although further studies are neccesary to clarify the mechanisms of microtubule disruption in relation to the cellular Ca overload, our observations may provide a new insight into the understanding of the cellular dysfuntion of failing hearts.

References

1. Dustin P (1984) Microtubules 2nd ed. Springer-Verlag
2. Iwai K, Hori M, Kitabatake A, Kurihara H, Uchida K, Inoue M, Kamada T (1990) Disruption of microtubules as an early sign of irreversible ischemic injury: Immunohistochemical study of in situ canine heart. Circ Res 67: 694-706
3. Sato H. Hori M, Iwai K, Kagiya T, Takashima S, Tada M (1990) Ca^{2+} overload disrupts microtubules in cultured rat cardiomyocytes. Circulation 82:III-297
4. Gwathmey JK, Copelas L, Mackinnon R, Schoen FJ, Feldman MD, Grossman W, Morgan JP (1987) Abnormal intracellular calcium handling in myocardium from patinets with end-stage heart failure. Circ res 61:70-76
5. Weisenberg R (1972) Microtubule formation in vitro in solutions containig low calcium concentration. Science 177: 1104-1105
6. Keith C, Dipaola M, Maxfield FR, Shelanski ML (1983) Microinjection of Ca^{++}-calmodulin causes a localized depolymerization of microtubules. J Cell Biol 97:1918-1924
7. Kusuoka H, Porterfield JK, Weisman HF, Weisfeldt ML, Marban E (1987) Pathophysiology and pathogenesis of stunned myocardium: Depressed Ca2+ activation of contraction as a consequence of reperfusion-induced cellular calcium overlod in ferret hearts. J Clin Invest 79:950-961
8. Marban E, Kitakaze M, Koretsune Y, Yue DT, Chacko VP, Pike MM (1990) Quantification of $[Ca^{2+}]_i$ in perfused hearts: Critical evaluation of 5F-Bapta and nuclear magnetic resonance method as applied to the study of ischemia and reperfusion. Circ Res 66: 1255-1267
9. Sato H, Iwai K, Kitakaze M, Kurihara K, Uchida K (1990) Disrupted cytoskeletal framework in the stunned myocardium. Circulation 82: III-444
10. Rona G, Chappel CI, Balazs T, Gaudry R (1959) An infarct-like myocardial lesion and other toxic manifestations produced by isproterenol in the rat. Arch Pathol 67: 443-455
11. Haft JI, Kranz PD, Albert FJ, Jani K (1972) Intravascular platelet aggregation in the heart induced by norepinephrine. Circulation 46: 698-708
12. Alderman J, Grossman W (1985) Are beta-adrenergic-blocking drugs useful in the treatment of dilated cardiomyopathy? Circulation 71: 854-857
13. Rona G (1985) Catecholamine cardiotoxity. J Mol Cell Cardiol 71: 854-857
14. Hori M, Sato H, Iwai K, Sato H, Inoue M, Kitabatake A, Kamada T. (1992) Norepinephrine disrupts cytoskeletal framework of microtubules in rat hearts. Jpn Circ J 56: 462-468
15. Sato H, Hori M, Iwai K, Kagiya T, Taskashima S, Kitabatake A, Inoue M (1990) ß-adrenergic stimulation disrupts microtubules in cultured rat cardiomyocytes through Ca^{2+} overload. Circulation 82: III-297
16. Iwai K, Hori M, Sato H, Takashima S, Hoki T, Fukunami M, Naka M, Kurihara H, Uchida K, Kitabatake A (1991) Disruption of microtubules in human cardiomyopathy. Circulation 84:II-440
17. Kelly RB (1990) Microtubules, membrane traffic, and cell organization. Cell 61:5-7

III: Signal Transduction in Myocardial Cells

GTP-binding Proteins and Bacterial Toxin-catalyzed ADP-ribosylation

TOSHIAKI KATADA, YOSHIHARU OHOKA, KATSUNOBU TAKAHASHI, and TAROH IIRI

Department of Life Science, Tokyo Institute of Technology, Kanagawa, 227 Japan

KEYWORDS: GTP-binding Proteins (G proteins), pertussis toxin, cholera toxin, ADP-ribosylation, membrane receptors

INTRODUCTION

GTP-binding proteins (G proteins)[1] are a family of signal-coupling proteins that carry signals from membrane receptors to effectors such as enzymes or ion channels [see refs. 1-3]. G proteins have been characterized as a common heterotrimeric structure consisting of $\alpha\beta\gamma$-subunits. The function of G proteins as the signal transducers is regulated cyclically by: (a) dissociation of bound GDP from the α-subunits; (b) association of GTP with the α-subunits; and (c) hydrolysis of GTP to GDP and P_i. Binding of GTP induces "activation" of the G proteins and consequently regulates the activity of the appropriate effectors, while hydrolysis of GTP initiates the deactivation of G proteins. An additional feature of G proteins is their susceptibilities to bacterial toxins. IAP catalyzes the transfer of an ADP-ribosyl moiety of NAD to the α-subunits of G_i, G_o and G_t. The site modified by IAP is a cysteine which is four amino acid residues away from the carboxyl terminus of the α-subunits. Since the carboxyl terminus region is responsible for the interaction with receptors, the ADP-ribosylation results in an uncoupling of the G proteins from receptors[4-5]; only receptor-mediated signalings are selectively abolished. On the other hand, cholera toxin ADP-ribosylates the α-subunits of G_s and G_t. The target amino acid residue for the toxin is an arginine which is located near the middle part of the α-subunits (*e.g.*, Arg^{173} of G_t-α). The ADP-ribosylation appears to result in a decrease in the intrinsic GTPase activity of the G proteins [6-7].

IAP-substrate G proteins such as G_i and G_o are not ADP-ribosylated by cholera toxin under usual conditions, though there is an amino acid sequence very much homologous to the cholera toxin site in these α-subunits. However, it has recently been reported that cholera toxin is also capable of ADP-ribosylating G_i-α in certain types of cell membranes under a condition that membrane receptors are stimulated by agonists [8-10]. The cholera toxin site on G_i-α, which was apparently differ from IAP site, appeared to be the postulated Arg residue corresponding to Arg^{201} of G_s-α [10]. In this report, we summarize characteristics of the two types of bacterial toxin-catalyzed ADP-ribosylation and investigate how the functions of IAP-substrate G proteins are modified by the cholera toxin-induced ADP-ribosylation.

MATERIALS AND METHODS

Preparation of Membranes from Differentiated HL-60 Cells and Purification of G Proteins

HL-60 cells were differentiated into neutrophil-like cells by treatment with dimethyl sulfoxide as described previously [10, 11]. Plasma membranes were obtained from the cells [12] and suspended at approximately 5 mg of protein/ml in buffer A consisting of 20 mM Tris-HCl (pH 7.5), 1 mM EDTA, 1 mM DTT, and 25 KIU/ml of aprotinin. The cell membranes were incubated with 100 μM NAD at

[1] Abbreviation. G protein, guanine nucleotide-binding protein; G_s and G_i, the guanine nucleotide regulatory components of adenylate cyclase that mediate stimulation and inhibition, respectively; G_o, a G protein of unknown function purified from brain tissues; G_t, a G protein purified from retina; GTPγS, guanosine 5′-(3-*O*-thio)triphosphate; Gpp(NH)p, guanosine 5'-(β,γ-imino)triphosphate; fMLP, formyl-Met-Leu-Phe; IAP, islet-activating protein or pertussis toxin; Chaps, 3-[(3-cholamido-propyl)dimethylammonio]-1-propanesulfate; DTT, dithiothreitol; Hepes, *N*-2-hydroxyethylpiperaine-*N'*-2-ethanesulfonic acid; SDS, sodium dodecyl sulfate.

30°C for 30 min in the presence (*cholera toxin-treated*) or absence (*control*) of preactivated cholera toxin [10] and then centrifuged at 40,000 x g for 15 min at 4°C. The membrane pellets were resuspended with buffer A containing 0.1 mM GDP and further incubated at 30°C for 2 min in order to exchange the Gpp(NH)p bound to G proteins with GDP. The membranes was further washed with buffer A and solubilized with 5 ml of buffer A containing 1% Chaps and 100 mM NaCl. After centrifugation at 200,000 x *g* for 30 min, each of the clear supernatants obtained from *cholera toxin-treated* and *control* membranes was applied to a column of DEAE-Toyopearl 650(S) and then eluted with a linear gradient of NaCl (50-250 mM) in buffer A containing 0.7% Chaps [13]. $G_{i\text{-}2}$ obtained from the column was fractionated on a Sephacryl S-300(HR) column in buffer A containing 0.5% sodium cholate, 1 μM GDP and 100 mM NaCl. Fractions containing $G_{i\text{-}2}$ activity from the column were further applied to a Mono Q HR5/5 column which had been equilibrated with 20 ml of buffer A containing 0.7% Chaps and 50 mM NaCl. The column was washed with 2 ml of the equilibration buffer and then eluted with a 20-ml linear gradient of NaCl (100-300 mM) in buffer A containing 0.7% Chaps. Fractions *C-I*, *C-II* and *T-I*, *T-II*, which had been purified from *control* and *cholera toxin-treated* membranes, respectively, were separately pooled and stored at -85°C until use for the following assays. Bovine brain G proteins were purified as described previously [14].

Guanine Nucleotide-binding and GTPase Assays

The purified $G_{i\text{-}2}$ (5-10 nM) was incubated at 25°C with 0.5 μM [^{35}S]GTPγS or 1 μM [γ-^{32}P]GTP in 20 mM Hepes-NaOH (pH 7.4), 10 mM $MgSO_4$, 1 mM EDTA, 1 mM DTT and 0.025% Lubrol-PX. At the indicated times, 25-μl aliquots of the mixture were withdrawn and subjected for the guanine nucleotide bindings as described previously [14,15]. For assay of the actual catalytic rate of GTP hydrolysis, the purified $G_{i\text{-}2}$ was incubated on ice for 5-6 h with 1 μM [γ-^{32}P]GTP in 200 μl of 20 mM Hepes-NaOH (pH 7.4), 10 mM EDTA, 1 mM dithiothreitol, and 0.025% Lubrol-PX. This incubation resulted in formation of a [γ-^{32}P]GTP-bound form of G proteins without releasing of $^{32}P_i$. The GTP hydrolysis was initiated at 20°C by the additions of $MgSO_4$ (at the final concentration of 6 mM). GTPγS at the final concentration of 10 μM was also added with $MgSO_4$ in order to prevent the further binding of [γ-^{32}P]GTP to $G_{i\text{-}2}$.

ADP-ribosylation of the Purified G_i by IAP

The purified $G_{i\text{-}2}$ (5-10 nM) was incubated at 25°C with 2 μM [α-^{32}P]NAD and 0.2-0.4 μg of activated IAP [10,13] in 200 μl of 20 mM Hepes-NaOH (pH 7.4), 10 mM $MgSO_4$, 1 mM EDTA, and 0.025% Lubrol-PX. At the indicated times, 25-μl aliquots of the reaction mixture were withdrawn for the assay of amount ADP-ribosylation by IAP as described previously [10].

Reconstitution of a High-affinity fMLP Binding by the Purified G Proteins

The differentiated HL-60 cells were cultured in the presence of 50 ng/ml of IAP for 20-24 h in order to effectively ADP-ribosylate the endogenous G proteins by IAP, and the plasma membranes were then prepared therefrom as described above. The treated membranes (15-25 μg of protein) were chilled on ice for 15 min with indicated amounts of the purified $G_{i\text{-}2}$ and then incubated at 30°C for 20 min with 80 nM [^{3}H]fMLP in 50 μl of 20 mM Hepes-NaOH (pH 7.4), 1 mM [ethylene-bis-(oxonitrilo)]tetraacetic acid, 0.2 mM $MgCl_2$, 0.1 mM EDTA, 1 mM dithiothreitol, and 50 KIU/ml of aprotinin. The reaction was terminated by dilution with 4 ml of an ice-cold buffer consisting of 20 mM Tris/HCl (pH 7.5) and 10 mM $MgCl_2$, and the specific binding of [^{3}H]fMLP was determined as described previously [16,17].

RESULTS AND DISCUSSION

Purification of Cholera Toxin ADP-ribosylated G_i from HL-60 Cell Membranes

HL-60 cells were differentiated into neutrophil-like cells by treatment with dimethyl sulfoxide, and plasma membranes were prepared from the cells. The membranes were incubated with NAD, Gpp(NH)p, Mg^{2+} and fMLP in the presence (*cholera toxin-treated*) or absence (*control*) of cholera toxin, and $G_{i\text{-}2}$-rich fractions were obtained from the two membranes by sequential column chromatographies of DEAE-Toyopearl and Sephacryl S-300. The $G_{i\text{-}2}$-rich fractions were further applied to a high-resolution Mono Q column. $G_{i\text{-}2}$ activity measured by GTPγS binding or IAP-catalyzed

ADP-ribosylation was recovered as a symmetrical peak from the Mono column to which the *control* G_{i-2}-rich fraction had been applied (Fig. 1A). However, there was an apparent shoulder in the descending portion of the activity, when the *cholera toxin-treated* fraction was applied and eluted from the column (Fig. 1B).

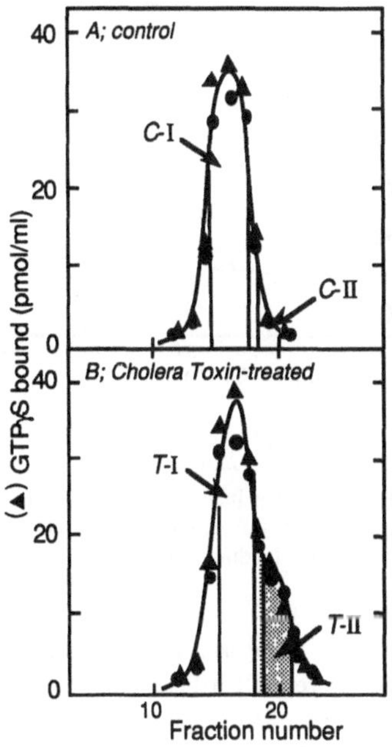

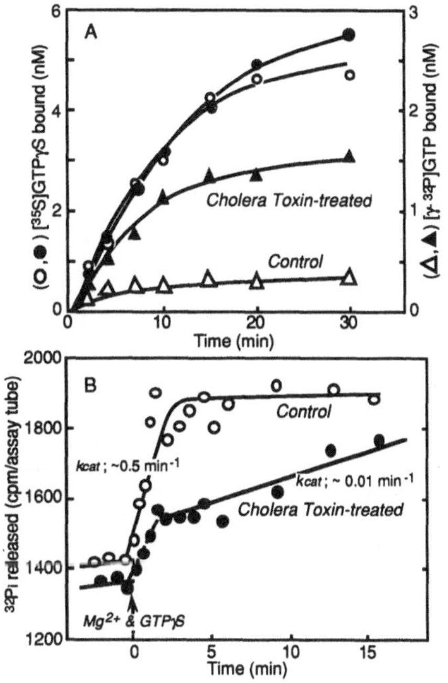

FIG. 1 (*left*). Mono Q chromatography of G_{i-2} originated from *control* (A) and *cholera toxin*-treated (B) HL-60 cell membranes. G_{i-2}-rich fractions obtained from the Sephacryl S-300 columns were applied to a Mono Q column.
FIG. 2 (*right*). Guanine nucleotide binding and GTP hydrolysis reactions. *Panel A*; the purified G_{i-2} (fraction of *T-II* or *C-I* in Fig. 1) was incubated with [^{35}S]GTPγS (O, ●) or [γ-^{32}P]GTP (Δ, ▲). *Panel B*; the purified G_{i-2} was incubated with [γ-^{32}P]GTP, and the GTP hydrolysis was then initiated by the additions of Mg^{2+}.

Characteristics of Cholera Toxin ADP-ribosylated G_i

Guanine nucleotide binding to the purified proteins was first investigated with two types of radiolabeled ligands. As shown in Fig. 2A, a non-hydrolyzable GTP analogue, [^{35}S]GTPγS, bound to the fractions of *C-I* and *T-II* in a time-dependent manner similar to each other. When [γ-^{32}P]GTP was used in the binding experiments, the radioactivity was more greatly retained in fraction *T-II* than in *C-I*. These results suggested that the hydrolysis of GTP bound to the α-subunit of G_{i-2} was selectively inhibited by its ADP-ribosylation by cholera toxin. A more direct evidence is shown in Fig. 2B where a single catalytic cycle of GTP hydrolysis was illustrated. The catalytic rate (k_{cat}) by fraction *C-I* that contained the unmodified G_{i-2} was estimated to be 0.5~1 min^{-1} under the present conditions. There were apparently two values of k_{cat} with fast and slow rates in GTP hydrolysis catalyzed by fraction *T-II*; the slow rate was calculated to be approximately 0.01 min^{-1}. Since fraction *T-II* contained both ADP-ribosylated and unmodified G_{i-2}, the slow k_{cat} value must be due to an entity of the ADP-ribosylated G_{i-2}. Thus, the catalytic rate of GTP hydrolysis was attenuated to less than one-fiftieth by cholera toxin-induced ADP-ribosylation of G_{i-2}.

Fig. 3 shows time courses of IAP-catalyzed [^{32}P]ADP-ribosylation of the two purified fractions. More than 90% of G_{i-2} in fraction *C-I* were ADP-ribosylated by IAP within 2 min under the present conditions. The time course of ADP-ribosylation of G_{i-2} in fraction *T-II*, however, displayed two different phases with rapid and slow reaction rates; the first half fraction was rapidly ADP-ribosylated as had been observed in fraction *C-I*, and ADP-ribosylation of the second half fraction was followed at a very slow rate. This implied that G_{i-2} once modified by cholera toxin resulted in a low substrate for IAP-catalyzed ADP-ribosylation, though the site to be modified by IAP was still intact.

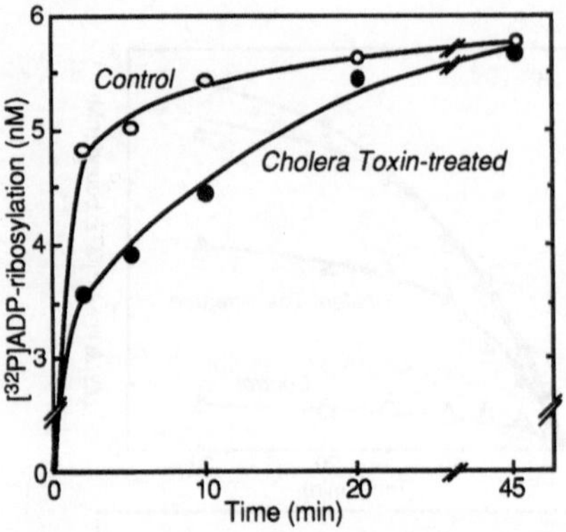

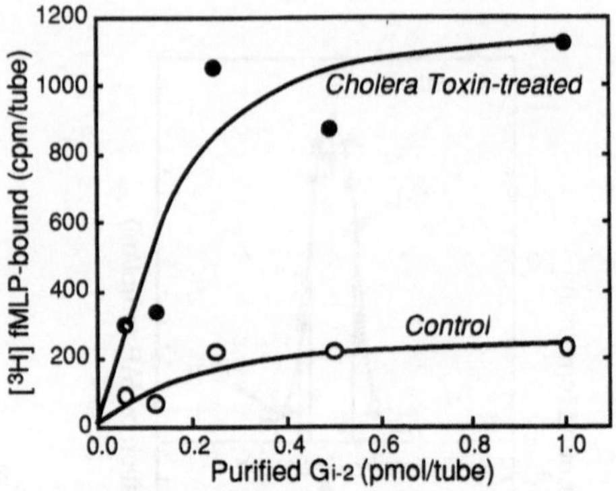

FIG. 3 (*left*). IAP-catalyzed ADP-ribosylation of the purified G_{i-2}. The purified G_{i-2} (the fraction of *T-II* or *C-I* in Fig. 1) originated from cholera toxin-treated (●) or control (○) membranes was incubated with $[^{32}P]NAD$ and IAP.
FIG. 4 (*right*). Reconstitution of a high-affinity fMLP binding by the purified G_{i-2}. The indicated amounts of the purified G_{i-2} (the fraction of *T-II* or *C-I* in Fig. 1) originated from cholera toxin-treated (●) or control (○) membranes were reconstituted into IAP-pretreated HL-60 cell membranes, and a high-affinity fMLP binding to the membranes was then assayed.

It is well established that there are two types of affinity with a high and a low for agonists in membrane receptors coupled to G proteins. When G proteins were ADP-ribosylated by IAP, they lost their abilities to interact with receptors, resulting in a conversion of the high-affinity receptors to the low-affinity ones. Therefore, we examined the interaction of fMLP receptors with the purified fractions by means of a reconstitution of the high-affinity receptors into HL-60 cell membranes in which the function of endogenous G proteins had been abolished by the ADP-ribosylation by IAP. There were progressive increases in the high-affinity fMLP binding, as the amounts of the purified proteins had been increased in the reconstitution experiments (Fig. 4). The degrees of the high-affinity fMLP binding reconstituted by fraction *T-II* were, however, much higher than those by fraction *C-I* at all the amounts of the purified proteins tested. Thus, cholera toxin ADP-ribosylated G_{i-2} appeared to be more effectively coupled with fMLP receptors than the unmodified protein.

Modification of G_i Functions by Cholera Toxin-catalyzed ADP-ribosylation

We have examined how the functions of G_i are modified by cholera toxin-catalyzed ADP-ribosylation, and the major findings obtained in the present study are summarized as follows. (*a*) The catalytic rate (k_{cat}) of GTP hydrolysis was inhibited by the toxin-induced ADP-ribosylation of G_{i-2} (see Fig. 2). (*b*) There was an increase in the apparent affinity of G_{i-2} for GDP (data not shown). (*c*) The ability of G_{i-2} to cause a high-affinity fMLP binding was enhanced by the toxin-catalyzed ADP-ribosylation (Fig. 4). (*d*) The activity of G_i as a substrate for IAP-catalyzed ADP-ribosylation was attenuated by its prior ADP-ribosylation by cholera toxin (Fig. 3). In other words, property of G_i for guanine nucleotides was doubly modified by the ADP-ribosylation, since there were not only a decrease in the k_{cat} of GTP hydrolysis but also an increase in the apparent affinity for GDP. In addition, the ability of G_{i-2} to produce a high-affinity agonist binding to receptors was also up-regulated by cholera toxin-catalyzed ADP-ribosylation. These properties would give the following advantages to the signal-transducing protein. Under resting conditions in the absence of receptor agonists, the modified G_i is tightly associated with GDP due to its higher affinity for GDP. This rigid formation of GDP-G_i complex may be required for a protection of the G protein from its spontaneous activation without receptor agonists. When agonists bind to the receptors, the modified G_i interacts very effectively with the activated receptors resulting in its high-affinity form for agonists, and GDP-GTP exchange reaction occurs on the α-subunit. The GTP-bound form of the modified G protein then acts as a long-life activator for effectors due to its low GTP-hydrolyzing activity. Thus, once cholera toxin ADP-ribosylates the α-subunit of G_{i-2}, the modified G protein would act as a rigid and efficient signal transducer between receptors and effectors.

A Possible Role of the Cholera Toxin-Site in G Protein-mediated Signal Transduction
Interestingly, new oncogenic G-α genes, termed *gsp* or *gip2*, in which the cholera toxin sites of Arg^{201} or Arg^{179} were replaced with Cys or His, have recently been discovered in several endocrine tumor tissues [18,19]. Since *gip* 2 actually promoted neoplastic transformation [20], the mutated G proteins will pathologically be involved in the oncogenesis. It is probable that these mutated G proteins and ADP-ribosylated G proteins at the cholera toxin site may share common functions [6,7]. If such an ADP-ribosylation occurs reversibly under physiological conditions, this type of post-translation modification may function as a novel regulatory mechanism in G protein-mediated signal transductions as well as phosphorylation-dephosphorylation pathways. Considering that the modified G_i is a candidate for undefined IAP less-sensitive G proteins in some cell types [21,22], we are tempted to speculate that the ADP-ribosylated G protein may function physiologically. Thus, the further studies of the modified G protein especially concerning its effector system is the next crucial step for its physiological significance.

ACKNOWLEDGMENTS

This work was supported by research grants from the Scientific Research Fund of the Ministry of Education, Science, and Culture of Japan, the Workshop for Cardiovascular System and Calcium Signal, and Yamanouchi Foundation for Research on Metabolic Disorders in Japan.

REFERENCES

1. Casey, P. J., and Gilman, A. G. (1988) *J. Biol. Chem.* **263**, 2577-2580
2. Ui, M. (1984) *Trends Pharmacol.* **5**, 277-279
3. Bourne, H. R., Sanders, D. A., and McCormick, F. (1990) *Nature* **348**, 125-132
4. Masters, S. B., Sullivan, K. A., Miller, R. T., Beiderman, B., Lopez, N. G., Ramachandran, J., and Bourne, H. R. (1988) *Science* **241**, 448-451
5. Katada, T., Oinuma, M., and Ui, M. (1986) *J. Biol. Chem.* **261**, 5215-5221
6. Freissmuth, M., and Gilman, A.G. (1989) *J. Biol. Chem.* **264**, 21907-21914
7. Masters, S. B., Miller, R. T., Chi, M. H., Chang, F. H., Beiderman, B., Lopez, N. G., and Bourne, H. R. (1989) *J. Biol. Chem.* **264**, 15467-15474
8. Gierscick, P., and Jakobs, K. H. (1987) *FEBS Lett.* **224,** 219-223
9. Milligan, G., and Mckenzie, F. R. (1988) *Biochem. J.* **252,** 369-373
10. Iiri, T., Tohkin, M., Morishima, N., Ohoka, Y., Ui, M., and Katada, T. (1989) *J. Biol. Chem.* **264**, 21394-21400
11. Tohkin, M., Iiri, T., Ui, M., and Katada, T. (1989) *FEBS Lett.* **225**, 187-190
12. Oinuma, M., Katada, T., and Ui, M. (1987) *J. Biol. Chem.* **262,** 8347-8353
13. Iiri, T., Ohoka, Y., Ui, M., and Katada, T. (1992) *J. Biol. Chem.* **267,** 1020-1026
14. Katada, T., Oinuma, M., and Ui, M. (1986) *J. Biol. Chem.* **261,** 8182-8191
15. Tomita, U., Inanobe, A., Kobayashi, I., Takahashi, K., Ui, M., and Katada, T. (1991) *J. Biochem. (Tokyo)* **109,** 184-189
16. Tohkin, M., Morishima, N., Iiri, T., Takahashi, K., Ui, M., and Katada, T. (1991) *Eur. J. Biochem.* **195,** 527-533
17. Iiri, T., Ohoka, Y., Ui, M., and Katada, T. (1991) *Eur. J. Biochem.* **202,** 635-641
29. Graziano, M. P., and Gilman, A. G. (1989) *J. Biol. Chem.* **264,** 15475-15482
18. Landis, C. A., Masters, S. B., Spada, A., Pace, A. M., Bourne, H. R., and Vallar, L. (1989) *Nature (London)* **340,** 692-696
19. Lyons, J., Landis, C. A., Harsh, G., Vallar, L., Grünewald, K., Feichtinger, H., Duh, Q. Y., Clark, O. H., Kawasaki, E., Bourne, H. R., and McCormick, F. (1990) *Science* **249,** 655-659
20. Pace, A. M., Wong, Y. H., & Bourne, H. R. (1991) *Proc. Natl. Acad. Sci. USA* **88,** 7031-7035
21. Ashkenazi, A., Winslow, J. W., Peralta, E. G., Peterson, G. L., Schimerlik, M. I., Capon, D. J., and Ramachandran, J. (1987) *Science* **238,** 672-675
22. Ashkenazi, A., Peralta, E. G., Winslow, J. W., Ramachandran, J., and Capon, D. J. (1989) *Cell* **56,** 487-493

Regulation of the G_s Protein in the Heart

PAUL INSEL, KAZUSHI URASAWA, DENIS LEIBER, DAVID ROTH, and H. KIRK HAMMOND

Departments of Pharmacology and Medicine, University of California, San Diego and VAMC-San Diego, CA 94305, USA

Key Words: G_s-protein, adenylyl cyclase, cyclic AMP, signal transduction

INTRODUCTION

The role of GTP-binding proteins (G proteins) as transducers of information across the plasma membrane is now well-established. A wide variety of hormones and neurotransmitters that regulate the heart and vascular system have been shown to produce their effects by the activation of such proteins (1). Acetylcholine released by postganglionic parasympathetic (vagal) neurons and norepinephrine released at postganglionic sympathetic neurons are the most physiologically important of these agonists. Norepinephrine and epinephrine, a circulating hormone principally derived from the adrenal medulla, activate cardiac β_1 and β_2-adrenergic receptors to produce chronotropic, dromotropic, lusitropic and inotropic actions. β-adrenergic receptors exert these actions via their ability to activate the stimulatory GTP binding protein, G_s. G_s, in turn, promotes the physiological responses via the regulation of effector molecules. In this article, we will address 4 questions regarding cardiac G_s: 1) What are the effector molecules regulated by G_s? 2) How much G_s is present in cardiac membrane preparations? 3) Is G_s exclusively localized to the cardiac sarcolemma? 4) Is G_s altered physiologically or during cardiac disease?

WHAT ARE THE EFFECTOR MOLECULES REGULATED BY G_s?

G_s was originally named because of its ability to stimulate adenylyl cyclase and thereby to increase cellular levels of cyclic AMP. There are several forms of cardiac adenylyl cyclase, but the most important ones that G_s regulates are not yet fully defined (2). Although certain results had suggested that G_s might link to other effectors, such as a Mg^{++} transporter [3], it was only within the past several years that work by Brown, Birnbaumer and colleagues have shown that G_s can also regulate voltage-sensitive calcium channels in the heart [4]. This action, which directly increases channel activity, may act in parallel with the indirect regulation of channel activity that occurs via a cyclic AMP/cyclic AMP-dependent protein kinase-mediated phosphorylation of voltage-sensitive calcium channels. The precise physiological contribution of these "direct" and "indirect" mechanisms of channel regulation is still under study. In addition, limited data have also been reported that G_s can directly inhibit cardiac sodium channels [5]. Thus, G_s appears to regulate multiple effectors in the heart.

HOW MUCH G_s IS PRESENT IN CARDIAC PREPARATIONS?

Quantitation of cardiac G_s has involved use of several different methods. These include assays that depend exclusively on amount of G_s, such as antibody-based methods (e.g., ELISA, quantitative immunoblotting) or others that are also measures of function of G_s (e.g. reconstitution into G_s-deficient membranes, such as those of cyc-S49 lymphoma cells, and cholera toxin-catalyzed ADP-ribosylation). Since the latter methods depend on factors in addition to amount of protein, they should be regarded as only semi-quantitative. Nevertheless, from a physiological perspective, those types of assays provide useful insights regarding the functional "state" of G_s.

Limited data are available regarding levels of cardiac G_s but ~10 pmol/mg protein is typically found in homogenates or crude sarcolemmal preparations (Table 1). This value is in contrast with the much (≤100 fold) lower concentration of β-adrenergic receptors found in parallel studies (e.g. 6,7). Such results suggest that the pharmacological concept of "spare receptors" (relatively to G_s) is not likely to be applicable to cardiac expression of receptors and G_s. Moreover, although precise quantitation of G_s-linked effector molecules is not yet possible, estimates suggest that these effectors are present at concentrations far below those observed for the G_s protein [8,9]. Thus, the heart appears to have a high concentration of G_s relative to both receptors and effectors.

Table 1: Cardiac G_s levels

Cardiac G_s levels

Species	Method	Region	G_s levels (pmol/mg protein)	Refs.
Dog	Cholera toxin-catalyzed ADP-ribosylation	left ventricle (sarcolemma)	7	[6]
Pig	ELISA	right atrium	11	[7]
		left ventricle (crude membrane)	6	
Pig	Quantitative Immunoblot	right atrium	11	this report
		left ventricle (crude membrane)	14	

IS G_S EXCLUSIVELY LOCALIZED TO THE CARDIAC SARCOLEMMA?

G_s, as other signal transducing G proteins, is comprised of 3 subunits, α, β, γ. Current thinking is that heterotrimeric G proteins are localized to the membrane via at least two mechanisms: 1) isoprenyl substitutions in Cys residues near the carboxy terminal of γ subunits and 2) myristoylation of Gly residues near the amino termini of α subunits [10]. It is of interest that α_s lacks a critical ser residue required for the latter acylation reaction and accordingly is not myristoylated. Moreover, data from non-cardiac cells have suggested that α_s may be released from the cell membrane by agonists or other activators [e.g. 11-13].

We have recently examined cardiac tissue and found that abundant portions (≥50%) of G_s is found in supernatant (relative to crude membrane) fractions prepared from porcine right atrium and left ventricle, as detected by immunoblotting and cholera toxin-catalyzed ADP ribosylation (14). However, in reconstitution studies, these supernatant fractions possessed only about 10-20% of cellular α_s activity. Thus, although a substantial portion of cardiac α_s can apparently be identified outside the sarcolemma, less than 50% of this α_s appears to be functional, at least with respect to ability to stimulate adenylyl cyclase. Further studies in other species will be necessary to confirm these findings but these data suggest that the notion that G_s is exclusively a sarcolemmal protein is not correct.

IS G_s ALTERED PHYSIOLOGICALLY OR DURING CARDIAC DISEASE?

Alterations in G_s might occur in several ways. The total amount of protein might change, the protein may be modified so as to alter its functional activity, or as suggested by the results just described, the protein may redistribute in cardiac cells. In turn, those ;eneral types of alterations could occur via multiple mechanisms: transcriptional, translational, post-translational, cellular modirications, etc. One example of physiological regulation is an increace in membrane levels of G_s (detected by ELISA) in pigs which undergo chronic dynamic exercise [7]. These increases, which were observed in both right atrium and left ventricle and were opposite to the exercise-promoted decrease in membrane content of β-adrenergic receptors in right atrium, occurred in parallel with an increase in β-adrenergic response (decreased EC_{50} for isoproterenol-stimulated chronotropic response).

Changes in the amount and/or function of G_s have been reported in several types of cardiac disease, including multiple types of cardiomyopathy, heart failure, and ischemic heart disease (as reviewed recently in ref. 1). Most of the available data are quite indirect, generally involving assay of adenylyl cyclase activity, although some results have been reported with more direct studies of G_s. With respect to disease in humans, heart failure (idiopathic dilated cardiomyopathy) seems not to be associated with major changes in levels of G_s, although because of increases in G_i the ratio of G_i/G_s increases (1). Other preliminary data suggest altered activation of G_s in dilated cardiomyopathy [15]. Together with decreases in the number of β-adrenergic receptors, such changes would produce decreases in sympathetic neuronal-mediated activation of the β-adrenergic receptor system in the failing heart.

The observation that G_s is in such great excess relative to receptors and effectors raises an intriguing question: Would modest changes in levels or functional modification of this protein have physiological consequences? The answer is not clear, but given the possibility of subcellular compartmentation of α_s and of an excess of G_s relative to effectors, one could imagine that redistributed G_s could be nonfunctional and that changing the ratio of G_s to effector could alter the rapidity and concentration dependence of response of effector systems to activation by agonists.

SUMMARY AND CONCLUSIONS

Recent work identifies several previously unknown features regarding cardiac G_s. Firstly, G_s appears to be multifunctional and can regulate

not only adenylyl cyclase activity but also voltage-sensitive calcium channels and perhaps sodium channels as well. Cardiac levels of G_s are ~10 pmol/mg protein and are in substantial excess of G_s-linked receptors, such as β-adrenergic receptors. A substantial portion of cardiac G_s can be found in supernatant fractions and not in crude membrane fractions. Physiologic and pathologic settings can be associated with changes in G_s, although mechanisms for these changes are poorly defined. The possibility that cardiac disease can alter distribution of G_s in subcellular compartments could provide a novel mechanism for the regulation of this key signal transducing protein.

REFERENCES

1. Urasawa K, Insel PA (1992) GTP-binding proteins and cardiovascular disease. In: G Milligan, M Wakelam (eds) G Proteins Signal Transduction and Disease. Acad Press, London pp. 47-85.
2. Katsushika S, Chen L, Kawabe J, Homcy J. Ishikawa Y (1992) Cardiac adenylyl cyclases, novel members of the cyclase superfamily. Clin Res 40: 191A.
3. Maguire ME and Erdos JJ (1980) Inhibition of magnesium uptake by β-adrenergic agonists and prostaglandin E_1 is not mediated by cyclic AMP. J Biol Chem 255: 1030-1035.
4. Birnbaumer L, Abramowitz J, Brown AM (1990) Receptor-effector coupling by G-proteins. Biochim Biophys Acta 1031: 163-224.
5. Schubert B, VanDongen AMJ, Kirsch GE, Brown AM (1989) Beta-adrenergic inhibition of cardiac sodium channels by dual G-protein pathways. Science 245: 516-519.
6. Longabaugh JP, Vatner DE, Vatner SF and Homcy CJ (1988) Decreased stimulatory guanosine triphosphate binding protein in dogs with pressure overload-left ventricular failure. J Clin Invest 81:420-424.
7. Hammond HK, Ransnäs LA, Insel PA (1988) Noncoordinate regulation of cardiac G_s protein and β-adrenergic receptors by a physiologic stimulus, chronic dynamic exercise. J Clin Invest 82: 2168-2171.
8. Alousi AA, Hilal-Dandan R, Insel PA, Brunton LL (1992) Quantitation of adenylyl cyclase in cardiac myocytes. FASEB J 6: A1562.
9. Kojima M, Ishima T, Taniguish N, Kimura K, Sada N, Sperelakis N (1990) Developmental changes in beta-adrenoceptors, muscarinic cholinoceptors and calcium channels in rat ventricular muscles. Br J Pharmacol 99: 334-339.
10. Milligan G. (1992) Guanine-nucleotide binding proteins in health and disease: an overview. In: G proteins, signal transduction and disease. G Milligan, M Wakelam (eds) Head Press, London pp. 1-28.
11. Ransnäs LA, Svoboda P, Jasper JR and Insel PA (1989) Stimulation of β-adrenergic receptors of S49 lymphoma cells redistributes the α-subunit of the stimulatory G protein between cytosol and membranes. Proc Nat Acad Sci USA 86: 7900-7903.
12. Milligan G and Unson C.G. (1989) Persistent activation of the alpha subunit of G_s promotes its removal from the plasma membrane. Bichem J 260: 837-841.
13. Negishi M, Hashimoto H, Ichikawa A (1992) Translocation of α-subunits of stimulatory guanine nucleotide-binding proteins through stimulation of the prostacyclin receptor in mouse mastocytoma cells. J Biol Chem 267: 2364-2369.
14. Roth DA, Urasawa K, Leiber D, Insel PA, Hammond HK (1992) A substantial portion of cardiac G_s is not associated with the plasma membrane. FEBS Lett 296: 46-50.
15. Ransnäs LA, Hjarlmarson A, Insel PA (1988) Dilated cardiomyopathy is associated with an impaired activation of the stimulatory G-protein, G_s, by GTP in heart membranes. Circulation 78(Suppl II): II-178.

Alterations in α_1-Adrenergic Receptors in Response to Myocardial Ischemia and their Role in Arrhythmogenesis

PETER B. CORR, THOMAS KURZ, and KATHRYN A. YAMADA
Departments of Medicine (Cardiology) and Molecular Biology and Pharmacology, Washington University, St. Louis, MO 63110, USA

KEYWORDS: ischemia; catecholamines

Several lines of clinical and experimental evidence indicate that catecholamines contribute substantially to the development of lethal ventricular arrhythmias during early myocardial ischemia [1-3]. There are at least two major mechanisms which underly the release of catecholamines during ischemia, the most prominent of which is local release from sympathetic nerve endings directly in the absence of any sympathetic neural activation [4]. In addition, there is also evidence to suggest that release of catecholamines occurs through enhanced central sympathetic neural outflow [1,2]. This heterogeneous release of catecholamines within the ischemic heart would be expected to lead to marked heterogeneity in the associated electrophysiologic responses and thereby enhance the evolution of lethal ventricular arrhythmias. Definitive experimental evidence has indicated that both reentrant as well as nonreentrant mechanisms contribute to the development of arrhythmias during early myocardial ischemia [5,6]. Thus, approaches to evaluate the electrophysiologic mechanisms underlying the arrhythmogenic effects of catecholamines should not only evaluate potential influences on electrophysiologic indices which would influence reentrant arrhythmias, but also indices which would contribute to nonreentrant or focal mechanisms. These would include normal and abnormal automaticity as well as triggered arrhythmias secondary to early or delayed afterdepolarizations. In this brief overview we will summarize the key elements underlying the electrophysiologic and biochemical influences of stimulation of α_1-adrenergic receptors on cardiac cells. The major emphasis will be on the appearance of enhanced α_1-adrenergic responsivity in the ischemic heart and how this might contribute to arrhythmogenesis. Although the influence of ß-adrenergic stimulation on the electrophysiologic properties of the myocardium are profound and certainly contribute to arrhythmogenesis in the ischemic heart in both animals and man, we have reviewed this topic elsewhere [1] and the present article will deal exclusively with the α-adrenergic component.

Electrophysiologic Effects of α_1-Adrenergic Stimulation

Alpha-adrenergic stimulation of the normal heart elicits a very modest increase in inotropy [7] as well as an increase in repolarization time and refractory period [8] and a decrease in automaticity in isolated Purkinje cells [9]. Although there is some evidence to suggest that α-adrenergic stimulation may lead to a delay in inactivation of the slow inward current (L-type calcium current) [10], it is more likely that the effect is secondary to an increase in intracellular calcium due to the lengthening of repolarization time. More recent findings have shown that activation of α_1-adrenergic receptors in isolated ventricular myocytes results in a suppression of the outward potassium current (I_K) with little or no influence on the L-type calcium current [11-13]. The effect to delay I_K appears to be secondary to a diacylglyerol stimulation of protein kinase C and thereby secondary phosphorylation of the channel mediating I_K since the effect can be reproduced by stimulation with phorbol esters [11]. Thus, the major effects of α-adrenergic stimulation would be analogous to that which might occur with a class III antiarrhythmic agent. However, the lengthening of repolarization may have important influences on impulse conduction, particularly if the effect is heterogenous leading to potential unidirectional conduction block in certain regions. Another potential arrhythmogenic effect of delaying I_K could be the development of early afterdepolarizations. In addition, an increase in repolarization time through α_1-adrenergic stimulation could also lead to an increase in intracellular calcium thereby activating the transient inward current (I_{Ti}) leading to the development of delayed afterdepolarizations and triggered rhythms.

The precise cellular mechanisms underlying the nonreentrant activity during ischemia and reperfusion are unknown [5,6]. However, because these focal activations are very rapid and at times accelerate leading to transition from ventricular tachycardia to ventricular fibrillation and appear in epicardial as well as endocardial regions suggests that they may be secondary to early or delayed afterdepolarizations leading to triggered rhythms. To investigate the underlying cellular mechanisms responsible, we developed procedures to assess the electrophysiologic influences of α_1-adrenergic stimulation in both normal and severely hypoxic adult ventricular myocytes. Initial studies demonstrated that α-adrenergic stimulation of normoxic myocytes leads to the expected dose-dependent increase in repolarization time [8], without the appearance of either early or delayed afterdepolarizations or any oscillatory membrane activity. More recently, we have demonstrated that exposure of hypoxic myocytes to α_1-adrenergic stimulation resulted in the development of delayed afterdepolarizations as well as triggered activity [14]. Interestingly, exposure to severe metabolic impairment inhibited the α-adrenergic induced induction of both afterdepolarizations and triggered activity [14], suggesting that there is a transient phase during early myocardial ischemia in which metabolic impairment is not profound and during which the α-adrenergic responsivity is enhanced. This would agree with the findings that α-adrenergic stimulation can elicit arrhythmias during very early myocardial ischemia as well as during subsequent reperfusion [15,16].

Antiarrhythmic Influence of α_1-Adrenergic Blockade During Myocardial Ischemia and Reperfusion

The antiarrhythmic effect of α_1-adrenergic blockade during ischemia and/or reperfusion has been demonstrated in a variety of different species including, guinea pig, cat, rat, and conscious and anesthetized dog [15-23]. Most of the evidence would suggest that the antiarrhythmic influence is not mediated through alterations in myocardial blood flow or favorable alterations in hemodynamics [16]. This is also supported by findings in which the α-agonist methoxamine can influence the incidence of ventricular tachycardia and fibrillation during ischemia and reperfusion in the isolated heart previously depleted of catecholamines, an effect which is specifically blocked by phentolamine rather than blockade of ß-adrenergic or histamine receptors [15]. Likewise, regional coronary infusion of methoxamine *in vivo* resulted in marked enhancement of the idioventricular rate during reperfusion, a response which did not occur in the absence of ischemia. These findings in the intact heart suggest an enhanced α-adrenergic response which contributes importantly to arrhythmogenesis.

Alterations in α_1-Adrenergic Receptors in Response to Ischemia

Over the past decade, several studies have indicated that myocardial ischemia is associated with an increase in α_1-adrenergic receptors which may, in part, contribute to the enhanced α-adrenergic responsivity discussed above. In 1981, we demonstrated that α_1-adrenergic receptors increased within 30 min of myocardial ischemia *in vivo* in the cat heart and returned rapidly to control values with sustained reperfusion [24]. A similar increase in α_1-adrenergic receptor density has been shown by others in response to ischemia in the guinea pig, cat, dog, and rat heart [24-29] although others have shown that the rat heart does not exhibit an increase in α_1-adrenergic receptor density during ischemia [25]. The major problem with this type of study is that during myocardial ischemia, a variety of metabolic events occur which could influence either the measurement of receptor density and/or assessment of coupling of receptors to intracellular events. These studies have relied on membrane preparations derived from ischemic tissue in which the "ischemic milieu" would be disturbed. This problem may explain the lack of measured α_1-adrenergic receptors until 30 min of ischemia despite the fact that a more rapid increase in α_1-adrenergic responsivity occurred in intact tissue in response to ischemia.

In an attempt to overcome these major methodologic problems, we have developed an *in vitro* system in which α_1-adrenergic receptors can be measured in intact adult canine ventricular myocytes under both normoxic as well as severely hypoxic conditions to replicate alterations in ß-oxidation typical of myocardial ischemia *in vivo*. This preparation exhibits a rapid increase in α_1-adrenergic receptors (2- to 3-fold) with 10 min of hypoxia at 37° with no change in receptor affinity [30], closely analogous to that which occurs during myocardial ischemia *in vivo*. It should be noted that this increase in α_1-adrenergic receptor density was reversible with reoxygenation and was not associated with any irreversible cellular injury as assessed using absence of release of CK or LDH [30].

Although ß-adrenergic receptors also increase in response to myocardial ischemia, the trafficking of the ß-adrenergic receptor appears to be markedly different than that for the α_1-adrenergic receptor. For example, Maisel and colleagues [27] have demonstrated that the increase in ß-adrenergic receptors in response to ischemia occurs secondary to a corresponding decrease in the density of receptors in an intracellular light vesicle fraction whereas the α-adrenergic receptor increases with no apparent change in the intracellular light vesicle compartment. Therefore, the changes in the density of the α_1-adrenergic receptors on the surface plasma membrane is not due to translocation from the same intracellular fraction from which the ß-receptors are derived [27]. At least two possibilities exist. First, the α_1-adrenergic receptor may reside in a different intracellular site under normal conditions or, alternatively, the α_1-adrenergic receptor may reside within or near the plasma membrane. Ischemia may induce an alteration in the plasma membrane or sarcolemma in which these sequestered receptors might then be exposed.

The very rapid increase in α_1-adrenergic receptors in response to ischemia or hypoxia excludes synthesis or degradation and recycling of the receptor, and indicates that externalization of an existing sequestered receptor is likely to be responsible. A substantial body of experimental evidence indicates that amphipathic metabolites, including lysophosphatidylcholine (LPC) and long-chain acylcarnitines, increase during early myocardial ischemia *in vivo* [31-37]. These amphiphiles have been shown to alter membrane function leading to a marked increase in membrane fluidity and to influence the kinetics of transmembrane ion channels, the activity of membrane bound enzymes and to influence ligand binding to receptors and coupling to intracellular events [for review, see 38,39]. Our work has focused most recently on the influence of long-chain acylcarnitine accumulation within the sarcolemma in response to hypoxia and whether this could influence exposure and/or coupling of the α_1-adrenergic receptor. We have shown that long-chain acylcarnitines increase 3.5-fold in ischemic myocardium selectively within 2 min [37]. In addition, we have shown using endogenous labeling of carnitine pools within myocytes and subsequent microscopic autoradiography that long-chain acylcarnitines increase 70-fold within the sarcolemma to a value of 1.4 mole%, at a time when α_1-adrenergic responsivity also increases 2-fold [40]. Most importantly, POCA, an inhibitor of carnitine acyltransferase I which completely prevents the increase in long-chain acylcarnitines also prevents the increase in α_1-adrenergic receptor number in response to hypoxia [30]. Likewise, exogenous addition of palmitoyl carnitine (1 μM) in normoxic myocytes also increases α_1-adrenergic receptor number [30]. Thus, there appears to be a relationship between the accumulation of long-chain acylcarnitines and the exposure of the α_1-adrenergic receptor. In the intact rat heart exposed to global ischemia, pretreatment with another inhibitor of carnitine acyltransferase I, 2-tetradecylglycidic acid (TGDA) also prevented the increase in α_1-adrenergic receptors [28]. These findings suggest that membrane alterations induced by accumulation of long-chain acylcarnitines into the sarcolemma, possibly mediated through an increase in membrane fluidity [41] leads to the exposure or externalization of the α_1-adrenergic receptor. Presumably, other amphiphiles, including LPC, could also contribute to the perturbation of the orderly packing of membrane phospholipids which may also result in a similar response.

Coupling of the α_1-Adrenergic Receptors During Hypoxia

There are substantial data available indicating that α_1-adrenergic receptors are coupled to phospholipase C which, when activated, results in cleavage of phosphatidylinositol 4,5-bisphosphate (PIP_2) to form inositol 1,4,5-trisphosphate (IP_3) and 1,2-diacylglycerol, both of which serve as intracellular second messengers to modulate a variety of intracellular responses. Diacylglycerol can stimulate protein kinase C which can phosphorylate a number of different cellular proteins including the L-type calcium channel. However, as indicated above, the modest positive inotropic effect of α_1-adrenergic stimulation does not appear to be secondary to direct activation of this L-type calcium current [42] but may be secondary to an inhibition of I_K. Other investigators have shown that protein kinase C can enhance Na^+/H^+ exchange which in turn activates Na^+/Ca^{2+} exchange resulting in an increase in intracellular calcium in cardiac myocytes exposed to hypoxia [43]. In a recent study in the canine heart *in vivo*, the concentration of diacylglycerol actually increases selectively in the ischemic zone within 5 min and was maintained during early reperfusion [44]. The fact that the α_1-adrenergic block attenuates this increase in diacylglycerol suggests that the effect was mediated through the α_1-adrenergic receptor. Additionally, it has been shown that norepinephrine can stimulate protein kinase C only in depolarized cardiac tissue [45] suggesting that the coupling to phospholipase C may in fact depend on membrane potential changes which occur in hypoxic or ischemic tissue. The α_1-adrenergic receptor may also be coupled to phospholipase A_2 [46] leading to the release of free fatty acids and lysophosphatidylcholine which also can contribute to arrhythmogenesis during early ischemia [39]. α_1-Adrenergic receptors have also been shown to stimulate cyclic AMP phosphodiesterase activity which may, in fact, decrease the effective ß-adrenergic mediated responsivity [47].

We have shown in adult cardiac myocytes that α_1-adrenergic stimulation can lead to an increase in IP_3 using mass measurements of inositol phosphates [48]. In normoxic cells, norepinephrine elicits a 3- to 4-fold increase in IP_3 within 30 sec returning to baseline by 60 sec with subsequent increases in in IP_2 and IP_1. We have also demonstrated that norepinephrine will result in a marked but transient increase in IP_4 in the same cell system [49]. Hypoxia for 10 min results in a 2- to 3-fold increase in α_1-adrenergic receptors and a 100-times lower concentration of norepinephrine required to elicit an increase in IP_3 and a 6-times lower EC_{50} for norepinephrine to elicit an increase in IP_3 [48]. The increase in IP_3 and IP_4 was completely blocked by an α_1-adrenergic blocking agent. These results suggest that an increase in coupling of the α_1-adrenergic receptor to phospholipase C occurs in response to hypoxia. Although the increase in receptor density during hypoxia may explain a portion of the increase in the IP_3 response, the fact that receptor density increased by only 2- to 3-fold whereas there was a 100-fold reduction in the threshold concentration required to elicit an increase in IP_3 strongly suggests that the coupling of the receptor to intracellular events can occur independent of an increase in receptor number *per se*.

Recent findings suggest that the α_1-adrenergic receptors can be divided into at least 2 pharmacologically distinct subtypes which are linked to different mechanisms for signal transduction [50]. The α_{1a}-subtype is characterized by a high affinity for WB-4101 and is not inactivated by the alkylating agent, chlorethylclonidine. Evidence to date suggests that only the α_{1b}-subtype (blocked by chlorethylclonidine) is linked to the formation of IP_3. However, in canine Purkinje fibers, the norepinephrine stimulated inositol phosphate accumulation is chlorethylclonidine insensitive and inhibited by WB-4101 suggesting differences in the coupling of the α_1-adrenergic receptor subtypes to intracellular signal transduction in different tissues and potentially different species. In addition, alterations in the 4 different subforms of phospholipase C described in rabbit myocardium [51] could influence the coupling of α_1-adrenergic receptors to second messengers in ischemic mycocardium.

SUMMARY

Based on findings from several laboratories, it is clear that α_1-adrenergic stimulation of the myocardium is altered in the presence of myocardial ischemia and probably under other pathophysiologic conditions including congestive heart failure. Future work will be required to clarify the precise mechanisms underlying the alterations in α_1-adrenergic receptors under hypoxic and ischemic conditions, whether specific receptor subtypes are involved, and whether the coupling to different subforms of phospholipase C influences intracellular responses. In addition, other membrane bound enzymes which could act as second messengers include phospholipase A_2 and phospholipase D both of which require further evaluation. A better understanding of the influence of α_1-adrenergic stimulation on ion channel function under hypoxic and simulated ischemic conditions will also be required. This information should lead to more efficient approaches for the prevention and treatment of lethal arrhythmias in patients with ischemic heart disease.

REFERENCES

1. Corr PB, Yamada KA, Witkowski FX (1986) Mechanisms controlling cardiac autonomic function and their relation to arrhythmogenesis. In: Fozzard HA, Jennings RB, Katz AM, Morgan HE (eds) The Heart and Cardiovascular System. Scientific Foundations. Raven Press. New York. pp 1343-1403
2. Malliani A, Schwartz PJ, Zanchetti A (1980) Neural mechanisms in life-threatening arrhythmias. Am Heart J 100: 705-715
3. Penny WJ (1984) The deleterious effects of myocardial catecholamines on cellular electrophysiology and arrhythmias during ischaemia and reperfusion. Eur Heart J 5: 960-973
4. Schoemig A (1990) Catecholamines in myocardial ischemia. Systemic and cardiovascular release. Circulation 82 (suppl II): II-13-II22
5. Pogwizd SM, Corr PB (1987) Reentrant and nonreentrant mechanisms contribute to arrhythmogenesis during early myocardial ischemia: Results using three-dimensional mapping. Circ Res 61:352-371
6. Pogwizd SM, Corr PB (1990) Mechanisms underlying the development of ventricular fibrillation during early myocardial ischemia. Circ Res 66: 672-695
7. Schuemann HJ, Wagner J, Knorr A, Reidemeister JC, Sadony V, Schramm B (1978) Demonstration in human atrial preparations of α-adrenoceptors mediating positive inotropic effects. Naunyn-Schmiedeberg's Arch Pharmacol 302: 333-336
8. Priori SG, Corr PB (1990) Mechanisms underlying early and delayed afterdepolarizations induced by catecholamines. Am J Physiol 258 (Heart Circ Physiol 27): H1796-H1805
9. Rosen MR, Hordof AJ, Ilvento JP, Danilo P Jr (1977) Effects of adrenergic amines on electrophysiologic properties and automaticity of neonatal and adult canine Purkinje fibres. Evidence for α- and ß-adrenergic actions. Circ Res 40: 390-400
10. Reuter H, Scholz H (1977) The regulation of the calcium conductance of cardiac muscle by adrenaline. J Physiol Lond 264: 49-62
11. Apkon M, Nerbonne JM (1988) α-Adrenergic agonists selectively suppress voltage-dependent K^+ current in rat ventricular myocytes. Proc Natl Acad Sci USA 85: 8756-8760
12. Fedida D, Shimoni Y, Giles WR (1989) A novel effect of norepinephrine on cardiac cells is mediated by α_1-adrenoceptors. Am J Physiol (Heart Circ Physiol) 256:H1500-H1504
13. Tohse N, Nakaya H, Hattori Y, Endou M, Kanno M (1990) Inhibitory effect mediated by α_1-adrenoceptors on transient outward current in isolated rat ventricular cells. Pfluegers Arch 415: 575-581
14. Priori SG, Yamada KA, Corr PB (1991) Influence of hypoxia on adrenergic modulationof triggered activity in isolated adult canine myocytes. Circulation 83:248-259
15. Culling W, Penny WJ, Cunliffe G, Flores NA, Sheridan DJ (1987) Arrhythmogenic and electrophysiological effects of alpha adrenoceptor stimulation during myocardial ischaemia and reperfusion. J Mol Cell Cardiol 19: 251-258
16. Sheridan DJ, Penkoske PA, Sobel BE, Corr PB (1980) α-Adrenergic contributions to dysrhythmia during myocardial ischemia and reperfusion in cats. J Clin Invest 65: 161-171
17. Wilber DL, Lynch JL, Montgomery DG, Lucchesi BR (1987) α-Adrenergic influences in canine ischemic sudden death. Effects of α_1-adrenoceptor blockade with prazosin. J Cardiovasc Pharmacol 10: 96-106
18. Benfey BG, Elfellah MS, Ogilvie RI, Varma DR (1984) Anti-arrhythmic effects of prazosin and propranolol during coronary artery occlusion and reperfusion in dogs and pigs. Br J Pharmacol 82: 717-725

19. Stewart JR, Burmeister WE, Burmeister J, Lucchesi BR (1980) Electrophysiologic and antiarrhythmic effects of phentolamine in experimental coronary artery occlusion and reperfusion in the dog. J Cardiovasc Pharmacol 2: 77-91
20. Williams LT, Guerrero JL, Leinbach RC (1982) Prevention of reperfusion dysrhythmias by selective coronary alpha-adrenergic blockade. Am J Cardiol 49: 1046
21. Thandroyen FT, Worthington MG, Higginson LM, Opie LH (1983) The effect of alpha- and beta-adrenoceptor antagonist agents on reperfusion ventricular fibrillation and metabolic status in the isolated perfused heart. J Am Coll Cardiol 1: 1056-1066
22. Schwartz PJ, Vanoli E, Zaza A, Zuanetti G (1985) The effect of antiarrhythmic drugs on life-threatening arrhythmias induced by the interaction between acute myocardial ischemia and sympathetic hyperactivity. Am Heart J 109: 937-948
23. Davey MJ (1980) Relevant features of the pharmacology of prazosin. J Cardiovasc Pharmacol 2 (Suppl 3): S287-S301
24. Corr PB, Shayman JA, Kramer JB, Kipnis RJ (1981) Increased α-adrenergic receptors in ischemic cat myocardium: A potential mediator of electrophysiological derangements. J Clin Invest 67: 1232-1236
25. Dillon JS, Gu XH, Nayler WG (1988) Alpha$_1$-adrenoceptors in the ischaemic and reperfused myocardium. J Mol Cell Cardiol 20: 725-735
26. Mukherjee A, Hogan M, McCoy K, Buja LM, Willerson JT (1980) Influence of experimental myocardial ischemia on alpha$_1$-adrenergic receptors. Circulation 64 (Suppl III):149
27. Maisel AS, Motulsky HJ, Ziegler MG, Insel PA (1987) Ischemia- and agonist-induced changes in α- and ß-adrenergic receptor traffic in guinea pig hearts. Am J Physiol 253: H1159-H1166
28. Allely MC, Brown CM (1988) The effects of POCA and TGDA on the ischaemia-induced increase in α_1-adrenoceptor density in the rat left ventricle. Br J Pharm 95: 705P
29. Butterfield MC, Chess-Williams R (1990) Enhanced α-adrenoceptor responsiveness and receptor number during global ischaemia in the Langendorff perfused rat heart. Br J Pharm 100: 641-645
30. Heathers GP, Yamada KA, Kanter EM, Corr PB (1987) Long-chain acylcarnitines mediate the hypoxia-induced increase in α_1-adrenergic receptors on adult canine myocytes. Circ Res 61: 735-746
31. Idell-Wenger JA, Grotyohann LW, Neely JR (1978) Coenzyme A and carnitine distribution in normal and ischemic hearts. J Biol Chem 253: 4310-4318
32. Liedtke AJ, Nellis S, Neely JR (1978) Effects of excess free fatty acids on mechanical and metabolic function in normal and ischemic myocardium in swine. Circ Res 43: 652-661
33. Shug AL, Thomsen JH, Folts JD, Bittar N, Klein MI, Koke JR, Huth PJ (1978) Changes in tissue levels of carnitine and other metabolites during myocardial ischemia and anoxia. Arch Biochem Biophys 187: 25-33
34. Snyder DW, Crafford WA Jr, Glashow JL, Rankin D, Sobel BE, Corr PB (1981) Lysophosphoglycerides in ischemic myocardium effluents and potentiation of their arrhythmogenic effects. Am J Physiol 241: H700-H707
35. Corr PB, Snyder DW, Lee BI, Gross RW, Keim CR, Sobel BE (1982) Pathophysiological concentrations of lysophosphatides and the slow response. Am J Physiol 243: H187-H195
36. Corr PB, Creer MH, Yamada KA, Saffitz JE, Sobel BE (1989) Prophylaxis of early ventricular fibrillation by inhibition of acylcarnitine accumulation. J Clin Invest 83: 927-936
37. DaTorre SD, Creer MH, Pogwizd SM, Corr PB (1991) Amphipathic lipid metabolites and their relation to arrhythmogenesis in the ischemic heart. J Mol Cell Cardiol 23: 11-22

38. Corr PB, Gross RW, Sobel BE (1984) Amphipathic metabolites and membrane dysfunction in ischemic myocardium. Circ Res 55: 135-154
39. Creer MH, Dobmeyer DJ, Corr PB (1990) Amphipathic lipid metabolites and arrhythmias during myocardial ischemia. In: Zipes DP, Jalife J (eds). Cardiac Electrophysiology: From Cell to Bedside. WB Saunders Co. Philadelphia. pp 417-433
40. Knabb MT, Saffitz JE, Corr PB Sobel BE (1986) The dependence of electrophysiological derangements on accumulation of endogenous long-chain acylcarnitine in hypoxic neonatal rat myocytes. Circ Res 58: 230-240
41. Fink KL, Gross RW (1984) Modulation of canine myocardial sarcolemmal membrane fluidity by amphiphilic compounds. Circ Res 55: 585-594
42. Hescheler J, Nawrath H, Tang M, Trautwein W (1988) Adrenoceptor-mediated changes of excitation and contraction in ventricular heart muscle from guinea-pigs and rabbits. J PHysiol 397: 657-670
43. Ikeda U, Arisaka H, Takayasu T, Takeda K, Natsume T, Hosoda S (1988) Protein kinase C activation aggravates hypoxic myocardial injury by stimulating Na^+/H^+ exchange. J Mol Cell Cardiol 20: 493-500
44. Kawai T, Okumura K, Hashimoto H, Ito T, Satake T (1990) Alteration of 1,2-diacylglycerol content in ischemic and reperfused heart. Mol Cell Biochem 99: 1-8
45. Kaku T, Lakatta E, Filburn CR (1986) Effect of α_1-adrenergic stimulation on phosphoinositide metabolism and protein kinase C (PK-C) in rat cardiomyocytes. Fed Proc 45: 209
46. Slivka SR, Insel PA (1987) Alpha$_1$-adrenergic receptor-mediated phosphoinositide hydrolysis and prostaglandin E_2 formation in Madin-Darby canine kidney cells. Possible parallel activation of phospholipase C and phospholipase A_2. J Biol Chem 262: 4200-4207
47. Buxton ILO, Brunton LL (1985) Action of the cardiac alpha$_1$-adrenergic receptor. Activation of cyclic AMP degradation. J Biol Chem 260: 6733-6737
48. Heathers GP, Evers AS, Corr PB (1989) Enhanced inositol trisphosphate response to α_1-adrenergic stimulation in hypoxic cardiac myocytes. J Clin Invest 83: 1409-1413
49. Heathers GP, Corr PB, Rubin LJ (1988) Transient accumulation of inositol (1,3,4,5)-tetrakisphosphate in response to α_1-adrenergic stimulation in adult cardiac myocytes. Biochem Biophys Res Commun 156: 485-492
50. Lefkowitz RJ, Kobilka BK, Caron MB (1989) The new biology of drug receptors. Biochem Pharm 38: 2941-2948

Enzyme-Specific Desensitization of Adenylyl Cyclase in Hypertrophied Heart in Monocrotaline-Treated Rats

KATSUYUKI TOBISE, HIROMITSU YOSHIE, KAZUMI UEKITA, MASAAKI FUJITA, and SOKICHI ONODERA

First Department of Internal Medicine, Asahikawa Medical College, Asahikawa, 078 Japan

KEYWORDS: hypertrophied heart, catalytic unit of adenylyl cyclase, homologous or heterologous desensitization

INTRODUCTION

Monocrotaline (MCT) is a toxic pyrrolizidine alkaloid isolated from the stem, foliage and seeds of Crotalaria spectabilis. Administration of MCT to rats results in pulmonary arterial hypertension, leading to a severe right ventricular hypertrophy and eventually to failure [1]. As reported in patients with heart failure caused by primary pulmonary hypertension, a chamber-specific decrease in the myocardial β-adrenoceptors was shown mostly in the failing right ventricle, while the β-adrenoceptor density in the left ventricle remained normal [2]. This phenomenon is explained as the down-regulation of the β-adrenoceptor due to an increased sympathetic nerve activity in a state of congestive heart failure. The goal of the present investigation was to determine whether the mechanism of the desensitization was mostly due to the downregulation of β-adrenoceptor or adenylyl cyclase activation in an experimental model of right ventricular failure. Although the phenomenon of desensitization, homologous or heterologous, has been recognized at the in vitro cultured cells, few studies have examined this phenomenon in the in vivo model of heart failure.

MATERIALS AND METHODS

Animal and Experimental Protocol

Male 5-weeks-old CD rats (Charles River Laboratories) were once injected subcutaneously with 2% MCT solution (40 mg/kg), and with saline (2 ml/kg) for the controls. An experimental protocol was performed at weekly intervals for 4 weeks after the MCT treatment. The right ventricular pressure and heart rate were measured. The ventricle was separated into the right ventricle (RV), septum (SEP) and left ventricle (LV), and then each ventricle was weighed. The weight ratios of RV/(LV+SEP) were used as an index of right ventricular hypertrophy.

Membrane Preparation

Crude cardiac membranes were prepared by the modified method of Jones and Besch [3]. Protein concentration was measured by the modified method of Lowry et al. [4]. The 5'-nucleotidase activity was measured according to the method of

Heppel and Hilmoe [5].

β–adrenoceptor Binding Studies

All studies were performed in the presence of Tris buffer. β–adrenoceptor antagonist binding was determined using 25 μl [^{125}I] cyanopindolol (New England Nuclear, 0.02–1.0 nM) in the presence or absence of 25 μl dl–propranolol (10^{-4} M) or buffer, and 100 μl (60–100 μg/assay). Assays were performed in duplicate, incubated at 37°C for 30 minutes, terminated by rapid filtration on Whatman GF/C filters, and counted in a gamma counter for 2 minutes. Specific binding was 60–70%. The density (Bmax) and dissociation constants (Kd) were calculated by the Scatchard analysis.

Toxin–catalyzed ADP Ribosylation or Immunoblot Analysis of Gs and Gi

Cholera toxin–catalyzed ADP ribosylation was performed as described by Longabaugh et al. [6]. Pertussis toxin–catalyzed ADP ribosylation of the GTP–binding protein was used according to the method of Bokoch et al. [7]. Immunoblotting was performed by using Gsα and Giα2 antiserum directed against a conserved sequence encoding residues.

Adenylyl Cyclase Assay

Adenylyl cyclase activity was assayed according to the method of Salomon [8]. The maximal adenylyl cyclase activity was assayed in the presence of 0.1 mM isoproterenol with 0.1 mM Gpp(NH)p, and 0.05 mM forskolin. The reaction was initiated by the addition of membranes and terminated after 15 minutes at 30° C with the addition of stopping solution. Cyclic AMP was separated by sequential chromatography on Dowex 50W–X4 cation exchange resins and on neutral alumina. Further, forskolin–stimulated adenylyl cyclase activities were obtained in the presence of 0.05 mM forskolin with $MnCl_2$.

A p value of <0.05 was considered statistically significant. All data were presented as mean±standard deviation (S.D.) of the mean.

RESULTS

Ventricular Weight, Hemodynamics and Membrane Marker Enzyme

The growth rates of MCT–treated rats were significantly decreased at 1 or 3 week after the treatment. The MCT–treated rats began to show tachypnea, white fibrosis of the lung, xanthochromic pleural and/or peritoneal effusions from 3 weeks after the treatment. The mortality rate was approximately 10% at 3 weeks, and 36% at 4 weeks after the treatment. Right ventricular systolic pressure in MCT–treated rats began to rise from 2 weeks after the treatment. The RV weight, RV/(LV+SEP) ratio and RV/BW ratio in MCT–treated rats were significantly increased compared with the controls from 2 weeks after the treatment. Although the 5'–nucleotidase activities in RV, SEP and LV in MCT–treated rats were significantly increased 4 weeks after the treatment, these activities were not significantly different among each ventricle. The final yield of cardiac membrane was approximately 50 mg of protein per 1 g of wet tissue. There was no difference of the yield between the control and MCT–treated rats.

β–adrenoceptor Density

Although the β–adrenoceptor density in RV in MCT–treated rats did not change 1 week after the treatment, it was significantly decreased by 27% 2 weeks after, by 43% 3 weeks after, and by 30% 4 weeks after the treatment. The β–adrenoceptor density in SEP did not change until 3 weeks after the treatment, but it was significantly decreased by 28% 4 weeks after. The β–adrenoceptor density in LV was not significantly decreased even 4 weeks after the treatment. There was no significant difference of the affinity (Kd) between the control and MCT–treated rats.

Amount of Gs and Gi by using bacteria toxin–catalyzed ADP–ribosylation or immunoblot analysis.

A molar amount of Gsα or Giα in the myocardial membranes from the control and the MCT–treated rats was made by labeling the 45 kDa Gsα or 40 kDa Giα substrate with ^{32}P–ADP ribosylation. Statistical analysis shows no significant difference in the level of Gsα and Gi in each ventricle between two groups. Immunoblotting using Gsα and Giα2 polyclonal antibody showed that the level of Gsα and Giα2 was almost similar to the results from bacteria–toxin catalyzed ADP–ribosylation.

Adenylyl Cyclase Activity

Although the basal activity in RV in MCT–treated rats did not change 1 or 2 weeks after the MCT treatment, it was significantly decreased by 59% 3 weeks after and by 56% 4 weeks after the treatment. The basal activity in SEP and LV did not significantly change even 4 weeks after the treatment. Four weeks after, the adenylyl cyclase activity stimulated by isoproterenol with Gpp(NH)p in the MCT–treated rats was lower in RV (−71.2%, $p<0.01$), in SEP (−54.2%, $p<0.05$), and in LV (−27.3%, $p<0.10$) than those of the control rats. The adenylyl cyclase activity stimulated by forskolin in the MCT–treated rats was significantly depressed in RV (−65.3%, $p<0.001$), in SEP (−40.9%, $p<0.01$), and even in LV (−40.5%, $p<0.05$). The basal adenylyl cyclase activity stimulated by manganese was significantly depressed in RV (−63.6%, $p<0.001$), in SEP (−39.1%, $p<0.001$) and in LV (−26.5%, $p<0.05$). The adenylyl cyclase activity stimulated by manganese plus forskolin was also significantly depressed in RV (−71.3%, $p<0.001$), in SEP (−47.2%, $p<0.01$) and in LV (−36.8%, $p<0.01$).

DISCUSSION

A progression of pulmonary hypertension produced by monocrotaline (MCT) is eventually followed by right ventricular hypertrophy and failure [1]. We determined the changes in β–adrenoceptor–adenylyl cyclase system with the development of right ventricular hypertrophy. The activity of 5'–nucleotidase in the hypertrophied RV was noted to be very similar to SEP or non–hypertrophied LV. The protein yield per gram of myocardial wet weight was almost identical in the control and MCT–treated rats, which suggested that the ventricular hypertrophy itself has little effect on the characteristics of the myocardial membrane used in the present study.

Adrenergic nervous system in part provides an important support to the progress of cardiac hypertrophy. Which type of desensitization to norepinephrine (NE), homologous or heterologous is observed in the model of congestive heart failure remains uncertain thoroughly. The reduced myocardial β–adrenoceptor density in chronic heart failure has been thought to be caused by agonist–induced homologous desensitization. Indeed, in this study the myocardial β–adrenoceptor density was significantly decreased in RV or SEP subjected to increased afterload, but not in LV. The level of plasma NE is eventually elevated in animals [9] and patients with congestive heart failure [10]. Thus, this decrease appears to be related to pressure overloading to the regional myocardial cells rather than to circulating factors, because both RV and LV are exposed to the same level of circulating NE.

The adenylyl cyclase activity stimulated by forskolin or $MnCl_2$ was significantly depressed in RV, SEP, and LV 4 weeks after MCT treatment. These reductions are principally associated with either diminished activation or enhanced inhibition by receptor–coupled G proteins, or the defective catalytic unit of adenylyl cyclase. The apparent change in the amount of Gs or Gi was not observed from bacteria toxin–catalyzed ADP–ribosylation or immunoblotting. However, the forskolin– or manganese–activated adenylyl cyclase activity in LV was depressed without reduction in the β–adrenoceptor density. This change is thought to be the same as heterologous desensitization observed in the in vitro cultured cells. For this explanation, the catalytic unit of adenylyl cyclase itself may be affected by β–adrenoceptor–coupled signal transduction. Very little evidence bearing on this hypothesis has been published. Both protein kinase A (PKA) and protein kinase C (PKC) can phosphorylate the catalytic unit of adenylyl cyclase in reconstitution assay system, leading to an impairment of Gpp(NH)p–stimulated activity by PKA or to an enhancement of this activity by PKC [11]. Therefore, the depressed activity of adenylyl cyclase may be associated with the change in the catalytic unit of adenylyl cyclase itself, or the PKA–dependent phosphorylation of the catalytic unit of adenylyl cyclase.

In conclusion, this study exhibited processes regulating the activation of the β–adrenoceptor transduction system. These results suggest that the signal transduction defects may be, at least in part, associated with the depressed catalytic unit of adenylyl cyclase rather than the β–adorenoceptor downregulation in a state of heart failure in MCT–treated rats.

REFERENCES

1. Hilliker KS, Bell TG, Roth R (1988) Pneumotoxicity and thrombocytopenia after single injection of monocrotaline. Am J Physiol 242: H573–H579
2. Bristow MR, Minobe W, Rasmussen R, Ginsburg R, Fowler M, Larrabee P (1985) Chamber-specific adrenergic abnormalities in isolated right ventricular failure in the human heart. Circulation 72 (Supp.III) :III–183
3. Jones LR, Besch HR Jr (1984) Isolation of canine cardiac sarcolemmal vesicles. Methods Pharmacol 5:1–12
4. Lowry OH, Rosebrough NJ, Farr AL, Randall RJ (1951) Protein measurement with the Folin phenol reagent. J Biol Chem 193:265–275
5. Heppel LA, Hilmoe RJ (1955) "5" Nucleotidases, In: Colowick SP, Kaplan NO (eds) Methods in Enzymology. Academic Press, New York, pp546–550
6. Longabaugh JP, Vatner DE, Graham RM, Homcy CJ (1986) NADP improves the efficiency of cholera toxin catalyzed ADP–ribosylation in liver and heart membranes. Biochem Biophys Res Commun 137: 328–333
7. Bokoch GM, Katada T, Northup JK, Ui M, Gilman AG (1984) Purification and properties of the inhibitory guanine nucleotide–binding regulatory component of adenylate cyclase. J Biol Chem 259:3560–3567
8. Salomon Y, Londos C, Rodbell M (1974) A highly sensitive adenylate cyclase assay. Anal Biochem 58:541–548
9. Liang C.–s., Fan T.–H. M, Sullebarger JT, Sakamoto S (1989) Decreased adrenergic neuronal uptake activity in experimental right heart failure. A chamber–specific contributor to beta–adrenoceptor downregulation. J Clin Invest 84:1267–1275
10. Swedberg K, Viquerat C, Rouleau J–L, Roizen M, Atherton B, Parmley WW, Chatterjee K (1984) Comparison of myocardial catecholamine balance in chronic congestive heart failure and in angina pectoris without failure. Am J Cardiol 54:783–786
11. Yoshimasa T, Bouvier M, Benovic JL, Amlaiky N, Lefkowitz RJ, Caron MG (1988) Regulation of the adenylate cyclase signalling pathway: Potential role for the phosphorylation of the catalytic unit by protein kinase A and protein kinase C, In McKerns KW, Chretien M (eds): Molecular Biology of Brain and Endocrine Peptide Systems. Plenum, New York, pp123–139

A Mechanism of Catecholamine Tolerance in Congestive Heart Failure

KAZUSHI URASAWA, KATSUHIKO SATO, YASUMI IGARASHI, HIDEAKI KAWAGUCHI, and HISAKAZU YASUDA

Department of Cardiovascular Medicine, Hokkaido University School of Medicine, Sapporo, 060 Japan

KEYWORDS: congestive heart failure, adenylyl cyclase system, GTP binding protein, desensitization

INTRODUCTION

Various diseases and clinical settings can induce congestive heart failure (CHF). As such, it is unlikely that a single mechanism can explain the cardiac dysfunction observed in CHF. However, CHF patients (or animals) share several similar features: reduced cardiac contractility, increased sympathetic nerve activity, and activation of several hormonal systems (e.g., renin-angiotensin system, vasopressin, and atrial natriuretic factor) to compensate for the impaired cardiac function. In this setting, cardiac receptor, GTP-binding proteins, and their effector molecules (adenylyl cyclase, phospholipase C, several ion channels) are inevitably exposed to chronically elevated neurohormonal stimulation. A widely recognized concept is that a chronic increase in such stimulation can desensitize target cell receptors and post-receptor signal transducing pathways (1). It is therefore likely that in CHF one or more types of desensitization contributes to a reduction in signal transducing efficiency in order to maintain intracellular homeostasis. To date, several laboratories have reported a decrease in β-adrenergic receptor (βAR) density in CHF patients and model animals (2-4, 5 for review). Recently, reports of several studies have indicated that the inhibitory GTP-binding protein (G_i) can be increased in CHF patients (6,7) and animal models (8). Although direct evidence for a change in the catalytic protein of adenylyl cyclase has not been available, limited information have suggested a reduced catalytic activity in terminally failing hearts (9). In this study, we have suggested changes of βAR, GTP-binding protein and catalytic protein using two different animal models with an emphasis on defining the kinetics for the desensitization process of adenylyl cyclase system.

MATERIALS AND METHODS

Materials

1) Cardiomyopathic Syrian hamsters, BIO53.58, were obtained from BIO Research Laboratory (USA). In this study, animals in two different ages (16- and 28-week-old) were used to examine the relation between severity of CHF and changes in various parameters. Hamsters in F1b were used as healthy control (four animals for each group). 2) A non-hypertensive-dose of norepinephrine (NE), 0.25μg/kg/min, was injected into Wistar Kyoto rats subcutaneously using implanted osmotic pumps (model 2002, Alzet, USA). Prior to this study, we conducted experiments to determine an optimal NE dose. We found that higher dose of NE (such as 1μg/kg/min) could increase blood pressure, promote cardiac hypertrophy, and reduce body weight, thus indicating potent cardiovascular and metabolic effects of NE. In order to focus on more localized effects of NE on the cardiac adenylyl cyclase system, we used a lower (non-hypertensive) dose (0.25μg/kg/min). In separate experiments, we measured plasma NE concentration at 7 days of injection; control group (n=6) 144.2±28.5 pg/ml, NE group (n=6) 1646.7±252.6 pg/ml. The NE injection was

maintained for 3 different durations, 3, 7 and 14 days (6 animals in each group). Physiological saline was injected into 6 WKY rats for 14 days using the same technique, and this group was used as control.

Methods

Membrane preparation
A crude membrane fraction was prepared as described previously (10). Briefly, hearts were minced in ice-cold K-phosphate buffer (pH7.5), homogenized by Polytron, and centrifuged at 1,250xg for 30min. The resultant supernatant fractions were centrifuged again at 100,000xg for 1hr, and the pellet fractions were suspended in the K-phosphate buffer and stored at -80°C until use. Protein concentration of the crude membrane fraction raged from 1 to 2mg/ml.

βAR binding experiments
^{125}I-cyanopindolol (ICYP, Amersham, USA) was used for the βAR binding experiments as described previously (10). The results were analyzed by Scatchard plot, and receptor density (Bmax) and dissociation constant for ICYP (Kd) were obtained.

ADP-ribosylation of GTP-binding proteins
Cholate extracted membrane fractions were incubated with [^{32}P]-NAD (Du pont NEN, USA) and preactivated bacterial toxin (cholera toxin for stimulatory GTP-binding protein, G_s, and pertussis toxin for G_i) as described previously (11). Radioactive products were precipitated by 6% trichloroacetic acid, filtered through nitrocellulose membranes (A025A025, Advantec, Japan), then counted in scintillation counter.

Assay of adenylyl cyclase activity
Forskolin (100μM)-stimulated cyclase activity was measured by conventional column chromatography methods using [α^{32}P]-ATP (Du pont NEN, USA) as substrate and [^{3}H]-cAMP (Du pont NEN, USA) as calibration standard (12).

Miscellaneous
Protein concentration was determined by Amido-black stain method (13). Bovine serum albumin was used as the protein standard. All experiments were performed in duplicate, and multiple observations were reported as the mean ± SD. Results were analyzed by *t*-test with $p<0.05$ considered to be statistically significant.

RESULTS AND DISCUSSION

Cardiomyopathic Syrian hamsters, BIO53.58, are characterized by progressive cardiac dilatation and early death with CHF within one year (14). The most prominent difference from strain BIO14.6, which has been widely used as an animal model for cardiomyopathy, is that BIO53.58 does not develop cardiac hypertrophy before CHF stage. Because of this characteristic feature, BIO53.58 may be a more suitable model than BIO14.6 to study dilated cardiomyopathy and CHF of humans.

The amount of G_i, measured by pertussis toxin-catalyzed ADP-ribosylation, was significantly increased in BIO53.58 compared to F1b at both ages (16-week-old ; F1b 0.51±0.05, BIO 0.95±0.25, 28-week-old ; F1b 0.57±0.13, BIO 1.37±0.33 pmol/mg protein). The amount of G_s, measured by cholera toxin-catalyzed ADP-ribosylation was not different between BIO53.58 and F1b at both ages (data not shown). So far, several laboratories have reported an increase of G_i in human CHF (6.7). Böhm *et al.* reported that the increase of G_i in dilated cardiomyopathic hearts was associated with reduced basal and GTP analogue-stimulated cyclase activity, and reduced responsiveness to isoprenaline (15). We also found that the increased G_i in BIO53.58 was functional and produced a greater activity in inhibiting adenylyl cyclase (data not shown).

There are several reports which indicate normal forskolin-stimulated cyclase activity in failing hearts (7.16). However, Harding *et al.* recently reported that atrial myocytes isolated from NYHA class IV patients show reduced amplitude in maximal contractile response to forskolin (9). This would suggest that the catalytic protein is also impaired in terminally failing hearts and such impairment could contribute to post-receptor dysfunction. Additionally, CHF induced by rapid ventricular pacing in pigs is also associated with a decrease of βAR density and reduction of catalytic activity (H. Kirk Hammond, personal communication). In our study, the catalytic activity of BIO53.58 was decreased even at the early stage of CHF (16-week-old; F1b 240±31.2, BIO 145±13.7 pmol cAMP/mg/min), and was impaired to a greater extent in the older age group (28-week-old; F1b 269.9±6.5, BIO 91.9±18.2 pmol cAMP/mg/min). In conjunction with the fact that increase of G_i in 28-week-old BIO53.58 was more prominent than that in 16-week-old BIO53.58, these alterations observed in post receptor components might be related to the severity of CHF.

Table 1. Effect of chronic norepinephrine infusion on adenylyl cyclase system of rat heart membranes.

group	βAR Bmax fmol/mg	βAR Kd pM	G_s pmol/mg	G_i pmol/mg	adenylyl cyclase pmol cAMP/mg/min
control	70.7 ± 6.2	100.1 ± 38.8	1.72 ± 0.26	6.02 ± 0.84	235.1 ± 47.7
3 days	51.4 ± 5.8 b	84.7 ± 12.6	1.41 ± 0.27	6.17 ± 0.74	174.1 ± 24.7 a
7 days	41.5 ± 7.2 c	91.9 ± 29.3	1.77 ± 0.44	8.08 ± 1.25 a	167.4 ± 31.2 a
14 days	49.5 ± 8.2 b	91.3 ± 18.8	1.77 ± 0.41	7.37 ± 1.18	128.1 ± 35.7 b

a; $p < 0.05$ b; $p < 0.01$ c; $p < 0.001$ vs control group

Catecholamine-induced down-regulation of βAR has been reported by several laboratories (17-19). Since most of these studies were conducted using isoproterenol as a stimulant, it is difficult to extrapolate from those results to the effect of an enhanced sympathetic nerve activity as would occur in CHF.

In the second models that we showed, a low dose (0.25μg/kg/min) of NE was chronically injected into WKY rats. The density of βAR was significantly reduced in all three treated groups (70.7±6.2, 51.4±5.8, 41.5±7.2 and 49.5±8.2 fmol/mg for control, 3-, 7- and 14-day group, respectively). The dissociation constant of βAR for ^{125}I-cyanopindolol was essentially the same in all four groups (100.1±38.8, 84.7± 12.6, 91.9±29.3 and 91.3±18.8 pM for control, 3-, 7- and 14-day group). Unlike our results, Vatner *et al.* reported an increase of βAR density after 4 weeks NE injection (0.5μg/kg/min) in dogs (20). Since we used nearly the same dose of NE and the same procedure (implanted osmotic pump) as those investigators, the reason for the differences in βAR regulation would likely reflect species difference.

The amount of G_i were 6.02±0.84, 6.17±0.74, 8.08±1.25 and 7.37±1.18 (pmol/mg protein) for control, 3- 7- and 14-day group, respectively, and significantly increased after 7-days treatment. There was no significant difference in the amount of G_s among the four groups. Thus chronic NE infusion also increased expression of G_i, but this response required a more persistent stimulation of adrenergic receptor than did the down-regulation of βAR. The catalytic activity of NE-infused rats was significantly decreased at 3 days of treatment, and maintained at a reduced level until 14 days of treatment (235.1±47.7, 174.1±24.7, 167.4±31.2 and 128.1±35.7 pmol cAMP/mg/min for control, 3-, 7- and 14-day group).

In this study, two different animal models were investigated: BIO53.58, a genetic model for CHF, and NE-infused rats, a model which simulates the neurohormonal milieu with respect to increased NE in human CHF. Alterations observed in each component of adenylyl cyclase system (a decrease of βAR density, increased amount of G_i, and decrease in catalytic activity) was quite similar in the two models, suggesting that those alterations in failing hearts might be secondary phenomena provoked by elevated plasma catecholamine concentrations. Moreover, there was a chronological order in development of the changes in adenylyl cyclase system: a rapidly responding element (βAR) and slowly responding elements (G_i and catalytic protein). In view of the time scale of response, the changes in post-receptor components (especially overexpression of G_i) might be a consequence of catecholamine-induced gene regulation, although no known sis-element has been reported in the genes of G_i family. In fact, Eschenhager *et al.* recently observed an isoprenaline-induced increase in $G_{i2}\alpha$ mRNA in rat hearts (21). One interpretation of the changes that occur in CHF is that they are part of compensatory reactions that protect the intracellular environment from βAR over stimulation by reducing signal transducing efficiency through this system. At the same time, however, these changes are somewhat counterproductive because the failing hearts are largely depending on adrenergic support to overcome its impaired pump function.

REFERENCES

1. Clark RB (1986) Advance in Cyclic Nucleotide and Protein Phosphorylation Research 20 (ed. by Greengard P and Robinson GA): 151-209, Raven Press, New York
2. Bristow MR, Ginsburg R, Minobe W, Cubicciotti RS, Sageman WS, Lurie K, Billingham ME, Harrison DC , Stinson EB (1982) N.Engl.J.Med. 307: 205-211
3. Dennis AR, Marsh JD, Quigg RJ, Gordon JB, Colucci WS (1982) Circulation 79: 1028-1034
4. Schwinger RH, Bohm M, Erdmann E (1990) J.Cardiovasc.Pharmacol. 15: 692-697
5. Brodde OE (1991) Pharmacol.Rev. 43: 203
6. Feldman AM, Cates AE, Veazey WB, Hershberger RE, Bristow MR, Baughman KL, Baumgartner WA, Van Dop C (1988) J.Clin.Invest. 82: 189-197
7. Böhm M, Gierschik P, Jakobs KH, Schnabel P, Kemkes B, Erdmann E (1989) Am.J.Cardiol. 64: 812-814
8. Urasawa K, Igarashi Y, Kawaguchi H, Yasuda H (1990) Jpn.Circ.J. 54: 980
9. Harding SE, Jones SM, O'gara P, Vescovo G, Poole-Wilson PA (1990) Am.J.Physiol. 259 (Heart Circ.Physiol. 28): H1009-H1014
10. Murakami T, Katada T, Yasuda H (1987) J.Mol.Cell Pharmacol. 19: 199-208
11. Katada T, Oinuma M, Ui M (1986) J.Biol.Chem. 261: 8182-8191
12. Salomon Y, Londos C (1974) Anal.Biochem. 58: 541-548
13. Schaffner W, Weissman C (1973) Anal.Biochem. 56: 502-514
14. Homburger F (1979) Ann.N.Y.Acad.Sci. 317: 2-17
15. Böhm M, Gierschik P, Jakobs KH, Pieske B, Schnabel P, Ungerer M, Erdmann E (1990) Circulation 82: 1249-1265
16. Fowler MB, Laser JA, Hopkins GL, Minobe W, Bristow MR (1986) Circulation 74: 1290-1302
17. Tse J, Powell JR, Baste CA, Priest RE, Kuo JF (1979) Endocrinol 105: 246-255
18. Chang HY, Klein RM, Kunos G (1982) J.Pharmacol.Exp.Ther. 221: 784-789
19. Maisel AS, Ziegler MG, Carter S, Insel PA, Motulsky HJ (1988) J.Clin.Invest. 82: 2038-2044
20. Vatner DE, Vatner SF, Nejima J, Uemura N, Susanni EE, Hintze TH, Homcy CJ (1989) J.Clin.Invest. 84: 1741-1748
21. Eschenhagen T, Mende U, Nose M, Schmitz W, Scholz H, Warnholtz A, Wüstel JM (1991) Naunyn-Schmiedeberg's Arch.Pharmacol. 343: 609-615

IV: Electrophysiological Abnormalities in Failing Heart

Regulation of Calcium Slow Channels in Myocardial Cells by Cyclic Nucleotides and Phosphorylation

NICHOLAS SPERELAKIS, NORITSUGU TOHSE, HIROSHI MASUDA, and JÁNOS MÉSZÁROS

Department of Physiology and Biophysics, College of Medicine, University of Cincinnati, Cincinnati, OH 45267-0576, USA

KEY WORDS: Cyclic nucleotide regulation of Ca channels; Cyclic AMP-cyclic GMP interactions; Whole-cell voltage clamp; Calcium channel regulation; Phosphorylation of Ca channels; Myocardial calcium channels

INTRODUCTION AND OVERVIEW

Considerable attention during the past few years has been given to phosphorylation of ion channels as a means whereby the activity of the ion channels can be regulated. This article will cover the evidence that cyclic nucleotides regulate the Ca^{2+} influx into the myocardial cells that occurs during each cardiac cycle. This regulation is presumably mediated by phosphorylation(s) of the Ca^{2+} slow channel protein (L-type) and/or of associated regulatory protein(s). In myocardial cells, phosphorylation of the slow Ca^{2+} channels (or of an associated regulatory protein) by cAMP-PK (Fig. 1) presumably (a) increases the number of Ca^{2+} slow channels available for voltage activation during the action potential (AP); (b) increases the probability of their opening, and (c) increases their mean open time. A greater density of available Ca^{2+} channels increases Ca^{2+} influx and inward Ca^{2+} slow current (I_{Ca}) during the AP, and so increases the force of contraction of the heart. Phosphorylation by cGMP-PK depresses the activity of the slow Ca^{2+} channels [1, 2, 3].

Besides the slow Ca^{2+} channel, a fast-type of Ca^{2+} channel (T-type) has been found in cardiac muscle and VSM cells on the basis of kinetics [e.g., 4, 5] These fast Ca^{2+} channels are much more rapidly inactivated than the slow Ca^{2+} channels, are active over a more negative voltage range, and are little affected by cAMP or Ca^{2+} antagonists (Table 1). Their function may be to trigger Ca^{2+} release from the SR (Ca-induced Ca release).

The Ca^{2+} slow channels in young (3-day-old) embryonic chick heart cells exhibited a high incidence of long openings, and the incidence was diminished by 17 days [6, 7]. Cyclic GMP inhibited these long openings [6].

In addition, a new type of Ca^{2+} channel was discovered in 18-day-old fetal rat ventricular cells [8]. A residual I_{Ca} remaining in the presence of a high concentration (3 μM) of nifedipine (nifedipine-resistant I_{Ca}) was not blocked by diltiazem, tetramethrine (T-type channel blocker), or ω-conotoxin (N-type channel blocker), and had a half-inactivation potential about 20 mV more negative than the nifedipine-sensitive (L-type channel) I_{Ca}.

TABLE 1. Summary of Major Differences Between the Slow (L-Type) and Fast (T-Type) Ca^{2+} Channels

Properties	Ca^{2+} Channels: Slow (L-Type)	Fast (T-Type)
Duration of current	Long-lasting (sustained)	Transient
Inactivation kinetics	Slower	Faster
Activation kinetics	Slower	Faster
Threshold	High (ca. -30 mV)	Low (ca. -50 mV)
Half-inactivation potential	ca. -20 mV	ca. -50 mV
Single-channel conductance	High (18-26 pS)	Low (8-10 pS)
Regulated by cAMP and cGMP	Yes	No
Regulated by phosphorylation	Yes	No
Blocked by Ca^{2+} antagonist drugs	Yes	No (slight)
Opened by Ca^{2+} agonist drugs	Yes	No
Permeation by Me^{2+}	Ba > Ca	Ba ≃ Ca
Inactivation by $[Ca]_i$	Yes	Slight (?)
Recordings in isolated patches	Runs down	Rel. stable

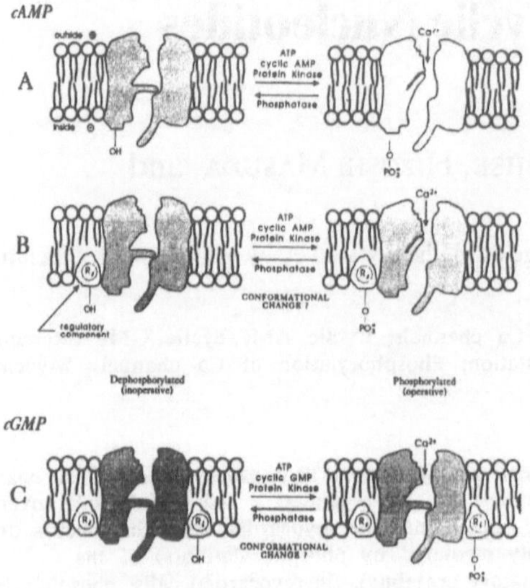

Fig. 1. Schematic model for a Ca^{2+} slow channel in myocardial cell membrane in two hypothetical forms: dephosphorylated (or electrically silent) form (left diagrams) and phosphorylated form (right diagram). The two gates associated with the channel are an activation gate and an inactivation gate. The phosphorylation hypothesis states that a protein constituent of the slow channel itself (A) or a regulatory protein associated with the slow channel (B) must be phosphorylated in order for the channel to be in a state available for voltage activation. Phosphorylation of a serine or threonine residue occurs by a cAMP-dependent protein kinase (PK-A) in the presence of ATP. Phosphorylation may produce a conformational change that effectively allows the channel gates to operate. The slow channel (or an associated regulatory protein) may also be phosphorylated by a cGMP-PK (C), thus mediating the inhibitory effects of cGMP on the slow Ca^{2+} channel. (Modified from Sperelakis & Schneider, 1976.)

CYCLIC AMP STIMULATION OF SLOW Ca^{2+} CHANNELS

The voltage- and time-dependent Ca^{2+} slow channels in the myocardial cell membrane are the major pathway by which Ca^{2+} ions enter the cell during excitation for initiation and regulation of the force of contraction of cardiac muscle. The slow channels have some special properties, including functional dependence on metabolic energy, selective blockade by acidosis, and regulation by the intracellular cyclic nucleotide levels. Because of these special properties of the slow channels, Ca^{2+} influx into the myocardial cell can be controlled by extrinsic factors (such as autonomic nerve stimulation or circulating hormones) and by intrinsic factors (such as cellular pH or ATP level).

Cyclic AMP (cAMP) modulates the functioning of the Ca^{2+} slow channels [9, 10, 11, 12, 13]. Histamine and β-adrenergic agonists, after binding to their specific receptors, lead to rapid stimulation of adenylate cyclase with resultant elevation of cAMP levels. Methylxanthines enter the myocardial cells and inhibit the phosphodiesterase, thus causing an elevation of cAMP. These positive inotropic agents also concomitantly induce Ca^{2+}-dependent slow APs by increasing I_{Ca}.

Additional evidence for the regulatory role of cAMP has been obtained. (a) The GTP analogue, GPP(NH)P, which directly activates adenylate cyclase, induced Ca^{2+}-dependent slow APs in heart cells [14]. (b) Forskolin, another highly potent activator of adenylate cyclase activity, exerted a strong positive inotropic effect and induced and potentiated slow APs [15, 16]. (c) cAMP iontophoretically microinjected into Purkinje fibers and ventricular muscle cells induced slow APs in the injected cells within seconds [17]. (d) Pressure injection of cAMP, GPP(NH)P, and cholera toxin (which irreversibly activates adenylate cyclase) rapidly induced and potentiated slow APs [18] (Fig. 2). (e) Liposome injection of cAMP into heart cells also induced slow APs [1].

Other results also support a role for cAMP in stimulating the slow inward Ca^{2+} current in myocardial cells (Table 2). (a) Injection of cAMP enhanced I_{Ca} in isolated single cardiac cells [19]. (b) A photochemical activation method for suddenly increasing the intracellular cAMP level enhanced I_{Ca} in bullfrog atrial cells [20]. (c) Noise analysis and patch clamp analysis suggest that cAMP increases the number of functional slow channels available in the sarcolemma and/or the probability of opening of a given channel [21, 22, 23]. Both actions would increase the number of slow channels open at any instant of time. Isoproterenol increased the mean open time of single Ca^{2+} channels and decreased the intervals between bursts; the conductance of the single channel was not increased [24]. Therefore, the increase in the slow Ca^{2+} current produced by isoproterenol could be produced by the observed increase in mean open time of each channel, as well as by an increase in the number of available channels.

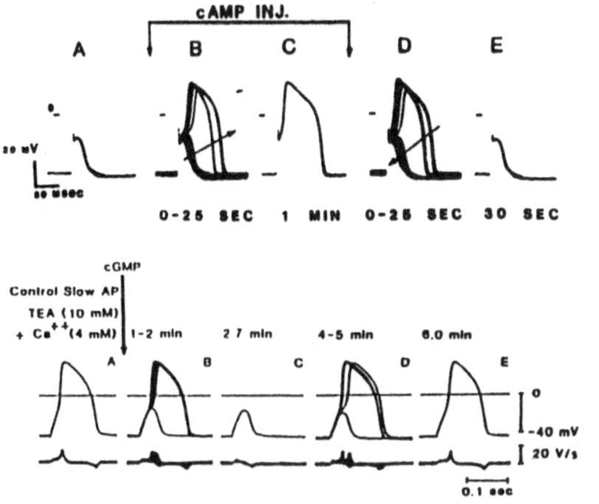

Fig. 2. Upper Row: Induction of Ca^{2+}-dependent slow action potentials (APs) in guinea-pig papillary muscle by intracellular pressure injection of cyclic AMP. The muscle was depolarized in 22 mM $[K]_o$ to voltage inactivate fast Na^+ channels. A: Small graded response (stimulation rate 30/min). B: Superimposed records showing the gradual appearance of slow APs upon cAMP injection over a 25-s period. C: Presence of stable slow APs after injection for 1 min. D: Gradual depression of slow APs over a period of 25 s after stopping injection. E: Complete decay of slow APs 30 s after cessation of cAMP injection. All records are from one impaled cell. Data taken from Li & Sperelakis, 1983. Lower Row: Transient abolition of Ca^{2+}-dependent slow APs by pressure injection of cGMP. A: Control slow AP induced by 10 mM TEA plus 4.0 mM $[Ca]_o$ in 25 mM K^+ to inactivate fast Na^+ channels. B-C: 1-2 min following the onset of cGMP injection (10 s duration), the slow APs were depressed and then abolished. D-E: At 4-6 min, the slow APs recovered spontaneously to control levels. All records from the same cell. (Taken from Wahler & Sperelakis, 1985.)

PHOSPHORYLATION HYPOTHESIS

Because of the relationship between cAMP and the number of available slow Ca^{2+} channels, and because of the dependence of the functioning of these channels on metabolic energy, it was postulated that the slow channel protein must be phosphorylated in order for it to become available for voltage activation [9, 10, 11, 22, 25]. Elevation of cAMP by a positive inotropic agent activates a cAMP-dependent protein kinase (cA-PK), which phosphorylates a variety of proteins in the presence of ATP. One protein that is phosphorylated might be the slow channel protein itself or a contiguous regulatory type of protein (Fig. 1).

Phosphorylation could make the slow channel available for activation by a conformational change that either allowed the activation gate to be opened upon depolarization. In this model, the phosphorylated form of the slow channel is the active (operational) form, and the dephosphorylated form is the inactive (inoperative) form. The dephosphorylated channels are electrically silent. Thus, phosphorylation increases the probability of channel opening with depolarization. An equilibrium would exist between the phosphorylated and dephosphorylated forms of the slow channels for a given set of conditions. Agents that elevate cAMP increase the fraction of the channels that are in the phosphorylated form, and hence readily available for voltage activation.

To test whether the regulatory effect of cAMP is exerted by means of the cA-PK and phosphorylation, intracellular injection of the catalytic subunit of the cA-PK was done. Such injections induced and enhanced the slow APs [26] and potentiated I_{Ca} [22, 27, 28]. Another test of the phosphorylation hypothesis was done by liposome injection of an inhibitor (protein) of the cA-PK into heart cells, and showing that it inhibited the spontaneous slow APs [26]. This protein kinase inhibitor also was shown to inhibit I_{Ca} of cardiac cells [29].

Based on the rapid decay of the response to injected cAMP (Fig. 2, top), the mean life span of a phosphorylated channel is likely to be only a few seconds at most, and it is possible that the channels are phosphorylated and dephosphorylated with every cardiac cycle [18]. Hence, agents which affect or regulate the phosphatase would affect the life span of the phosphorylated channel. Thus, channel stimulation can be produced either by increasing the rate of phosphorylation (by cA-PK) or by decreasing the rate of dephosphorylation (inhibition of the phosphatase) [30]. For example, the Ca^{2+}-dependent phosphatase, calcineurin, inhibits slow APs in 3-day-old embryonic chick hearts [31]. Phosphatases have been shown to decrease the Ca^{2+} current in neurons [32] and ventricular myocardial cells [33]. The catalytic subunit of the protein phosphatases 1 and 2A inhibited the Ca^{2+} channel, and okadaic acid, a protein phosphatase inhibitor, enhanced the amplitude of the I_{Ca} pre-stimulated by β-adrenergic agents [34].

Consistent with the phosphorylation hypothesis, it has been found that the slow Ca^{2+} channel activity disappears within 90 sec in isolated membrane inside-out patches [35], and was restored by applying catalytic subunit of cA-PK and Mg-ATP [36]. This is consistent with the washing away of regulatory components of the slow channels or of the enzymes necessary to phosphorylate the channel. Even in whole-cell voltage clamp, there is a progressive run-down of the slow Ca^{2+} current, which is slowed or partially reversed by conditions that enhance cA-PK phosphorylation [32].

Some agents that affect the force of contraction of the heart may do so without increasing the level of cyclic AMP. For example, fluoride ion (<1 mM) is a potent positive inotropic agent and potentiates the Ca^{2+}-dependent slow APs and Ca^{2+} influx (I_{si}), but yet does not elevate cAMP [30]. Fluoride may act by inhibiting the phosphatase which dephosphorylates the slow channel protein (or associated regulatory protein). This would prolong the life span of the phosphorylated channel, resulting in potentiation of I_{si} and contraction. In contrast, it is possible that some negative inotropic drugs depress the rate of phosphorylation. It might be difficult to distinguish between a drug that depressed phosphorylation of the slow Ca^{2+} channel and one that physically blocked the channel.

cAMP also has effects on other types of ion channels. For example, the following channels of heart are stimulated by cAMP: (a) delayed rectifier K^+ channel [28, 37], (b) hyperpolarization-activated Na-K I_f (I_h) channel [38], and (c) catecholamine-activated Cl^- channel [39]. The fast Na^+ channel was reported to be inhibited by cAMP [40]. The delayed rectifier K^+ current was also stimulated by cGMP, presumably by PDE inhibition [41], and the catecholamine-activated Cl^- current was also stimulated by cGMP [42].

CYCLIC GMP INHIBITION OF SLOW Ca^{2+} CURRENT

The physiological role of cyclic GMP on cardiac function is still controversial. 8-Br-cGMP (10^{-4} M) shortened the action potential duration in rat atria accompanied by a negative inotropic effect, and it was suggested that cyclic GMP might decrease the Ca^{2+} conductance [43]. ACh and 8-Br-cGMP reduced upstroke velocity and duration of the Ca-dependent slow action potential in guinea-pig atria [44]. The abbreviation of action potential duration was also observed following pressure injection of cGMP into isolated guinea-pig cardiomyocytes [28].

It has been proposed that cGMP plays an antagonistic role to that of cAMP, namely that there was a "Yin-Yang" relationship between cAMP and cGMP [45]. Superfusion of isolated ventricular muscle with 8-Br-cGMP abolished the Ca^{2+}-dependent slow APs and accompanying contractions within 7-20 min [2]. A similar inhibition by cGMP was shown for the slow APs of atrial muscle and Purkinje fibers [44, 46]. Intracellular pressure injection of cGMP into ventricular cells transiently depressed or abolished slow APs much more quickly (e.g., 1-2 min) [2] (Fig. 2, bottom). Injection of cGMP into heart cells by the liposome method also abolished the slow APs [1]. It was also demonstrated that 8-Br-cGMP inhibits the basal I_{Ca} (unstimulated by cAMP) in voltage-clamped ventricular myocytes [3] (Fig. 3).

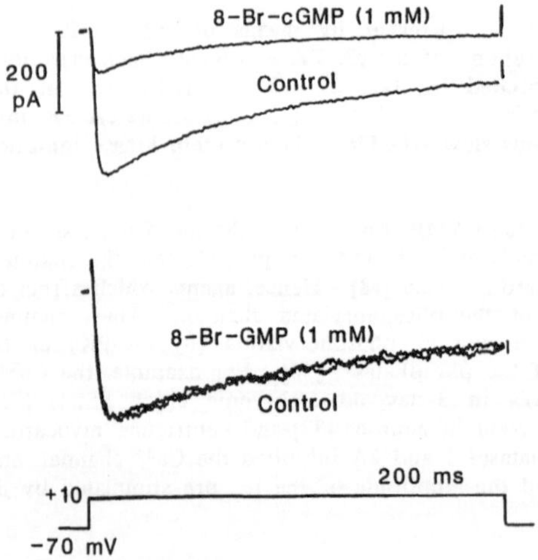

Fig. 3. Effect of 8-Br-cGMP on the slow inward Ca^{2+} current in two cultured embryonic chick ventricular myocytes. Upper Traces: Currents elicited by depolarizing pulses from -70 mV to +10 mV in the control bath solution and following 10 min superfusion with a solution containing 1 mM 8-Br-cGMP. Note the large inhibition of $I_{Ca(s)}$. Lower Traces: Currents elicited by depolarizing pulses in the control bath solution and following 10 min superfusion with a solution containing 1 mM 8-Br-GMP, the non-cyclic analog of 8-Br-cGMP. The bath solution (20-22° C) included (in mM): 10 $BaCl_2$ and 135 TEA-Cl; the pipette solution included: 150 Cs-glutamate, 5 MgATP, 1 EGTA. (Reproduced from Wahler et al., 1990.)

We recently demonstrated cGMP inhibition of Ca^{2+} slow channel activity at the single-channel level [47]. Cyclic GMP did not change unit amplitude and slope conductance of the Ca^{2+} channel, but prolonged the closed times and shortened the open times. Because 8-Br-cGMP is a potent activator of G-kinase and does not stimulate cAMP hydrolysis, cGMP-induced inhibition of the basal activity of the Ca^{2+} channels (not pre-stimulated by cAMP) may be mediated by G-kinase. Similar observations were made by Tohse et al. [48] on isolated rabbit ventricular myocytes.

In 3-day-old embryonic chick heart cells, the Ca^{2+} slow channels often exhibited long-lasting openings (e.g., for 300 ms) under normal conditions, especially at the more positive command potentials [6]. That is, the Ca^{2+} slow channels naturally possessed mode 2 behavior, in the absence of any added Ca^{2+} channel agonist such as the dihydropyridine, Bay-K-8644. Addition of Bay-K-8644 did not further prolong the open times, but appeared to recruit silent Ca^{2+} channels [49]. Long-lasting openings were much less frequently observed in 17-day-old embryonic cells [47]. Addition of 8-Br-cGMP to the bath of 3-day cells exhibiting long openings completely inhibited Ca^{2+} slow channel activity (Fig. 4).

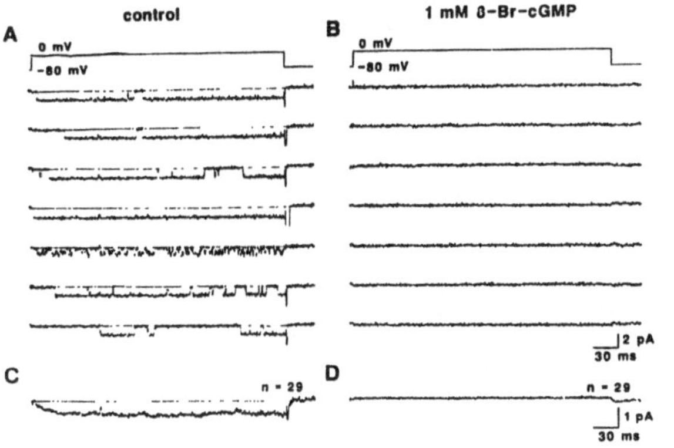

Fig. 4. Current recordings from a cell-attached patch showing effect of 8-Br-cGMP on the Ca^{2+} slow channel activity in a single myocardial cell isolated from a 3-day-old embryonic chick heart. Single-channel currents were evoked by depolarizing voltage pulses to 0 mV from a holding potential of -80 mV, at a duration of 300 msec and repetition rate of 0.5 Hz. A and B: Examples of original current recordings from the same patch, before (A) and after (B) superfusion with 1.0 mM 8-Br-cGMP. C and D: Ensemble-averaged currents calculated from the current recordings (n = 29). The current tracings were low-pass filtered at 1 kHz and corrected for leakage and capacitive currents. (Data taken from Tohse & Sperelakis, 1991a.)

In preliminary whole-cell voltage clamp experiments on single ventricular cardiomyocytes from 17-day embryonic chicks, it was demonstrated that the stimulation of $I_{Ca(s)}$ produced by 1.0 mM 8-Br-cAMP added to the bath could be completely reversed by the addition of 1.0 mM 8-Br-cGMP (Fig. 5A) (Meszaros et al., unpublished). The I/V curves showed that cGMP did not alter the voltage for maximum current (+10 mV) or the reversal potential (V_{rev}; +80 mV). Figure 5B gives a graphic plot of the concentration/response curve for 8-Br-cAMP in presence of four different concentrations of 8-Br-cGMP. Note that there was almost no stimulation or inhibition of basal I_{Ca} when the ratio of the two cyclic nucleotides was 1.0. In similar experiments on early neonatal (2-day) rat ventricular myocytes, similar results were obtained, namely 8-Br-cGMP antagonized the stimulation of $I_{Ca(s)}$ by 8-Br-cAMP (Fig. 6) (Masuda et al., unpublished). Therefore, it appears that the ratio of cAMP/cGMP determines the degree of stimulation of $I_{Ca(s)}$, and that even the basal I_{Ca} is inhibited by cGMP, at least in the case of chick.

Therefore, cGMP regulates the functioning of the myocardial Ca^{2+} slow channels in a manner that is antagonistic to that of cAMP (Fig. 7). It is possible that the Ca^{2+} slow channel protein has a second site that can be phosphorylated by cG-PK and which, when phosphorylated, inhibits the slow channel. Another possiblity is that there is a second type of regulatory protein that is inhibitory when phosphorylated (Fig. 1).

In further preliminary studies, G-kinase was added to the patch pipette for diffusion into the cell during whole-cell voltage clamp. It was found that basal I_{Ca} was inhibited markedly and rapidly by the G-kinase, maximum inhibition being reached in about 1.0 min (Figs. 8B and 9). Data from 17-day chick cardiomyocytes are illustrated in Figure 8 (Meszaros et al., unpublished). The control with no G-kinase to demonstrate the lack of significant I_{Ca} rundown in 2 min. is shown in Fig. 8A, and the effect of G-kinase (25 nM in pipette) is shown in Fig. 8B. Note that inhibition of basal I_{Ca} began within about 20 sec. after breaking into the cell. Similar effects of G-kinase infusion were observed in early neonatal rat ventricular myocytes, as illustrated in Figure 9 (Masuda et al., unpublished). As can be seen, there was a very rapid and prominent inhibition of the basal I_{Ca} by G-kinase (25 nM) following breaking into the cell. Addition of H-7 (a blocker of protein kinases including G-kinase) to the bath caused a rapid restoration of I_{Ca} to about the original basal level, and this action was reversed upon washout (Fig. 9). Addition of 1 mM 8-Br-cAMP to the bath was capable of producing a small stimulation of I_{Ca} in the continued presence of G-kinase (Fig. 9). Therefore, these findings indicate that the inhibitory effects of cGMP on I_{Ca} are mediated by activation of PK-G (G-kinase) and resultant phosphorylation, and that the *basal* I_{Ca} is inhibited.

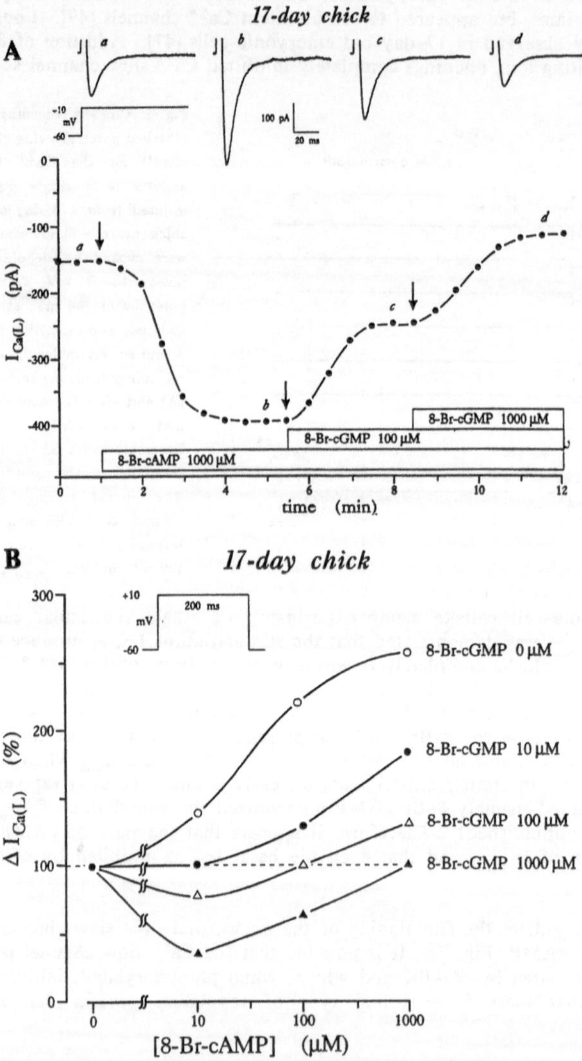

Fig. 5. A: Antagonism of the stimulating effect of 8-Br-cAMP on $I_{Ca(s)}$ by 8-Br-cGMP in a single 17-day-old embryonic chick heart cell. Upper tracings show the original current recordings of $I_{Ca(L)}$ taken at the time-points shown by the corresponding letters in the lower graph. $I_{Ca(L)}$ was elicited by 200 ms depolarizing pulses to +10 mV from a holding potential of -60 mV. Temperature was 35 °C; $[Ca]_o$ was 2.5 mM. B: Effect of the different concentration ratios of 8-Br-cAMP/8-Br-cGMP on $I_{Ca(L)}$ in 4 different cells. (Meszaros et al., unpublished)

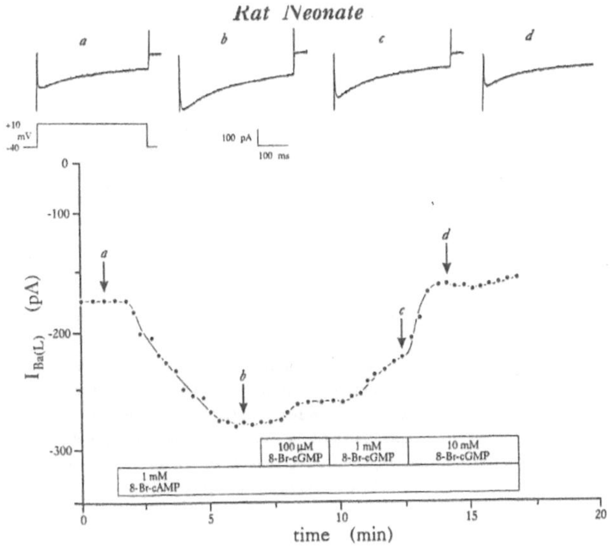

Fig. 6. Antagonism of the stimulating effect of 8-Br-cAMP in $I_{Ca(s)}$ by 8-Br-cGMP in a single young neonatal rat ventricular myocyte. Upper tracings show four original current recordings of I_{Ca} corresponding to the four time-points labelled in the lower graph. $I_{Ca(s)}$ was elucited by 300 ms depolarizing pulses to +10 mV from a holding potential of -40 mV. Ba $^{2+}$ (2.0 mM) was used as the charge carrier. At room temperature of 25° C (Masuda et al., unpublished).

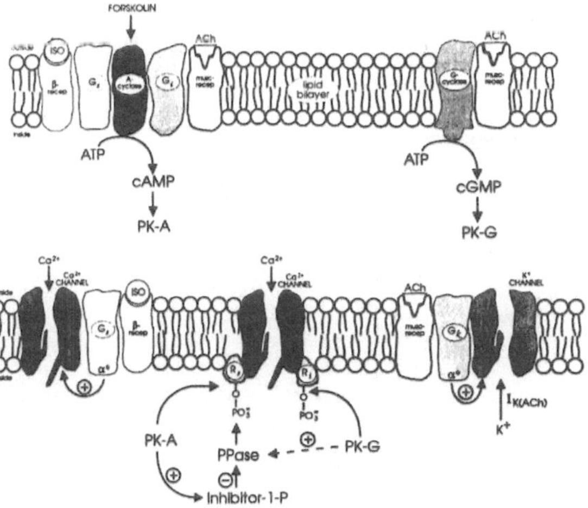

Fig. 7. Diagrammatic summary of the regulation of the Ca^{2+} slow channels in the myocardial cell membrane and the mechanisms of action of some inotropic agents. The B-adrenergic agonists and histamine H_2 agonists act via their receptors on a GTP-binding protein (G_s) to stimulate adenylate cyclase and cAMP production. The voltage-dependent myocardial slow Ca^{2+} channels are stimulated by cAMP, presumably because the channel (or an associated regulatory protein) must be phosphorylated in order for it to be in a form that is available for voltage activation. cGMP-dependent phosphorylation also regulates the slow channel in a manner antagonistic to cAMP, namely producing inhibition. Thus, the muscarinic receptor activated by ACh can produce inhibition of Ca^{2+} influx by at least the four mechanisms depicted: (a) reversal of adenylate cyclase stimulation produced by B-agonists or H_2 agonists; (b) stimulation of guanylate cyclase and production of cGMP; (c) activation of a K^+ channel ($I_{K(ACh)}$) that produces an outward K^+ current which depresses excitability and terminates the AP earlier, and thereby voltage deactivates the Ca^{2+} slow channels earlier; and (d) stimulation of a phosphatase (PPase) by cGMP and PK-G. Mechanism (c) may be absent in ventricular myocardial cells.

A single protein has been found to be specifically phosphorylated by cG-PK in guinea pig sarcolemmal preparations [50]. In the presence of the purified kinase plus 10^{-5} M cGMP or 8-Br-cGMP, a protein of approximately 47 kD was phosphorylated. Thus, this substrate, the identity of which is unknown, may be a possible mediator of cGMP-mediated control of cardiac function.

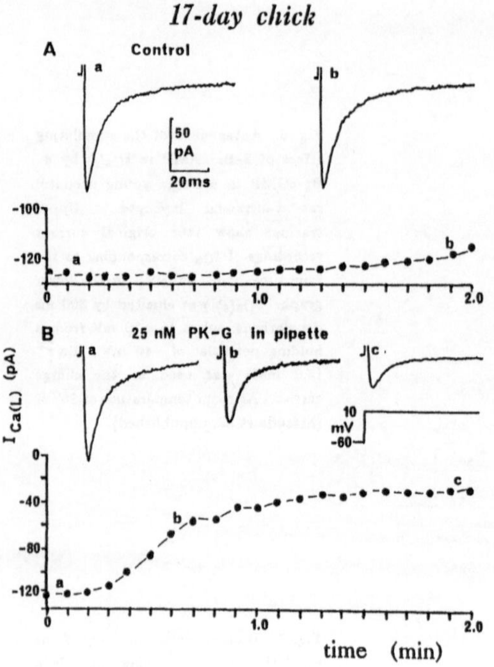

Fig. 8. Inhibition of basal I_{Ca} by G-kinase (25 nM) present in the patch pipette in a 17-day embryonic chick cardiomyocyte for diffusion into the cell during whole-cell voltage clamp. A: Control experiment in a cell with no G-kinase present in the pipette. There was very little rundown of the basal I_{Ca} over the 2-min. period. The two current tracings illustrated correspond to the time-points labelled a and b. B: Experiment in a cell with G-kinase in the pipette. Inhibition of basal I_{Ca} began within 30 sec after breaking into the cell, and reached maximum at about 60 sec. The three current tracings illustrated correspond to the time-points labelled a, b, and c in the graph. Experiments were done at 35° C, and $[Ca]_o$ was 2.5 mM. (Meszaros et al., unpublished.)

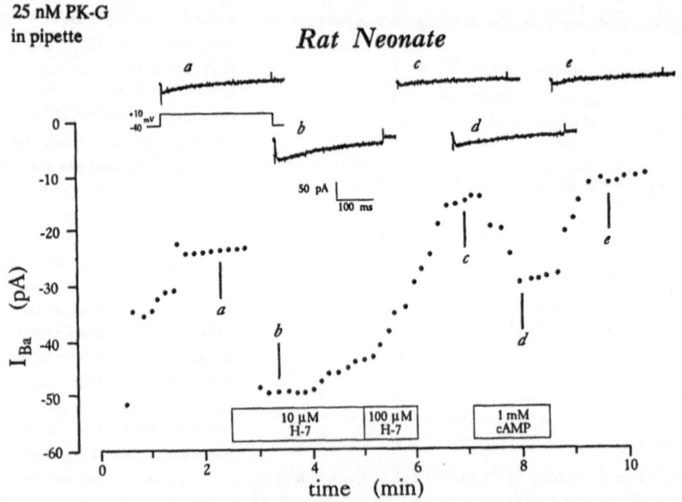

Fig. 9. Inhibition of basal I_{Ca} by G-kinase (25 nM) present in the patch pipette in a ventricular myocyte from an early (2-day) neonatal rat heart. Very shortly after breaking into the cell, there was a marked decrease in I_{Ca}. This inhibition by G-kinase was reversed by application of the kinase inhibitor H-7 to the bath, and this action could be reversed by washout of H-7. 8-Br-cAMP (1 mM) added to the bath produced a small stimulation of I_{Ca} (in the continued presence of G-kinase), and this action of the cyclic nucleotide was reversed by washout. The five current tracings illustrated correspond to the five time-points labelled a, b, c, d, and e in the graph. Experiments were done at room temperature (ca. 25° C), with 2.0 mM Ba^{2+} as the charge carrier. (Masuda et al., unpublished.)

Another mechanism proposed for cGMP inhibition is based on cGMP depression of the cAMP level. Intracellular application of cGMP inhibited I_{Ca} of frog ventricular myocytes, but only after the cAMP levels had been increased; i.e., there was no effect of cGMP on the basal I_{Ca} [51, 52, 53]. It was concluded that cGMP inhibited I_{Ca} by stimulating a phosphodiesterase, resulting in increased degradation of cAMP. However, in a later study on guinea pig and rat cardiomyocytes, this same group reported a direct inhibition of I_{Ca} by cGMP and a direct cG-PK [53, 54]. In addition, 8-Br-cAMP inhibition of slow APs in mammalian cardiac muscle occurs without a decrease in cAMP levels [55]. Thus, it appears that in mammalian ventricular muscle, cGMP inhibits I_{Ca} directly through a cGMP-mediated phosphorylation (8-Br-cGMP is a potent activator of cG-PK) of some protein involved in the functioning of the slow Ca^{2+} channels (Fig. 1).

It has been proposed that muscarinic agonists also act to inhibit the Ca^{2+} slow channel by cG-PK stimulation of a phosphatase (Type I) that dephosphorylates the channel [56, 57] (Fig. 7). This would have the effect of lowering the fraction of channels in the phosphorylated form, and therefore the Ca^{2+} influx. In this mechanism, the rate of phosphorylation is unaffected, but the rate of dephosphorylation is increased. Muscarinic agonists are known to elevate cGMP [58]. However, it was reported that ACh was ineffective in reducing the basal I_{Ca} [59], and that cGMP actually potentiated the stimulating effect of ISO on I_{Ca}, perhaps mediated by PDE inhibition [41]. Elevation of intracellular cGMP by photo-activation of a derivative had no effect on the L-type Ca^{2+} current (I_{Ca}) in isolated rat ventricular cells [20].

The parasympathetic neurotransmitter acetylcholine (ACh) exerts a negative inotropic effect on ventricular myocardium pre-stimulated by β-adrenergic agonists. Activation of the muscarinic receptor by ACh exerts an inhibitory effect on adenylate cyclase and cAMP levels, via the G_i (inhibitory) coupling protein, to reverse the stimulation of adenylate cyclase produced by means of the G_s coupling protein due to, for example, activation of the β-adrenoceptor (Fig. 5). Thus, ACh may depress Ca^{2+} influx and contraction by reversing cAMP elevation produced by various agonists. For example, in cultured chick ventricular cells, ACh depressed I_{Ca} that had been stimulated by isoproterenol [14]. ACh also reverses the electrophysiological effects of direct adenylate cyclase stimulation by forskolin [16]. Additionally, in ventricular cells, ACh may inhibit the slow Ca^{2+} channels due, in part, to elevation of cGMP levels [60]. Adenosine exerts effects similar to those of ACh.

CALMODULIN-PROTEIN KINASE AND PROTEIN KINASE C

Inhibitors of calmodulin (trifluoperazine and calmidazolium) inhibit the slow APs of heart cells [61, 62, 63]. Subsequent injection of calmodulin reverses the inhibition produced by calmidazolium. It appears that maximal activation of the slow channels requires two separate phosphorylation steps (calmodulin-dependent and cAMP-dependent). These may be on the same protein or on two separate proteins.

High concentration of the α-adrenergic agonist, phenylephrine, causes a positive inotropic effect in cardiac muscle [64]. The α-adrenoceptor agonists stimulate the phosphatidyl inositol cycle and generation of inositol trisphosphate (IP_3) and diacyl glycerol (DAG). IP_3 acts as a second messenger to release stored Ca^{2+} from the sarcoplasmic reticulum (SR). DAG and Ca^{2+} activate PK-C, which phosphorylates a number of proteins. It is presently controversial whether PK-C is involved in regulation of the myocardial slow Ca^{2+} channels. One group reported that phorbol ester and ang-II stimulated I_{Ca} [65], whereas another group did not observe such stimulation [66]. There have been variable findings with respect to the effect of activation of α-adrenoceptor agonists on elevation of cAMP.

SUMMARY AND CONCLUSIONS

The slow Ca^{2+} channels of the heart are stimulated by cAMP. Elevation of cAMP produces a very rapid increase in number of slow channels available for voltage activation during excitation. The probability of a slow channel opening and the mean open time of the channel are increased. Therefore, any agent that increases the cAMP level of the myocardial cell will tend to potentiate I_{si}, Ca^{2+} influx, and contraction.

The myocardial slow Ca^{2+} channels are also regulated by cGMP, in a manner that is opposite to that of cAMP. The effect of cGMP may be mediated by means of phosphorylation of a protein, as for example, a regulatory protein (inhibitory-type) associated with the slow channel. In addition, cGMP may act by stimulating a phosphatase that dephosphorylates the Ca^{2+} channel.

Preliminary data suggest that calmodulin also may play a role in regulation of the myocardial slow Ca^{2+} channels, possibly mediated by the Ca^{2+}-calmodulin-protein kinase and phosphorylation of some regulatory-type of protein.

Thus, it appears that the slow Ca^{2+} channel is a complex structure, including perhaps several associated regulatory proteins, which can be regulated by a number of extrinsic and intrinsic factors (Fig. 7).

SUMMARY

The effects of cAMP and cGMP on the slow Ca^{2+} channels in cardiac muscle, VSM, and skeletal muscle fibers are summarized in Table 2. As shown, in cardiac muscle, cAMP stimulates and cGMP inhibits. In VSM, both cAMP and cGMP inhibit. In skeletal muscle, both cAMP and cGMP stimulate.

TABLE 2. Summary of Effect of Cyclic Nucleotides on Ca^{2+} Slow Channels in Cardiac Muscle, Vascular Smooth Muscle, and Skeletal Muscle

	Cardiac Muscle	Vascular Smooth Muscle Cells	Skeletal Muscle†
cAMP	Stimulation	Inhibition	Stimulation
cGMP	Inhibition	Inhibition	Stimulation

†From bullfrog (Kokate et al., unpublished)

ACKNOWLEDGEMENTS

These research projects were supported by N.I.H. Grants HL-31942 and HL-22619. We would like to thank Rhonda S. Hentz for typing this manuscript, and Glenn Doerman for making some figures, and Anthony Sperelakis for photography.

REFERENCES

1. Bkaily G, Sperelakis N (1985) Injection of cyclic GMP into her cells blocks the slow action potentials. Am J Physiol (Heart Circ Physiol) 248: H745-H749.
2. Wahler GM, Sperelakis N (1985) Intracellular injection of cyclic GMP depresses cardiac slow action potentials. J Cyclic Nucleo Prot Phos Res 10: 83-95.
3. Wahler GM, Rusch NJ, Sperelakis N (1990) 8-bromo-cyclic GMP inhibits the calcium channel current in embryonic chick ventricular myocytes. Can J Physiol Pharm 68: 531-534.
4. Bean B (1985) Two kinds of calcium channels in canine atrial cells. Differences in kinetics, selectivity, and pharmacology. J Gen Physiol 86: 1-30.
5. Nilius B, Hess P, Lansman JB, Tsien RW (1985) A novel type of cardiac calcium channel in ventricular cells. Nature 316: 443-446.
6. Tohse N, Sperelakis N (1990) Long-lasting openings of single slow (L-type) Ca^{2+} channels in chick embryonic heart cells. Am J Physiol 259: H639-H642.
7. Tohse N, Meszaros J, Sperelakis N (1992) Developmental changes in long-opening behavior of L-type Ca^{2+} (slow) channels in embryonic chick heart cells. Circ Res (in press).
8. Tohse N, Masuda H, Sperelakis N (1992) Novel isoform of Ca^{2+} channel in rat fetal cardiomyocytes. J Physiol (Lond) (in press).
9. Shigenobu K, Sperelakis N (1972) Ca^{2+} current channels induced by catecholamines in chick embryonic hearts whose fast Na^{+} channels are blocked by tetrodotoxin or elevated K^{+}. Circ Res 31: 932-952.
10. Tsien RW, Giles W, Greengard P (1972) Cyclic AMP mediates the action of adrenaline on the action potential plateau of cardiac Purkinje fibers. Nature 240: 181-183.
11. Sperelakis N, Schneider JA (1976) A metabolic control mechanism for calcium ion influx that may protect the ventricular myocardial cell. Am J Cardiol 37: 1079-1085.

12. Schneider JA, Shigenobu K, Sperelakis N (1976) Valinomycin inhibition of the inward slow current of cardiac muscle. In: Recent Advances in Studies on Cardiac Structure and Metabolism, 33-52.
13. Reuter H, Scholz H (1977) The regulation of the calcium conductance of cardiac muscle by adrenaline. J Physiol (Lond) 264: 49-62.
14. Josephson I, Sperelakis N (1978) 5'-Guanylimidodiphosphate stimulation of slow Ca^{2+} current in myocardial cells. J Mol Cell Cardiol 10: 1157-1166.
15. Spah F (1984) Forskolin, a new positive inotropic agent, and its influence on myocardial electrogenic cation movements. J Cardiovasc Pharm 6: 99-106.
16. Wahler GM, Sperelakis N (1986) Cholinergic attenuation of the electrophysiological effects of forskolin. J Cyclic Nucleo Prot Phosph Res 11: 1-10.
17. Vogel S, Sperelakis N (1981) Induction of slow action potentials microiontophoresis of cyclic AMP into heart cells. J Mol Cell Cardiol 13: 51-64.
18. Li T, Sperelakis N (1983) Stimulation of slow action potentials in guinea pig papillary muscle cells by intracellular injection of cAMP, Gpp(NH)p, and cholera toxin. Circ Res 52: 111-117.
19. Irisawa H, Kokobun S (1983) Modulation by intracellular ATP and cyclic AMP of the slow inward current in isolated single ventricular cells of the guinea-pig. J Physiol 338: 321-327.
20. Nargeot J, Nerbonne JM, Engels J, Lester HA (1983) Time course of the increase in the myocardial slow inward current after a photochemically generated concentration jump of intracellular cAMP. Proc Natl Acad Sci 80: 2395-2399.
21. Cachelin AB, dePeyer JE, Kokubun S, Reuter H (1983) Ca^{2+} channel modulation by 8-bromo-cyclic AMP in culture heart cells. Nature 304: 462-464.
22. Trautwein W, Hoffman F (1983) Activation of calcium current by injection of cAMP and catalytic subunit of cAMP-dependent protein kinase. Proc Internat Union Physiol Sci 15: 75-83.
23. Bean BP, Nowycky MC, Tsien RW (1984) Beta-adrenergic modulation of calcium channels in frog ventricular heart cells. Nature 307: 371-375.
24. Reuter H, Stevens C-F, Tsien RW, Yellen G (1982) Properties of single calcium channels in cardiac cell culture. Nature 297: 501-504.
25. Sperelakis N (1988) Regulation of calcium slow channels of cardiac muscle by cyclic nucleotides and phosphorylation. J Mol Cell Cardiol 20: 75-105.
26. Bkaily G, Sperelakis N (1984) Injection of protein kinase inhibitor into cultured heart cells blocks calcium slow channels. Am J Physiol 246: H630-H634.
27. Osterrieder W, Brum G, Hescheler J, Trautwein W, Flockerzi V, Hofmann F (1982) Injection of subunits of cyclic AMP-dependent protein kinase into cardiac myocytes modulates Ca^{2+} current. Nature 298: 576-578.
28. Trautwein W, Taniguchi J, Noma A (1982) The effect of intracellular cyclic nucleotides and calcium on the action potential and acetylcholine response of isolated cardiac cells. Pflugers Arch 392: 307-314.
29. Kameyama M, Hofmann F, Trautwein W (1986) On the mechanism of β-adrenergic regulation of the Ca^{2+} channel in the guinea-pig heart. Pflugers Arch 405: 285-293.
30. Vogel S, Sperelakis N, Josephson J, Brooker G (1977) Fluoride stimulation of slow Ca^{2+} current in cardiac muscle. J Mol Cell Cardiol 9: 461-475.
31. Tripathi O, Sperelakis N (1991) Effects of 8-Bromo cyclic GMP on slow channel mediated action potentials of 3-days-old embryonic chick ventricle. J Dev Physiol 16: 309-316.
32. Chad JE, Eckert RJ (1986) An ezymatic mechanism for calcium current inactivation in dialysed Helix neurones. J Physiol 378: 31-51.
33. Hescheler J, Kameyama M, Trautwein W, Mieskes G, Soling HD (1987) Regulation of the cardiac calcium channel by protein phosphatases. Eur J Biochem 165: 261-266.
34. Hescheler J, Mieskes G, Ruegg JC, Takai A, Trautwein W (1988) Effects of a protein phosphatase inhibitor, okadaic acid, on membrane currents of isolated guinea-pig cardiac myocytes. Pflugers Arch 412: 248-252.
35. Reuter H (1983) Calcium channel modulation by neurotransmitters, enzymes, and drugs. Nature 301: 569-574.
36. Armstrong D, Eckert R (1987) Voltage-activated calcium channels that must be phosphorylated to respond to membrane depolarization. Proc Natl Acad Sci USA, 84: 2518-2522.
37. Yazawa K, Kameyama M (1990) Mechanism of receptor-mediated modulation of the delayed outward potassium current in guinea-pig ventricular myocytes. J Physiol 421: 135-150.
38. DiFrancesco D, Tromba C (1988) Muscarinic control of the hyperpolarization-activated current (i_f) in rabbit sino-atrial node myocytes. J Physiol (Lond) 405: 493-510.
39. Ehara T, Ishihara K (1990) Anion channels activated by adrenaline in cardiac myocytes. Nature 347: 284-286.

40. Ono K, Kiyosue T, Arita M (1989) Isoproterenol, DBcAMP, and forskolin inhibit cardiac sodium current. Am J Physiol 256: C1131-C1137.
41. Ono K, Trautwein W (1991) Potentiation by cyclic GMP of β-adrenergic effect on Ca^{2+} current in guinea-pig ventricular cells. J Physiol 443: 387-404.
42. Tareen FM, Ono K, Noma A, Ehara T (1991) β-adrenergic and muscarinic regulation of the chloride current in guinea-pig ventricular cells. J Physiol 440: 225-241.
43. Nawrath H (1977) Does cyclic GMP mediate the negative inotropic effect of acetylcholine in the heart? Nature 267: 72-74.
44. Kohlhardt M, Haap K (1978) 8-Bromo-guanosine-3',5'-monophosphate mimics the effect of acetylcholine on slow response action potential and contractile force in mammalian atrial myocardium. J Molec Cel. Cardiol 10: 573-578.
45. Goldberg ND, Haddox MK, Nicol SE, Glass DB, Sanford CH, Kuehl FA Jr, Estensen R (1975) Biological regulation through opposing influences of cyclic GMP and cyclic AMP: The Yin Yang hypothesis. Adv Cyclic Nucleo Res 5: 307-330.
46. Mehegan JP, Muir WW, Unverferth DV, Fertel RH, McGuirk SM (1985) Electrophysiological effects of cyclic GMP on canine cardiac Purkinje fibers. J Cardiovasc Pharmacol 7: 30-35.
47. Tohse N, Sperelakis N (1991) Cyclic GMP inhibits the activity of single calcium channels in embryonic chick heart cells. Circ Res 69: 325-331.
48. Tohse N, Nakaya H, Takeda Y, Kanno M (1992) Jpn J Pharmacol 58: 184P.
49. Tohse N, Conforti L, Sperelakis N (1991) Bay K 8644 enhances Ca^{2+} channel activities in embryonic chick heart cells without prlongation of open times. Eur J Pharmacol 203: 307-310.
50. Cuppoletti J, Thakkar J, Sperelakis N, Wahler G (1988) Cardiac sarcolemmal substrate of the cGMP-dependent protein kinase. Memb Biochem 7: 135-142.
51. Hartzell HC, Fischmeister R (1986) Opposite effects of cyclic GMP and cyclic AMP on Ca^{2+} current in single heart cells. Nature 323: 273-275.
52. Fischmeister R, Hartzell RC (1987) Cyclic guanosine 3',5'-monophosphate regulates the calcium current in single cells from frog ventride. J Physiol 387: 455-472.
53. Levi RC, Alloatti G, Fischmeister R (1989) Cyclic GMP regulates the Ca-channel current in guinea pig ventricular myocytes. Pflugers Arch 413: 685-687.
54. Mery PF, Lohmann SM, Walter U, Fischmeister R (1991) Ca^{2+} current is regulated by cyclic GMP-dependent protein kinase in mammalian cardiac myocytes. Proc Natl Acad Sci 88: 1197-1201.
55. Thakkar J, Tang S, Sperelakis N, Wahler G (1988) Inhibition of cardiac slow action potentials by 8-bromo-cyclic GMP occurs independent of changes in cyclic AMP levels. Can J Physiol Pharamcol 66: 1092-1095.
56. Ahmad Z, Green FJ, Subuhi HS, Watanabe AM (1989) Purification and characterization of a Alpha 1,2-mannosidase involved in processing asbaragine linked olig saccharides. J Biol Chem 264: 3859-3863.
57. Watanabe AM, Green F, Ahmad Z (1989) Studies on the cellular mechanisms of action of positive and negative inotropic agents. Basic Res Cardiol 84: 19-22.
58. George WJ, Polson JB, O'Toole AG, Goldberg ND (1970) Elevation of guanosine 3',5'-cyclic phosphate in rat heart after perfusion with acetylcholine. Proc Natl Acad Sci 66: 398-403.
59. Hescheler J, Kameyama M, Trautwein W (1986) On the mechanism of muscarinic inhibition of the cardiac Ca current. Pflugers Arch 407: 182-189.
60. MacLeod KM, Diamond J (1986) Effects of the cyclic GMP lowering agent LY83583 on the interaction of carbachol with forskolin in rabbit isolated cardiac preparations. J Pharmacol Exp Therap 238: 313-318.
61. Johnson JC, Wittenauer LA, Nathan RD (1983) Calmodulin, Ca^{2+}-antagonists and Ca^{2+}-transporters in nerve and muscle. J Neural Trans Suppl 18: 97-111.
62. Bkaily G, Sperelakis N, Eldefrawi M (1984) Effects of the calmodulin inhibitor, trifluoperazine, on membrane potentials and slow action potentials of cultured heart cells. Eur J Pharm 105: 23-31.
63. Bkaily G, Sperelakis N (1986) Calmodulin is required for a full activation of the calcium slow channels in heart cells. J Cyclic Nucleo Prot Phosph Res 11: 25-34.
64. Bruckner R, Scholz H (1984) Effects of alpha-adrenoceptor stimulation with phenylephrine in the presence of propranolol on force of contraction, slow inward current and cyclic AMP content in the bovine heart. Br J Pharmacol 82: 223-232.
65. Dosemeci A, Dhalla RS, Cohen NM, Lederer WJ, Rogers TB (1988) Phorbol ester increases calcium current and stimulates the effects of angiotensin II on cultured neonatal rat heart myocytes. Circ Res 62: 347.
66. Tohse N, Kameyama M, Sakiguchi K, Shearman MS, Kanno M (1990) Protein kinase C activation enhances the delayed rectifier K^+ current in guinea-pig heart cells. J Mol Cell Cardiol 22: 725-734.

Electrophysiological Abnormalities in Cardiac Hypertrophy

SHINICHI KIMURA[1], ARTHUR L. BASSETT[2], and ROBERT J. MYERBURG[1]

Department of Medicine (Division of Cardiology)[1] and Department of Molecular and Cellular Pharmacology[2], University of Miami School of Medicine, Miami, FL 33101, USA

The myocardial cell hypertrophies as an adaptive response to a mechanical overload. However, cardiac hypertrophy induced by chronic pressure overload results in a variety of structural and functional changes. These include alterations in morphology, metabolism, hemodynamics, contraction, and electrophysiology. Despite these adaptations, or because of these alterations, patients with left ventricular hypertrophy have high risk of cardiovascular morbidity and mortality. Electrophysiological abnormalities may be partly responsible for the increased mortality rate with left ventricular hypertrophy. Several recent clinical studies have demonstrated an increased incidence of ventricular arrhythmias and sudden cardiac death presumably due to ventricular fibrillation or tachycardia in association with left ventricular hypertrophy (1-3). In addition, superimposition of ischemia enhances arrhythmogenesis in hypertrophied hearts. Experimentally, it has been demonstrated that the incidence of ischemia- and reperfusion-induced ventricular fibrillation and sudden death are significantly higher in rats and dogs with left ventricular hypertrophy (4-6). However, the precise mechanisms of electrophysiological abnormalities and enhanced arrhythmogenesis in cardiac hypertrophy remain unsettled.

Electrophysiological Alterations in Hypertrophy

The characteristic feature of cellular electrophysiological changes in most experimental models of cardiac hypertrophy induced by chronic pressure overload is action potential prolongation at the plateau level. The early electrophysiological studies of pressure overload-induced hypertrophy used the cat model of right ventricular hypertrophy via pulmonary artery occlusion, which revealed prolonged action potential, depressed plateau, reduced resting potential, and decreased upstroke velocity, depending on the severity and duration of pressure overload (7-9). Left ventricular hypertrophy has been studied in rats with renal hypertension by Aronson (10) and Gulch (11); they found action potential prolongation without significant changes in resting potential, action potential amplitude, overshoot, or maximum rate of rise of the upstroke. We also demonstrated that left ventricular hypertrophy induced by aortic banding or renal hypertension in rats and cats is associated with action potential lengthening (4, 12, 13).

Action potential duration is determined by the balance between the inward and outward currents passing through the membrane at the plateau phase. These include the L-type Ca^{2+} current, inward rectifier and delayed rectifier K^+ currents, Na^+ window current, Na^+-Ca^{2+} exchange current, and probably Na^+-K^+ pump current. Alteration in either or both the maximal conductance or the kinetics of channel gating of these currents may affect the action potential duration and could be a factor responsible for action potential prolongation in hypertrophied cells. Recently a voltage-clamp approach was brought to bear on the ionic basis for action potential prolongation in hypertrophied cells. TenEick et al. (14) suggested that outward repolarizing currents were reduced in magnitude in hypertrophied feline myocardium in multicellular papillary muscle preparations. Subsequently, Kleiman and Houser (15), using the patch clamp technique, demonstrated that chronic right ventricular pressure overload induced by partial occlusion of the pulmonary artery resulted in altered characteristics of Ca^{2+} and K^+ currents in cats. They found that the magnitude of the Ca^{2+} current, when corrected by surface area, was not different for myocytes obtained from normal and hypertrophied right ventricles, but the inactivation of the Ca^{2+} current was delayed. They also demonstrated that the magnitude of the delayed rectifier K^+ current was reduced, its activation was slower, and its deactivation was enhanced in myocytes from hypertrophied right ventricles (16). These abnormalities of the Ca^{2+} current and the delayed rectifier K^+ current may contribute to the prolongation of action potential duration which characterizes pressure-overload cardiac hypertrophy.

Little information is available for the ionic mechanisms of action potential changes in left ventricular hypertrophy. Keung (17) showed increased amplitude of the L-type Ca^+ current in hypertrophied rat left ventricular cells, while Scamps et al. (18) reported that the magnitude of the Ca^{2+} current, when corrected for increased cellular size of hypertrophied myocytes, was similar for normal and hypertrophied cells. In our laboratory, patch-clamp experiments are underway to study ionic mechanisms of action potential prolongation in myocytes isolated from hypertrophied feline left ventricles induced by aortic constriction. Our preliminary studies showed that the amplitude of the L-type Ca^{2+} current, when corrected by surface area, was similar for myocytes isolated from normal and hypertrophied left ventricles. However, inactivation of the current was slower in hypertrophied cells. The time course of inactivation of the Ca^{2+} current was fitted to a two exponential function. Although the fast component was not changed, the slow component was delayed in hypertrophied cells. Also, our preliminary studies suggest that the magnitude of the delayed rectifier K^+ current was reduced, its activation was slower, and its deactivation was enhanced. These findings are similar to those from right ventricular hypertrophy reported by Kleiman and Houser (15, 16). Alterations in Ca^{2+} current kinetics and magnitude and kinetics of the delayed rectifier K^+ current appear to be major factors responsible for action potential lengthening in both right and left ventricular hypertrophy induced by sustained pressure overload. Abnormalities at single Ca^{2+} channel levels are under investigation in our laboratory, and preliminary studies indicate that the channel kinetics are altered in hypertrophied cells.

Enhanced Arrhythmogenesis in Hypertrophy During Ischemia

The presence of left ventricular hypertrophy is associated with increased incidence of arrhythmias (1-3). Superimposition of ischemia further enhances arrhythmogenesis in hypertrophied hearts. Kohya et al. (4) have demonstrated that the incidence of ventricular fibrillation during coronary artery ligation increases with the severity of left ventricular hypertrophy as estimated by the left ventricular weight to body weight ratio in rats. Ventricular fibrillation developed in all rats with severe left ventricular hypertrophy (left ventricular weight/body weight ratio > 3.0). Koyanagi et al. (5) have also demonstrated that the presence of left ventricular hypertrophy increases the incidence of ventricular fibrillation and sudden death in dogs. Although the precise mechanisms of enhanced ischemic arrhythmogenesis in hypertrophied hearts are not well understood, it has been shown that electrophysiological responses to ischemia are greater in hypertrophied hearts (19). Kohya et al. (4) have demonstrated that action potentials shorten to a greater extent in hypertrophied rat left ventricles during simulated ischemia. Together with prolonged action potentials in the normal zone and greater action potential shortening in the ischemic zone, hypertrophied hearts may have greater dispersion of action potential duration between the normal and ischemic zone during ischemia, a condition which facilitates reentrant arrhythmias. Also, it is conceivable that conduction abnormalities may be exaggerated in hypertrophied hearts with larger mass during ischemia, which may also contribute to the development of reentrant arrhythmias.

Ionic Basis for Enhanced Electrophysiological Responses to Ischemia in Hypertrophied Hearts

As mentioned above, shortening of action potential duration during ischemia is greater in hypertrophied hearts. In preliminary studies, we found that even in isolated single myocytes, with no electronic influence from neighboring cells and no restricted extracellular space, action potentials shorten to a greater extent during simulated ischemia in myocytes from hypertrophied left ventricles. These findings indicate that enhanced electrophysiological responses to ischemia in hypertrophied cells are due, at least in part, to alterations in cell membrane properties (i.e., ionic mechanisms).

The ionic mechanisms of action potential shortening during ischemia have been the subject of extensive studies, but still remain unsettled. Possible membrane currents responsible for ischemia-induced action potential shortening are L-type Ca^{2+} current, delayed rectifier K^+ current, transient outward K^+ current, and ATP-sensitive K^+ current. Recently, much attention has been focused on the role of the ATP-sensitive K^+ (K_{ATP}) current in action potential shortening during ischemia and hypoxia, since this current is activated by ATP depletion (20), a major component of ischemia and hypoxia. In addition, Cuevas et al. (21) have demonstrated that K_{ATP} channel activity is enhanced by lowering intracellular pH, a phenomenon which occurs in ischemic myocardium; these data further support the hypothesis that K_{ATP} currents are involved in ischemia-induced action potential shortening. Furthermore, Cameron et al. (22) showed that the sensitivity of the channel to ATP was lower in patches obtained from hypertrophied feline left ventricles induced by aortic banding. That is, more ATP is required to suppress K_{ATP} channel activity in hypertrophied cells. These findings indicate that I_{ATP-K} may be activated to a greater extent in hypertrophied cells during ischemia, which, in turn, enhances action potential shortening. A detail characterization of K_{ATP} channels in hypertrophied cells is underway in our laboratory. Preliminary data on the open-state probability and gating kinetics of the channel at various pH lead us to suggest that the baseline activity of the K_{ATP} channel is higher in hypertrophied cells.

The L-type Ca^{2+} current and the delayed rectifier K^+ current may also be involved in action potential shortening during ischemia. Intracellular ATP influences the Ca^{2+} current. It has been shown that the magnitude of the Ca^{2+} current decreases in a concentration-dependent manner over the concentration range of 0-5 mM ATP when guinea pig single ventricular cells are dialyzed with various ATP-deficient internal solutions (23). It is conceivable that the magnitude and/or kinetics of the Ca^{2+} current are influenced to a greater extent in hypertrophied cells during ischemia. Experiments are underway to examine the effect of metabolic inhibition induced by CN^+ on action potentials and L-type Ca^{2+} current in myocytes obtained from normal and hypertrophied feline left ventricles. Preliminary data indicate that action potentials shorten more during metabolic inhibition in hypertrophied cells. The magnitude of the Ca^{2+} current is reduced more in hypertrophied cells along with shortening of the time course of inactivation of the Ca^{2+} current; the latter did not occur in normal cells. It appears that L-type Ca^{2+} current also may contribute to enhanced shortening of action potential duration in hypertrophied cells during ischemia.

Conclusion

Chronic pressure overload prolongs action potential repolarization of cardiac muscle, which may be beneficial by compensating for depressed mechanical activity. Several ionic currents appear to be involved in persistent action potential changes in cardiac hypertrophy. In particular, alterations in the magnitude and kinetics of the L-type Ca^{2+} current and the delayed rectifier K^+ current are involved in action potential prolongation, although other membrane currents also may contribute.

Myocardial ischemia further enhances arrhythmogenesis in hypertrophied hearts. Greater electrophysiological dispersion expected to occur in hypertrophied hearts during ischemia would facilitate reentrant arrhythmias. The precise ionic mechanisms of enhanced arrhythmogenesis in hypertrophied cells during ischemia remain uncertain. However, it is suggested that altered characteristics of the L-type Ca^{2+} and ATP-sensitive K^+ currents contribute to the enhanced electrophysiological responses to ischemia in hypertrophy.

References

1. Levy D, Anderson KM, Savage DD Balkus SA, Kannel WB, Castelli WP (1987) Risk of ventricular arrhythmias in left ventricular hypertrophy (The Framingham Heart Study). Am J Cardiol 60:560-565
2. McLenachan JM, Henderson E, Morris KI, Dargie HJ, (1987) Ventricular arrhythmias in patients with hypertensive left ventricular hypertrophy. N Engl J Med 317:787-792
3. Messerli FH, Ventura HO, Elizardi DJ, Dunn FG, Frolisch ED (1984) Hypertension and sudden death: increased ventricular ectopic activity in left ventricular hypertrophy. Am J Med 77:18-22
4. Kohya T, Kimura S, Myerburg RJ, Bassett AL (1988) Susceptibility of hypertrophied rat hearts to ventricular fibrillation during acute ischemia. J Mol Cell Cardiol 20:159-168
5. Koyanagi S, Eastham G, Marcus ML (1982) Effects of chronic hypertension and left ventricular hypertrophy on the incidence of sudden death after coronary artery occlusion in conscious dogs. Circulation 65:1192-1197
6. Taylor AL, Winter R, Thandroyen F, Murphree S, Buja LM, Eckels R, Pastor P, Kremers M (1990) Potentiation of reperfusion-associated ventricular fibrillation by left ventricular hypertrophy. Circ Res 67:501-509
7. Bassett AL, Gelband H (1973) Chronic partial occlusion of the pulmonary artery in cats: change in ventricular action potential configuration during early hypertrophy. Circ Res 32:15-26
8. Tritthart H, Leudcke H, Bayer R, Sterle H, Kauffmann R (1975) Right ventricular hypertrophy in the cat: An electrophysiological anatomical study. J Mol Cell Cardiol 7:163-174
9. TenEick RE, Houser SR, Bassett AL (1989) Cardiac hypertrophy and altered cellular electrical activity of the myocardium. In: Physiology and Pathophysiology of the Heart. edited by Sperelakis N, Kluwer Academic Publishers, Boston, p.573-594
10. Aronson RS (1980) Characteristics of action potentials of hypertrophied myocardium from rats with renal hypertension. Circ Res 47:443-454
11. Gulch RW (1980) The effect of chronic loading on the action potential of mammalian myocardium. J Mol Cell Cardiol 12:425-420
12. Cameron JS, Myerburg RJ, Wong SS, Gaide MS, Epstein K, Alvarez TR, Gelband H, Guse PA, Bassett AL (1983) Electrophysiologic consequences of chronic experimentally-induced left ventricular pressure overload. J Am Coll Cardiol 2:481-487
13. Cameron JS, Linda SM, Kimura S, Kaiser CJ, Campbell DR, Kozlovskis PL, Gaide MS, Myerburg RJ, Bassett AL (1986) Systemic hypertension induces disparate localized left ventricular action potential lengthening and altered sensitivity to verapamil in left ventricular myocardium. J Mol Cell Cardiol 18:169-175
14. Ten Eick RE, Bassett AL, Robertson LL (1983) Possible electrophysiological basis for decreased contractility associated with myocardial hypertrophy in the cats: a voltage clamp approach. In: Perspectives in Cardiovascular Research. Myocardial Hypertrophy

and Failure, edited by Alpert NR. New York, Raven, vol. 7, p.245-259
15. Kleiman RB, Houser SR (1988) Calcium currents in normal and hypertrophied isolated feline ventricular myocytes. Am J Physiol 255 (Heart Circ Physiol 24):H1434-1442
16. Kleiman RB, Houser SR (1989) Outward currents in normal and hypertrophied feline ventricular myocytes. Am J Physiol 256 (Heart Circ Physiol 25):H1450-1461
17. Keung EC (1989) Calcium current is increased in isolated adult myocytes from hypertrophied rat myocardium. Circ Res 64:753-763
18. Scamps F, Mayoux E, Charlemagne D, Vassort G (1991) Calcium current in single cells isolated from normal and hypertrophied rat heart: Effects of β-adrenergic stimulation. Circ Res 67:199-208
19. Cameron JS, Bassett AL, Gaide MS, Wong SS, Lodge NJ, Kozlovskis PL, Myerburg RJ (1987) Cellular electrophysiological effects of coronary artery ligation in chronically pressure overloaded cat hearts. Int J Cardiol 14:155-168
20. Noma A (1983) ATP-regulated K^+ channels in cardiac muscle. Nature 305:147-148
21. Cuevas J, Bassett AL, Cameron JS, Furukawa T, Myerburg RJ, Kimura S (1991) Effect of H^+ on ATP-regulated K^+ channels in feline ventricular myocytes. Am J Physiol 261 (Heart Circ Physiol 30):H755-H761
22. Cameron JS, Kimura S, Jackson-Burns DA, Smith DB, Bassett AL (1988) ATP-sensitive K^+ channels are altered in hypertrophied ventricular myocytes. Am J Physiol 255 (Heart Circ Physiol 24):H1254-H1258
23. Noma A, Shibasaki T (1985) Membrane current through adenosine-triphosphate-regulated potassium channels in guinea-pig ventricular cells. J Physiol 363:463-480

Altered Responsiveness to Humoral Factors in Cardiac Myocytes of Cardiomyopathic Syrian Hamsters

HARUAKI NAKAYA[1], TAKEHIRO YAMASHITA[2], NORITSUGU TOHSE[1], HISAKAZU YASUDA[2], AKIRA KITABATAKE[2], and MORIO KANNO[1]

Department of Pharmacology[1], Department of Cardiovascular Medicine[2], Hokkaido University School of Medicine, Sapporo, 060 Japan

KEYWORDS: cardiomyopathic hamster, α-adrenoceptor, angiotensin II receptor, action potential, ion currents

INTRODUCTION

It has been considered that neurohumoral factors, such as catecholamines and renin angiotensin system, may play an important role in the development of cardiomyopathy [1-4]. Previous studies have demonstrated that α-adrenergic stimulation and angiotensin II (Ang II) receptor stimulation result in increased protein synthesis and cell hypertrophy [5-7]. In addition, α-adrenergic stimulation reportedly causes intracellular Ca^{2+} overload in myocytes of cardiomyopathic hamsters [8]. On the other hand, these neurohumoral factors may also play a role in the maintenance of cardiac performance in failing heart, in which β-adrenoceptor-mediated positive inotropic response is compromised [9-11]. α-Adrenergic stimulation and Ang II receptor stimulation are reported to produce positive inotropic responses in human failing myocardium [12,13]. The Syrian hamster of genetic cardiomyopathy is a widely utilized model of congestive cardiomyopathy [14]. Since BIO 14.6 strain develops hypertrophy at 85-150 days of age before the appearance of overt congestive heart failure [14], it has been used as a model of hypertrophic cardiomyopathy. In contrast, BIO 53.58 develops a dilated cardiomyopathy, which is characterized by thin ventricular walls and dilated chambers, throughout most of its life, and is used as a model of the idiopathic congestive cardiomyopathy [15]. In the present study we evaluated electromechanical responses to α-adrenoceptor and Ang II receptor stimulation in these two models of cardiomyopathy using conventional microelectrode techniques. In addition, we evaluated the ionic mechanisms underlying the difference of the electromechanical responses in isolated ventricular myocytes of the hamsters using patch clamp techniques.

MATERIALS AND METHODS

Hamster Strains

Syrian hamsters 14-20 weeks of age with either hypertrophic (BIO 14.6) and dilated cardiomyopathy (BIO 53.58) were used for the study. Age-matched inbred normal Syrian hamsters (F1B) served as controls. All the hamsters were purchased from BIO Breeders, Inc. (Fitchburg, Mass., U.S.A.).

Action Potential Experiments

The heart was immersed in an oxygenated Tyrode solution, and papillary muscles (PMs) were dissected from the left ventricle. The preparations were pinned to the bottom of a tissue chamber and continuously superfused with the modified Tyrode solution equilibrated with 95% O_2 and 5% CO_2. The composition of the solution was as follows (in mM): NaCl, 125; KCl, 4; NaH_2PO_4, 1.8; $MgCl_2$, 0.5; $CaCl_2$, 2.7; $NaHCO_3$, 25; and glucose, 5.5. The bath temperature was kept constant at 30°C. Transmembrane potentials and developed tension (DT) were simultaneously recorded from PMs, as previously described [16]. In brief, one end of the preparation was hooked to the lever arm of a transducer and the other was pinned to the bottom of the tissue chamber. Resting tension was progressively increased to 200 mg. The preparations were stimulated at 0.5 Hz through platinum field electrodes. Stimuli were rectangular pulses of 1 ms duration at twice the diastolic threshold. Transmembrane action potentials were recorded using glass microelectrodes filled with 3 M KCl.

Patch Clamp Experiments

Single ventricular myocytes were obtained from hamsters by enzymatic dispersion, as described previously [17]. Briefly, hearts, removed from pentobarbital-anesthetized hamsters, were Langendorff-perfused and digested using collagenase. Single ventricular cells were placed in a recording chamber attached to an inverted microscope and superfused with the HEPES-Tyrode solution at 36°C. The composition of the normal HEPES-Tyrode solution was (mM): NaCl, 143; KCl, 5.4; $CaCl_2$, 1.8; $MgCl_2$, 0.5; NaH_2PO_4, 0.33; glucose, 5.5 and HEPES-NaOH buffer (pH 7.4), 5. Whole-cell membrane currents were recorded with the patch clamp method, using glass patch pipettes with a diameter of 3-4 μm. The resistance of the pipette was 1-2 megohms when filled with an internal solution composed of KOH 110, KCl 20, $MgCl_2$ 1, K_2ATP 5, K_2 creatinine phosphate 5, aspartic acid 90-100, HEPES 5, EGTA 10 (in mM).

Drugs

The following drugs were used: phenylephrine hydrochloride (Sigma), angiotensin II (Sigma), dl-propranolol hydrochloride (Sigma), prazosin hydrochloride (Pfizer).

Statistics

All data are expressed as the mean ± S.E. and were evaluated for statistical significance by Student's paired *t*-test or two-way ANOVA whichever was appropriate. Differences with probability values less than 0.05 were considered significant.

RESULTS

Cardiac Pathology

The ratio of heart weight to body weight was higher in BIO 14.6 hamsters than F1B hamsters. However, it was lower in BIO 53.58 than in F1B hamsters. Macroscopically ventricular hypertrophy was noted in the hearts of BIO 14.6, and thinning of ventricular wall and enlarged cavities were observed in those of BIO 53.58.

Baseline Characteristics of Action Potential and Developed Tension

There were no significant differences in the resting membrane potential and action potential amplitude among preparations of cardiomyopathic and control hamsters. Action potential duration at 50% and 90% repolarization (APD_{50} and APD_{90}) in PMs of BIO 14.6 were shorter than those in PMs of BIO 53.58 and F1B (Fig. 1). Basal DT, which was corrected for muscle cross sectional area (XS), in PMs of BIO 14.6 and BIO 53.58 was smaller than that in F1B PMs.

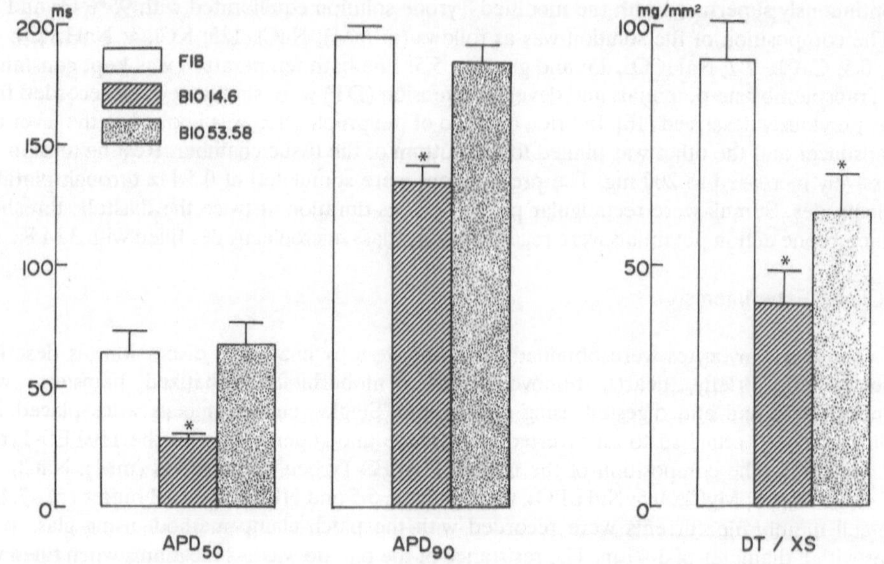

Fig.1 Basal values of APDs and DT/XS in PMs of normal and cardiomyopathic hamsters. *p<0.05 vs F1B PMs.

Changes in Action Potentials and Developed Tension during α-Adrenoceptor and Angiotensin II Receptor Stimulation

Phenylephrine (3×10^{-7} - 3×10^{-5} M) in the presence of propranolol (10^{-6} M) produced concentration-dependent increases in DT and APD in PMs of both control and cardiomyopathic hamsters. Increases in APD and DT in response to 3×10^{-5} M phenylephrine in BIO 14.6 PMs were significantly greater than those in F1B PMs (Fig. 2). However, the α-adrenoceptor-mediated increases in DT and APD in BIO 53.58 PMs were comparable to those observed in F1B PMs (Fig. 2). Ang II (10^{-8} - 10^{-6} M) also produced concentration-dependent increases in APD and DT in propranolol (10^{-6}M) and prazosin (10^{-6} M)-treated PMs of control and cardiomyopathic hamsters. In contrast with electromechanical responses to α-adrenergic stimulation, Ang II produced a significantly smaller increase in DT in BIO 14.6 PMs than F1B ones, concomitantly with a smaller increase in APD (Fig. 2). The Ang II-induced increase in DT in BIO 53.58 PMs was also smaller than that in F1B PMs (Fig. 2). Thus, two cardiomyopathic models, i.e., hypertrophic and dilated cardiomyopathic hamsters, showed disparate electromechanical responses to α-adrenoceptor stimulation and depressed responses to Ang II receptor stimulation.

Changes in Membrane Currents during α-Adrenoceptor and Angiotensin II Receptor Stimulation

Since PMs of BIO 14.6 showed a significant greater electromechanical response to α-adrenergic stimulation and a significantly smaller response to Ang II receptor stimulation than F1B PMs, we evaluated underlying ionic mechanisms in single ventricular myocytes isolated from BIO 14.6 and F1B hamsters. Membrane currents were elicited by 300-ms test pulses to various potentials from a holding potential of -38 mV. On depolarization to +2 mV, an inward current with rapid activation and slow inactivation was observed. Amplitude of the calcium current (I_{Ca}) was obtained by

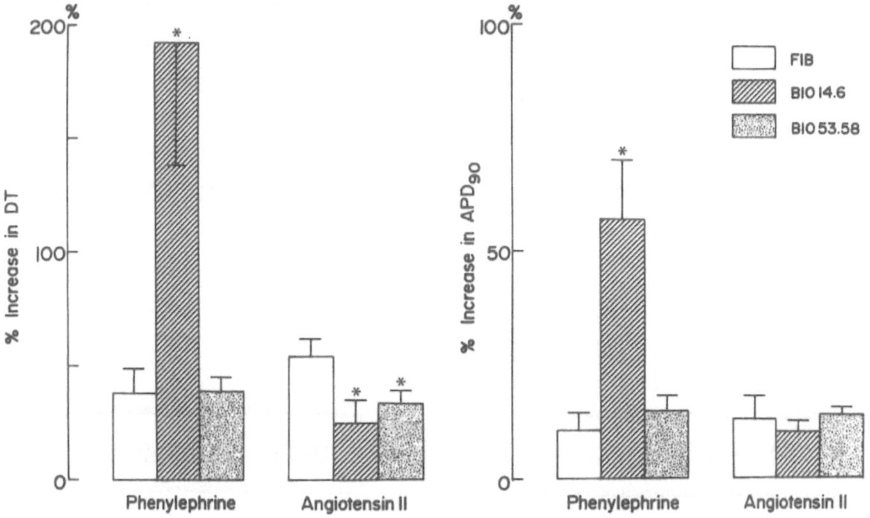

Fig.2 α-Adrenoceptor and Ang II receptor-mediated changes in DT and APD_{90} in PMs of normal and cardiomyopathic hamsters. *p<0.05 vs F1B PMs.

subtracting the late current from the initial peak current. Phenylephrine (3×10^{-5} M) failed to increase I_{Ca} in both BIO 14.6 and F1B myocytes. On hyperpolarization to -58 mV, the time-independent outward current (the inward rectifier K^+ current, I_{K1}) almost reached its maximum value. Phenylephrine at a concentration of 3×10^{-5} M decreased I_{K1} by 32 ± 7 % in BIO 14.6 myocytes although it decreased I_{K1} only by 3 ± 1 % in F1B cells. Depolarizing pulses from a holding potential of -68 mV in the presence of 2 mM $CoCl_2$ induced a 4-aminopyridine-sensitive transient outward current (I_{to}). In both F1B and BIO 14.6 myocytes, the amplitude of I_{to}, the difference between the peak current and the current at the end of the 300 ms pulse to +12 mV, was reduced by phenylephrine. The decrease in I_{to} in BIO 14.6 myocytes (26 ± 9 %) was comparable to that in F1B myocytes (20 ± 4 %). Thus, the greater inhibition of I_{K1} by phenylephrine in BIO 14.6 myocytes seems to be mainly responsible for the greater prolongation of APD in BIO 14.6 PMs. In contrast with α-adrenergic stimulation, Ang II receptor stimulation increased I_{Ca}. The Ang II (10^{-6} M)-induced increase in I_{Ca} in F1B myocytes (85 ± 25 %) was greater than that in BIO 14.6 myocytes (46 ± 5 %). Ang II slightly decreased I_{K1} and I_{to} in both F1B and BIO 14.6 myocyte. Thus, the smaller increase in I_{Ca} in BIO 14.6 myocytes may be at least in part responsible for the depressed positive inotropic response.

DISCUSSION

Consistent with previous reports [18,19], the contractile function of left papillary muscles isolated from hypertrophic (BIO 14.6) and dilated cardiomyopathic hamsters (BIO 53.58) was significantly depressed. In the present study, APDs recorded from BIO 14.6 PMs were shorter than those of PMs of age-matched control hamsters (F1B) whereas APDs of BIO 53.58 PMs were comparable to those of F1B PMs. These results are, however, conflicting with previous reports [18-20], which

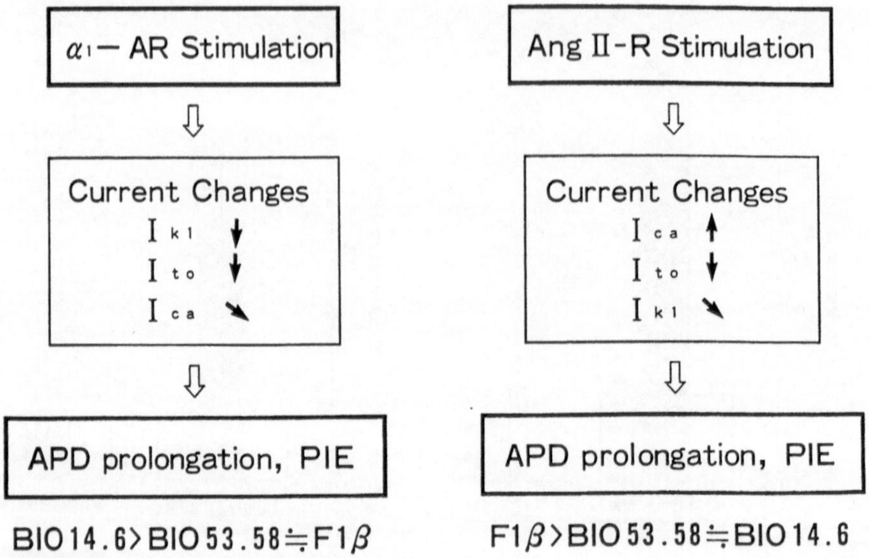

Fig.3 Electromechanical responses to α-adrenoceptor and Ang II receptor stimulation in normal and cardiomyopathic hamsters.

showed prolonged APD in ventricular muscles of cardiomyopathic hamsters. The inconsistency might stem from the differences in experimental conditions such as stimulation frequency. Previous studies [21,22] have demonstrated that the positive inotropic response to α-adrenergic stimulation is enhanced in hypertrophic cardiomyopathy. Although the increased mechanical responsiveness to α-adrenergic stimulation was observed in BIO 14.6 PMs, the α-adrenoceptor mediated positive inotropic response in BIO 53.58 PMs was comparable to that in F1B PMs, indicating the enhanced α-adrenergic responsiveness is observed only in hypertrophic cardiomyopathy (Fig. 3). The α-adrenoceptor-mediated increase in APD was in parallel with the positive inotropic response and the APD prolongation was greater in BIO 14.6 PMs than F1B ones (Fig. 3). In this study we examined effects of phenylephrine on the membrane current system in F1B and BIO 14.6 ventricular cells. Phenylephrine inhibited I_{to} in these hamster myocytes. Similar α-adrenoceptor-mediated inhibition of I_{to} has been observed in rat [17,23] and rabbit cardiac cells [24]. However, there was little difference in the magnitude of I_{to} inhibition between F1B and BIO 14.6 myocytes. We failed to detect an increase in I_{Ca} during α-adrenergic stimulation in both BIO 14.6 and F1B cardiac myocytes, which is consonant with the reports from our [17] and other's laboratory [25] using ventricular cells of several other species. Therefore, the phenylephrine-induced APD prolongation cannot be ascribed to changes in I_{Ca}. Recently, it has been reported that α-adrenergic stimulation inhibited I_{K1}, leading to APD prolongation [26,27]. In the present study, α-adrenergic stimulation decreased I_{K1} in hamster myocytes, especially in BIO 14.6 cells. Therefore, the greater inhibition of I_{K1} may partly explain the potentiated APD prolongation during α-adrenergic stimulation. The enhanced APD prolongation might result in an indirect increase in Ca^{2+} influx during plateau phase and the potentiated positive inotropic response (Fig. 3). In terms of Ang II receptor-mediated inotropic response in cardiomyopathic hamsters (BIO 14.6), conflicting results have been reported. Moravec et al.[13] reported the depressed positive inotropic response, but Hirakata et al.[28] demonstrated the enhanced positive inotropic response to Ang II in BIO 14.6 hearts. Consistent with the former report, Ang II-induced positive inotropic response was depressed in BIO 14.6 PMs in this study. The present study also revealed the Ang II-induced positive inotropic response was also depressed in PMs of dilated cardiomyopathic hamsters. The depressed responsiveness to Ang II in BIO 14.6 and BIO 53.58 PMs was accompanied by the smaller increases in APD. Ang II has been reported to increase I_{Ca} in cultured neonatal rat heart myocytes [29] and human atrial myocytes [30]. In contrast with α-adrenergic stimulation, stimulation of Ang II receptors increased I_{Ca} in isolated hamster ventricular cells. The Ang II-induced increase in I_{Ca} was greater in control (F1B) myocytes than hypertrophic cardiomyopathic cells (BIO 14.6). Therefore, the smaller increase in I_{Ca} appears to explain the depressed inotropic response to Ang II. In addition, the present study has reported for the first time that Ang II inhibits I_{to} and I_{K1} in similar fashion to α-adrenergic stimulation. It is noteworthy that physiological responses to α-adrenergic stimulation were enhanced but those to Ang II receptor stimulation were depressed in hypertrophic cardiomyopathic hamsters. α-Receptor density was reported to increase in cardiac membrane of BIO 14.6 [3]. The present findings may indicate that Ang II receptor density is decreased and/or the coupling of receptor and effector system is compromised in BIO 14.6 myocytes. It has been postulated that the increased breakdown of plasma membrane inositol phospholipids may be involved in the physiological responses mediated by α-adrenoceptors [31] and Ang II receptors [29]. However, stimulation of Ang II receptors but not α-receptors increased I_{Ca} in hamster myocytes. Therefore, it would be difficult to make a straightforward conclusion that the increase in phosphoinositide hydrolysis,inositol trisphosphate production and C-kinase activation, can increase I_{Ca} in heart cells. Further studies are needed to clarify the signal transduction system of these receptors in normal and cardiomyopathic hearts.

REFERENCES

1. Sole MJ, Liew CC (1988) Catecholamines, calcium and cardiomyopathy. Am J Cardiol 62:20G-24G
2. Ikegaya, Nishiyama T, Kobayashi A, Yamazaki N (1988) Role of α_1-adrenergic receptors and the effect of bunazosin on the histopathology of cardiomyopathic Syrian hamsters of strain BIO 14.6. Jpn Circ J 52:181-187
3. Kagiya T, Hori M, Iwakura K, Iwai K, Watanabe Y, Uchida S, Yoshida H, Kitabatake A, Inoue M, Kamada T (1991) Role of increased α_1-adrenergic activity in cardiomyopathic hamster. Am J Physiol 260:H80-H88
4. Urata H, Healy B, Stewart RW, Bumpus M, Husain A (1990) Angiotensin II-forming pathways in normal and failing human hearts. Circ Res 66:883-890
5. Simpson P (1985) Stimulation of hypertrophy of cultured neonatal rat heart cells through an α_1-adrenergic receptor and induction of beating through an α_1 and β_1-adrenergic receptor interaction: Evidence for independent regulation of growth and beating. Circ Res 56:884-894
6. Ikeda U, Tsuruga Y, Yaginuma T (1991) α_1-Adrenergic stimulation is coupled to cardiac myocyte hypertrophy. Am J Physiol 260:H953-H956
7. Baker KM, Aceto JF (1990) Angiotensin II stimulation of protein synthesis and cell growth in chick heart cells. Am J Physiol 259:H610-H618
8. Hano O, Lakatta EG (1991) Diminished tolerance of prehypertrophic, cardiomyopathic Syrian hamster hearts to Ca^{2+} stresses. Circ Res 69:123-133
9. Bristow MR, Minobe W, Rasmussen R, Hershberger RE, Hoffman BB (1989) α_1-Adrenergic receptors in the nonfailing and failing human heart. J Pharmacol Exp Ther 247:1038-1045
10. Bristow MR, Kowtrowitz NE, Ginsburg R, Fowler MB (1985) β-Adrenergic function in heart muscle disease and heart failure. J Mol Cell Cardiol 17(Suppl 2):41-52
11. Urata H, Healy B, Stewart RW, Bumpus FM, Husain A (1989) Angiotensin II receptors in normal and failing human hearts. J Clin Endocrinol Metab 69:54-66

12. Böhm M, Diet F, Feiler G, Kemkes B, Erdmann E (1988) α-Adrenoceptors and α-adrenoceptor-mediated positive inotropic effects in human myocardium. J Cardiovasc Pharmacol 12:357-364
13. Moravec CS, Schluchter MD, Paranandi L, Czerska B, Stewart RW, Rosenkranz E, Bond M (1990) Inotropic effects of angiotensin II on human cardiac muscle in vitro. Circulation 82:1973-1984
14. Gertz EW (1972) Cardiomyopathic Syrian hamster:A possible model of human disease. Prog Exp Tumor Res 16:242-260
15. Whitmer JT (1987) L-Carnitine treatment improves cardiac performance and restores high-energy phosphate pools in cardiomyopathic Syrian hamsters. Circ Res 61:396-408
16. Nakaya H, Tohse N, Kanno M (1987) Electrophysiological derangements induced by lipid peroxidation in cardiac tissue. Am J Physiol 253:H1089-H1097
17. Tohse N, Nakaya H, Hattori Y, Endou M, Kanno M (1990) Inhibitory effect mediated by alpha1-adrenoceptors on tran sient outward current in isolated rat ventricular cells. Pflügers Arch 415:575-581
18. Capasso JM, Olivetti G, Anversa P (1989) Mechanical and electrical properties of cardiomyopathic hearts of Syrian hamsters. Am J Physiol 257:H1836-H1842
19. Capasso JM, Sonnenblick EH, Anversa P (1990) Chronic calcium channel blockade prevents the progression of myocardial contractile and electrical dysfunction in the cardiomyopathic Syrian hamster. Circ Res 67:1381-1393
20. Rossner KL (1978) Electrophysiological study of Syrian hamster hereditary cardiomyopathy. Cardiovasc Res 12:436-443
21. Karliner JS, Alabaster C, Stephens H, Barnes P, Dollery C (1981) Enhanced noradrenaline response in cardiomyopathic hamsters: Possible relation to changes in adrenoceptors studied by radioligand binding. Cardiovasc Res 15:296-304
22. Böhm M, Mende U, Schmitz W, Scholz H (1988) Increased responsiveness to stimulation of α- but not β-adrenoceptors in the hereditary cardiomyopathy of the Syrian hamster: Intact adenosine and cholinoceptor-mediated isoprenaline antagonistic effect. Eur J Pharmacol 128:195-203
23. Apkon M, Nerbonne JM (1988) α_1-Adrenergic agonists selectively suppress voltage-dependent K^+ currents in rat ventricular myocytes. Proc Natl Acad Sci USA 85:8756-8760
24. Fedida D, Shimoni Y, Giles WR (1989) A novel effect of norepinephrine on cardiac cells is mediated by α_1-adrenoceptors. Am J Physiol 256:H1500-H1504
25. Hescheler J, Nawrath H, Tang M, Trautwein W (1988) Adrenoceptor-mediated changes of excitation and contraction in ventricular muscle from guinea pigs and rabbits. J Physiol (Lond) 397:657-670
26. Shah A, Cohen IS, Rosen MR (1988) Stimulation of cardiac α-receptors increases Na/K pump current and decreases gK via a pertussis toxin-sensitive pathway. Biophy J 54:219-225
27. Fedida D, Braun AP, Giles WR (1991) α_1-Adrenoceptors reduce background K^+ current in rabbit ventricular myocytes. J Physiol (Lond) 441:673-684
28. Hirakata H, Fouad-Tarazi FM, Bumpus M, Khosla M, Healy B, Husain A, Urata H, Kumagai H (1990) Angiotensins and the failing heart: Enhanced positive inotropic response to angiotensin I in cardiomyopathic hamster heart in the presence of captopril. 66:891-899
29. Allen IS, Cohen NM, Dhallan RS, Gaa ST, Lederer WJ, Rogers TB (1988) Angiotensin II increases spontaneous contractile frequency and stimulates calcium current in cultured neonatal rat heart myocytes: Insights into the underlying biochemical mechanisms. Circ Res 62:524-534
30. Grand BL, Hatem S, Deroubaix E, Couetil JP, Coraboeuf E (1991) Calcium current depression in isolated human atrial myocytes after cessation of chronic treatment with calcium antagonists. 69:292-300
31. Kawaguchi H, Shoki M, Sano H, Kudo T, Sawa H, Okamoto H, Sakata Y, Yasuda H (1991) Phospholipid metabolism in cardiomyopathic hamster heart cells. Circ Res 69:1015-1021

Stretch-Activated Current in Rabbit Cardiac Myocytes

NOBUHISA HAGIWARA, NAOKI MATSUDA, MORIO SHODA, HIROSHI KASANUKI, SAICHI HOSODA, and HIROSHI IRISAWA

The Heart Institute of Japan, Tokyo Women's Medical College, Tokyo, 162 Japan

KEYWORDS: sinoatrial node , atrial cell, membrane stretch, Cl^- current

INTRODUCTION

The stretch-activated (SA) ion channels have been widely observed in various excitable cell membranes [1-3], and SA channels are now considered to play an important role in mechano-transduction. In cardiac myocytes, existence of SA channels has not yet been identified both in the whole-cell voltage clamp and single channel current. In the present study, we found a Cl^- conductance in response to membrane stretch in isolated sinoatrial node and atrial cells. The Cl^--conductance activated by stretch was determined from reversal potential measurements, and from the blocking effect of various Cl^- channel blockers. The only Cl^- currents described in detail so far are the catecholamine-induced Cl^- current [4-6] and the Ca^{2+}-activated Cl^- current [7] in cardiac cells. The stretch-activated Cl^- current is different from the Cl^- currents which were activated by catecholamine or intracellular Ca^{2+}. Since mechanical stimulations are continuously present in the intact cardiac tissue, stretch-activated Cl^- current may contribute to the action potential of cardiac myocytes under physiological conditions.

MATERIALS AND METHODS

Cell isolation and current recording

Single cells were isolated from the sinoatrial node and right atrial region of albino rabbit according to the chopping method of Hagiwara et al [8]. Albino rabbit was fully anesthetized with an intravenous injection of sodium pentobarbitone (40 mg/kg) under heparinization (300 U/kg). The heart was dissected out and the sinoatrial node region was isolated, cut into pieces and incubated in a warm Ca^{2+}-free Tyrode solution for 10 min. The strips were then transferred to a nominally Ca^{2+}-free Tyrode solution containing 350 U/ml collagenase with 0.5 mg/ml elastase for 60 min at 37° C. The collagenase was then washed out by rinsing with high-K^+, low-Cl^- solution and the digested tissue was stored in the same solution at 4 °C until used in experiments. A portion of the atrium was separated from the sinoatrial node region, and was incubated in the same solution as employed for the sinoatrial node cells. The membrane currents were measured using methods similar to those described by Hamill et al [9]. From the holding potential of -30 mV, ramp pulses of $\pm$ 70 mV (0.93 V/sec) or $\pm$ 90 mV (1.2 V/sec) amplitude were applied every 10 sec. Five to seven I-V curves were averaged for illustrations.

Solutions

The normal Tyrode solution contained (in mM) NaCl 136.9, KCl 5.4, $CaCl_2$ 1.8, $MgCl_2$ 0.5, NaH_2PO_4 0.33, glucose 5 and HEPES 5 (pH 7.4 with NaOH). Standard 150 mM Na^+ external solution contained (in mM) NaCl 150, $MgCl_2$ 1 and HEPES 5. The following blockers were added: $BaCl_2$ 1 (to block the delayed rectifier K^+ current, I_K); CsCl 2 (hyperpolarization activated current, I_f); $NiCl_2$ 2 (Ca^{2+} current and Na-Ca exchange current) and ouabain 10 μM (Na-K pump current). Ca^{2+} was not added to this external solution, and the pH was adjusted to 7.4 with Tris base. The total Cl^- concentration of the standard external solution was 160 mM. Under these conditions, time-dependent currents were blocked and the remaining conductance showed only time-independent currents as described before [8].

The composition of the standard NMG internal solution was (in mM): N-methyl-D-glucamine (NMG) 150, EGTA 10, MgATP 5, K_2 creatine phosphate (CrP) 5, $MgCl_2$ 2 and HEPES 5. This solution was titrated to pH 7.4 with HCl and the total Cl^- concentration of this solution was 110 mM. When the Cl^- concentration of the pipette solution was reduced, Cl^- was replaced with equimolar concentration of aspartate.

Drugs
Anthracene-9-carboxylate (9AC), the stilbene derivatives, 4-acetamide-4'-isothiocyano stilbene 2, 2' disulfonic acid (SITS) and 4-4'-dinitrostilbene -2,2' disulfonic acid (DNDS) were used for the Cl^- channel blockers. 1-(5-Isoquinolyl sulphonyl) -2-methyl piperazine dihydrochloride (H-7) was dissolved in distilled water as a 10 mM stock solution. Cyclic AMP-dependent protein kinase inhibitor was directly dissolved in the pipette solution.

Methods for applying membrane stretch
To apply the membrane stretch in the single sinoatrial node and atrial cells, we employed the following two different methods: (1) Positive pressure was applied to the patch electrode during the whole-cell voltage clamp recording, by mouth, through a long polyethylene tube. The steady state pressure was 5 -20 cm H_20 when measured near the patch electrode. (2) Superfusing the cell with hypoosmotic external solution. The cell volume and the cross sectional area were increased by both stimuli. Figure 1 shows the cell inflation method using positive pressure of 10 cm H_20 through the patch pipette in sinoatrial node cell. The cross sectional area (the relative surface area) of this cell increased by 20 % (Fig. 1B). All statistical data are given as mean $\pm$ S.D.

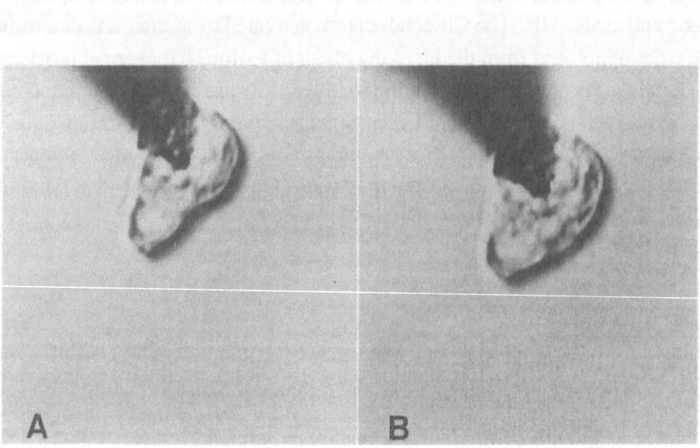

Fig. 1 The cell inflation method by applying positive pressure through the patch pipette. **A** is the control and **B** is after inflation of the cell. The relative cross sectional area was increased by 20 % after inflation.

RESULTS

Inflation and swelling activated membrane current
Time-dependent currents, such as the Ca^{2+} current, the delayed rectifier K^+ current and the hyperpolarization activated current were all blocked by superfusing the myocytes with 150 mM Na^+ , K^+-free external solution containing 2 mM Ni^{2+}, 1 mM Ba^{2+} and 2 mM Cs^+. The atrial cell showed only a small amplitude of background conductance in response to voltage pulses. The application of positive pressure (10 cm H_2O) through the patch pipette, both the cell size and the membrane conductance were increased. The membrane conductance at 40 mV in the control was 0.9 nS (Fig. 2-1a), and it increased to 12 nS after inflation (Fig. 2-1b). The difference current (Fig. 2-2, b-a) showed an outward rectification and time-independent changes. The membrane slope conductance increased from 0.5 $\pm$ 0.2nS to 11.0 $\pm$ 5.8 nS (n=32) at 40 mV in atrial cells.

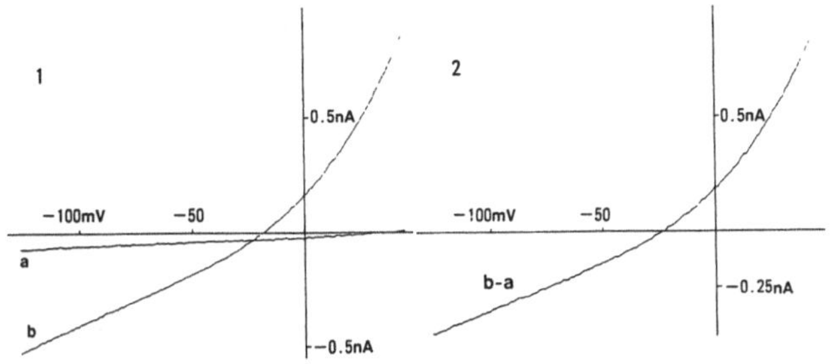

Fig. 2 Inflation-activated current in atrial cell. **1**: From the holding potential of -30 mV, ramp pulses of ± 90 mV amplitude were applied. The I-V relations before (a) and after inflation of the cell (b). **2**: (b-a) is the difference current between (a) and (b), indicating the inflation-activated current. The reversal potential of the inflation-activated current was -23 mV.

We also identified an activation of similar current changes by superfusing the cell with hypoosmotic external solution. Figure 3 shows swelling-activated current in sinoatrial node cells. The membrane slope conductance was 0.7 nS in the control (Fig. 3-1a), and it was 4.1 nS after an application of 60% hypoosmolar external solution (Fig. 3-1b). These current changes resumed to the control level when we applied negative pressure to the patch pipette or changed to normal osmotic solution. The reversible nature of the current indicates the membrane conductance changes were not due to the change in the seal resistance.

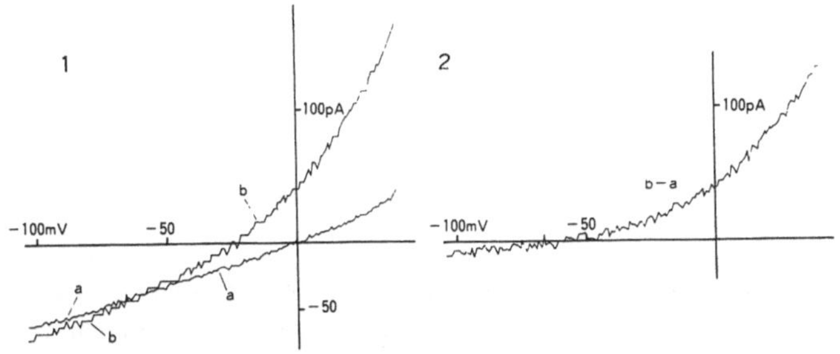

Fig. 3 The swelling-activated current induced by hypoosmolar external solution in sinoatrial node cell. **1**: The I-V relation before (a) and after an application of 60 % hypoosmolar external solution (b). **2** is the difference current between (a) and (b). The reversal potential was -50 mV in this condition.

<u>Effect of pipette Cl^- concentration and Cl^- channel blockers on the stretch- activated current</u>

The pipette solution contained large molecular NMG and other cations were not added, therefore, the outward component of stretch-activated current was suggested to be carried by anion. The I-V relation of the stretch-activated current intersected at -23 mV in Fig. 2 and at -50 mV in Fig. 3. In these conditions, the external solution contained 160 mM Cl^- and the pipette solution contained 50 mM Cl^-,(Fig. 2) and 24 mM Cl^- (Fig. 3). The distribution of Cl^- gives E_{Cl} of -30 and -47 mV, respectively, suggesting the inflation- or swelling-activated current is predominantly Cl^- selective. To confirm that the stretch-activated current is carried by Cl^- ions, we changed the pipette Cl^- concentration. The reversal potentials of the stretch-activated current were -65 mV in 10 mM pipette Cl^- and it was -5 mV in 110 mM pipette Cl^- concentration. These values are closely equal to the expected values of E_{Cl}. Moreover, the amplitude and the reversal potential of the stretch-activated current were not change in Na^+-free NMG external solution. To further demonstrate that the stretch-activated current is Cl⁻ selective, we applied several Cl⁻ channel blockers. The stretch-activated current was blocked by external application of 5 mM DNDS (Fig. 4-c). Other Cl⁻ channel blockers, such as SITS, DIDS or A9C effectively reduced the stretch-activated current. All these results indicate their Cl⁻ selective nature.

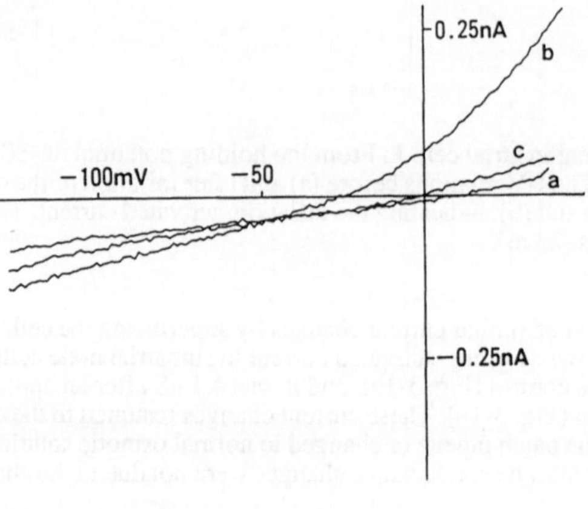

Fig. 4 Effect of DNDS on the stretch-activated current. A: I-V relation in control (**a**) 2.5 min. after inflation (**b**) and (**c**) after an administration of 5 mM DNDS.

<u>Comparison of other cardiac Cl⁻ current</u>

In cardiac myocytes, it has been known that the intracellular c-AMP dependent protein kinase [4-6] and Ca^{2+} [7] can activate the Cl⁻ current. However, involvement of intracellular Ca^{2+} for the activation of this Cl⁻ current is unlikely, because the pipette solution contained 10 mM EGTA and Ca^{2+} was not added. The known Ca^{2+}-activated Cl⁻ channel blockers such as furosemide failed to affect the stretch-activated Cl⁻ current.

The stretch-activated Cl⁻ current was not affected by extracellular application of 20 μM H-7, a blocker of non-specific protein kinase inhibitor or intracellular application of 50 μM specific c-AMP dependent protein kinase inhibitor. These results indicate that the stretch-activated Cl⁻ current is different type of Cl⁻ currents which activated by c-AMP dependent protein kinase or intracellular Ca^{2+}.

CONCLUSION

The Cl⁻ currents have been postulated to contribute to the action potential of cardiac myocytes through the transient outward current. However, the existence of Cl⁻ currents themselves in the heart muscle appeared to be in doubt until recently, when Bahinski et al., Harvey et al. and Matsuoka et al [4-6] found cathecolamine-activated Cl⁻ currents and Zygmunt & Gibbons reconfirmed a Cl⁻ component in the transient outward current [7].

Many Cl⁻ channels are known to be activated by an increase in intracellular Ca^{2+} or protein kinases such as protein kinase A or protein kinase C [10]. The present stretch-activated Cl⁻ current is unlikely to depend on intracellular Ca^{2+} or protein kinases, since this current is activated in the absence of internal Ca^{2+}, and it was unaffected by known protein kinase inhibitors. The application of positive pressure through the patch pipette, both the cell size and the membrane conductance were increased, and it decreased to control level on a subsequent application of a negative pressure. These results suggest that the Cl⁻ current obtained in the present study is not mediated by intracellular signal-transduction, but is activated purely by mechanical stretch of the membrane or deformation of cell cytoskeleton.

Many arrhythmias are known to be triggered by mechanical stretch in some pathological status, such as pressure or volume overloaded diseases. The membrane potential will depolarize and it causes an abnormal automaticity, if stretch-activated Cl^- current is activated in such cases. Moreover, the mechanical stress is continuously exist in the intact heart, this current may supply an inward current during normal pacemaker potential in sinoatrial node cells.

REFERENCES

1. Guharay F, Sachs F (1984) Stretch-activated single ion channel currents in tissue-cultured embryonic skeletal muscle. J Physiol 352: 685-701
2. Guharay F, Sachs F (1985) Mechano transducer ion channels in chick skeletal muscle: the effects of extracellular pH. J Physiol 363: 119-134
3. Morris C.E. (1990) Mechanosensitive ion channels. J Memb Biol 113: 93-107
4. Bahinski A, Nairn A C, Greengard P, Gadsby D C (1989) Chloride conductance regulated by cyclic AMP-dependent protein kinase in cardiac myocytes. Nature 340: 718-721
5. Harvey R.D, Clark C D, Hume J R (1990) Chloride current in mammalian cardiac myocytes. Novel mechanism for autonomic regulation of action potential duration and resting membrane potential. J G Physiol 95: 1077-1102
6. Matsuoka S, Ehara T, Noma A (1990) Chloride-sensitive nature of the adrenaline induced current in guinea-pig cardiac myocytes. J Physiol 425: 579-598
7. Zygmunt A C, Gibbons W R (1991) Calcium-activated chloride current in rabbit ventricular myocytes. Circ Res 68: 424-437
8. Hagiwara N, Kasanuki H, Hosoda S,Irisawa H (1992) Background current in the sinoatrial node cells of the rabbit heart. J Physiol 448: 53-72
9. Hamill O P, Marty A, Neher E, Sakmann B, Sigworth F J (1981) Improved patch clamp techniques for high-resolution current recording for cells and cell-free membrane patches. Pflugers Archiv 391: 85-100
10. McCann J D, Welsh M J (1990) Regulation of Cl and K+ channels in airway epitheliums. An Rev Physiol 52: 115-135

V: Drug Therapy of Failing Heart

Evaluation of Functional Capacity of Patients with Congestive Heart Failure

SHIGETAKE SASAYAMA, HIDETSUGU ASANOI[2], SHINJI ISHIZAKA[2], and KYOKO MIYAGI[2]

Third Division, Department of Internal Medicine, Kyoto University, Kyoto, 606 Japan[1] and
The 2nd Department of Internal Medicine, Toyama Medical and Pharmaceutical University, Toyama, 930-01 Japan[2]

KEYWORDS: NYHA criteria, peak oxygen consumption, specific activity scale, anaerobic threshold

Traditionally, the clinical syndrome of heart failure has been viewed as a pathophysiologic state in which ventricular performance is depressed and leads to symptoms related to low cardiac output and elevated left ventricular filling pressure. It would seem logical to assess the patients with heart failure by hemodynamic evaluation, however, hemodynamic measures are not always abnormal in the failing heart. More recently, heart failure has been defined as a syndrome in which cardiac dysfunction is associated with reduced exercise tolerance, a high incidence of ventricular arrhythmias and shortened life expectancy.

1. NEW YORK HEART ASSOCIATION (NYHA) FUNCTIONAL CLASSIFICATION

Because congestive heart failure is a clinical syndrome, the most direct approach to its evaluation is to inquire about symptoms of dyspnea and fatigue at rest and on exertion. The severity of cardiovascular disability has been classified most often into four categories according to the criteria proposed by a committee of NYHA. This classification is based on the patients report of the amount of activity the patient can sustain without experiencing symptoms. This classification, though simple and widely adopted in numerous clinical studies, has several major disadvantages in reporting patients' cardiac functional states. 1) the classification is subjective and nonparametric, 2) its large stepwise gradations preclude to denote important transitions from one state to another, 3) this classification does not provide distinctions in different types of activity, 4) this concerns with the patients' condition at only a single point in time [1].

Franciosa and co-workers compared clinical classification by NYHA criteria with exercise classification in 44 patients with DCM, and found these two classifications agreed in only 16 patients [2].

Goldman et al [3] reported that reproducibility as interobserver agreement and validity of the NYHA criteria as the agreement with the objective measures of exercise tolerance were 56% and 51%

respectively, suggesting that this system is not adequate to evaluate patients' response to therapy or to compare one patient to another. These authors also showed that the reproducibility and validity increased significantly when the Canadian Cardiovascular Society (CCS) criteria with greater details in definition of cardiac function were adopted.

2. EXERCISE CAPACITY

Patients with congestive heart failure are usually more symptomatic during exertion. Therefore, it has been widely accepted that the functional state is reasonably indicated by exercise capacity. Engler et al emphasized an importance of symptom score by showing that functional status is reliably represented by treadmill performance or symptoms, but not by measurements of left ventricular function at rest [4].

Maximal oxygen uptake has been proposed as a reliable index which allows for the quantification of maximal exercise capacity. Measurement of this variable (max $\dot{V}O_2$) requires that a plateau in oxygen uptake should be demonstrated despite further increments in exercise work load. However, patients with congestive heart failure cannot achieve a plateau in oxygen uptake during graded exercise because they are limited by symptoms. Therefore, the observed peak $\dot{V}O_2$ has been used by many investigators to quantify exercise capacity.

Anaerobic threshold has been proposed as an useful objective measure to evaluate functional capacity of patients with chronic heart failure. However, in severe heart failure, the early occurrence of anaerobic metabolism or an abnormal ventilatory response to graded exercise precluded the reliable detection of anaerobic threshold.

3. SPECIFIC ACTIVITY SCALE

The tests of functional capacity mentioned above are designed to evaluate exercise performance at maximal work loads, but daily activities do not generally require an energy expenditure in the maximal range.

In the clinical research, many investigators challenged to transform clinical data into useful clinical scales. Katz et al [5] developed a graded scale according to overall performance in the daily life. Data obtained from more than 2,000 evaluations of 1,001 individuals confirmed the usefulness of such quantitative information as a survey instrument as an objective guide to the course of chronic illness, as a tool for studying the aging process and as an aid in rehabilitation teaching. Feinstein and Wells [6] have proposed a new taxonomy for rating transitions in functional capacity in patients with ischemic heart disease as noted in three kinds of functional performance: occupation, customary activities and sporadic activities. The combined single global rating of changes in these three activities was shown to be more pertinent for the clinical challenge of choosing and evaluating the agents used in patient care. A subjective sensation is difficult to evaluate by physiologic measurements. Mahler et al [7] developed new indexes to improve the clinical rating of dyspnea by rating the severity of dyspnea at a single state (a baseline dyspnea index) and by denoting changes from baseline (a transition dyspnea). The both scores consisted of three categories; functional impairment, magnitude of task, and magnitude of effort. This direct rating of dyspea also has been shown to provide important information not disclosed by customary physiologic tests.

The categorical values for severity of patient's symptoms are subjective and bitemporal transition of a particular phenomenon from one state to another is expressed in a dimensional scale simply as a relative change to a measurement of the basic entity.

In contrast to such scales which depend on subjective symptom and are prone to be modified by psychological factors, there are some attempt to develop a specific activity scale (SAS) according to the matabolic costs of individual activities. Taylar and colleagues [8] developed a new questionnaire for evaluation of energy expended in variety of leisure time activities and found a clear and statistically significant relationship between each exercise endpoint and the sum of energy expenditures. Goldman et al [3] estimated metabolic costs of a variety of personal care, housework, occupational and recreational activities based on available data. They demonstrated that though their SAS could not improve upon the reproducibility attained by the CCS criteria, it was significantly more valid especially for the evaluation of true class II patients and was significantly less likely to underestimate treadmill performance.

We actually measured metabolic costs of various types of physical activity and prepared questionnaires for specific physical activities which a patient would perform either customarily or sporadically in daily life (Table I).

Table I. Questionnaires for Sepecific Activity Scale

1. Can you have a comfortable sleep at night? (1 Met or less)
2. Do you feel comfortable in the lying position? (1 Met or less)
3. Can you take meals or wash your face by yourself? (1.4 Mets)
4. Can you go to the bathroom by yourself? (2 Mets)
5. Can you change your clothes by yourself? (2-2.3 Mets)
6. Can you do kitchen work or sweep the room with a broom?(2-3 Mets)
7. Can you make your bed by yourself? (2-3 Mets)
8. Can you swab the floor? (3-4 Mets)
9. Can you have a shower without any trouble? (3-4 Mets)
10. Can you practice radio gymnatic exercises without any trouble? (3-4 Mets)
11. Can you walk 100 to 200 m of level ground at the same speed as healthy persons do (4km/hr) without any trouble? (3-4 Mets)
12. Can you garden (weeding for a brief time, etc.) without any

trouble? (4-5 Mets)
13. Can you take a bath by yourself? (4-5 Mets)
14. Can you go upstairs at the same speed as healthy persons do without any trouble? (5-6 Mets)
15. Can you do light farming (digging the garden, etc.)? (5-7 Mets)
16. Can you walk 200 m of level ground at a quick pace without any trouble? (6-7 Mets)
17. Can you remove snow? (6-7 Mets)
18. Can you practice tennis (or ping pong) without any trouble? (6-7 Mets)
19. Can you practice jogging (at about 8km/hr) over a distance of 300 to 400 m without any trouble? (7-8 Mets)
20. Can you practice swimming without any trouble? (7-8 Mets)
21. Can you practice rope skipping without any trouble? (≥8 Mets)

A patient was asked to specify whether he/she could perform each type of activity without symptomatic limitation or not. Summarizing the questionnaire data, a given number of metabolic costs (SAS) was derived for each patient regarding the self-perceived exercise tolerance. Interobserver variation in estimating SAS in 20 patients was very small with mean difference of 0.4±0.5 Mets (Fig 1). The relations between SAS and peak $\dot{V}O_2$ were examined in 51 patients. The correlation coefficient between them was 0.78; $p<0.001$ (Fig 2).

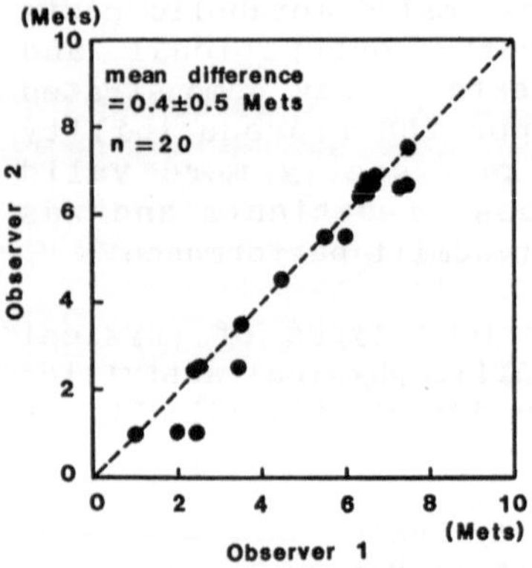

Fig 1. Reproducibility in estimating SAS

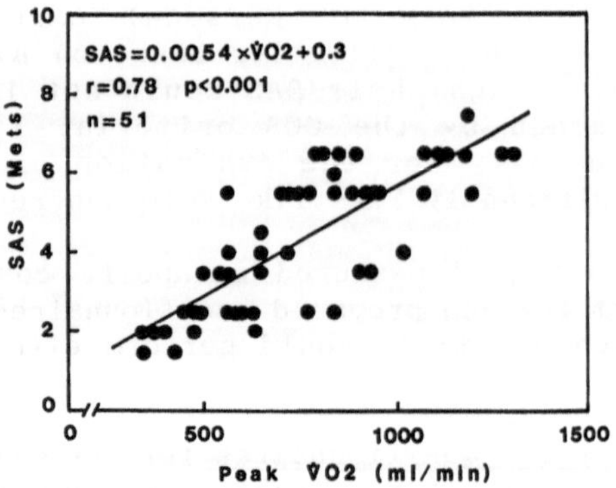

Fig 2. Relationship between SAS and peak $\dot{V}O_2$

In 60 patients, cardiopulmonary test was performed with electronically braked bicycle ergometer and breath-by-breath analysis of respiratory gas. Questions related to the SAS was also asked in these patients. Patients were divided into four classes according to the peak $\dot{V}O_2$: >1000 ml/min (A, n=16), 800-999 ml/min (B, n=14), 500-799 ml/min (C, n=21) and <500 ml/min (D, n=9). Measurement of anaerobic threshold was achieved in 100% in A, 71% in B, 37% in C and 0% in D, while SAS was determined in 63% in A, 86% in B, 95% in C and 100% in D. Therefore, SAS was more likely to be reliable means of estimating functional capacity in patients with severe heart failure (Fig 3).

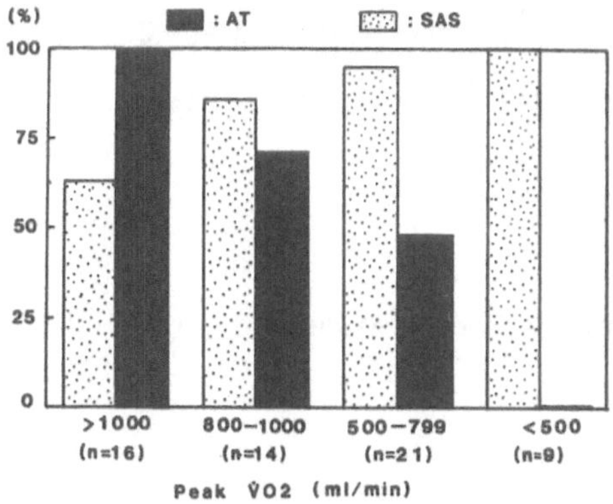

Fig. 3
The detection rates of SAS (dotted bars) and anaerobic threshold (solid bars)

Subsequently, we monitored alterations in the status of 14 patients with heart failure by medical therapy over 3 month period. As a result of sustained therapy peak $\dot{V}O_2$ was augmented in all patients (from 649$\pm$195 (SD) to 860$\pm$216 ml/min). These changes were accompanied by comparable improvements of SAS, while NYHA Class remained unchanged in 8 of 14 patients. Since the difference between NYHA Class II and Class III is extremely subjective and arbitariry, these ratings are too coarse to denote important changes that can be produced by the treatment. On the contrary, SAS appears to have advantages over NYHA classification system as a useful objective tool in reporting cardiac disability.

REFERENCES

1. Selzer A, Cohn K (1972) Functional classification of cardiac disease: a critique. Am J Cardiol 30: 306-308
2. Franciosa JA, Ziesche S, Wilen M (1979) Functional capacity of patients with chronic left ventricular failure. Relationship of bicycle exercise performance to clinical and hemodynamic characterization. Am J Med 67: 460-466
3. Goldman L, Hashimoto B, Cook EF, Loscalzo A (1981) Comparative reproducibility and validity of systems for assessing cardiovascular functional class: advantages of a new specific activity scale. Circulation 64: 1227-1234
4. Engler R, Ray R, Higgins CB, McNally C, Buxton WH, Bhargava V, Shabetai R (1982) Clinical assessment and follow-up of functional capacity in patients with chronic congestive cardiomyopathy. Am J Cardiol 49: 1832-1837
5. Kats S, Ford AB, Moskowitz RW, Jackson BA, Jaffe MW (1963) Studies of illness in the aged. The index of ADL: a standardized measure of biological and psychosocial function. JAMA 185: 94-919
6. Feinstein AR, Wells CK (1977) A new clinical taxonomy for rating change in functional activities of patients with angina pectoris. Am Heart J 93: 172-182
7. Mahler DA, Weinberg DH, Wells CK, Feinstein AR (1984) The measurement of dyspnea. Contents, interobserver agreement, and physiologic correlates of two new clinical indexes. Chest 85:751-758
8. Taylor HL, Jacobs DR, Schucker B, Knudsen J, Leon AS, Debacker G (1978) A questionnaire for the assessment of leisure time physical activities. J Chron Dis 31:741-755

Progress of Treatment and Changing Views on the Role of Compensatory Mechanisms in Chronic Heart Failure

MASAHIKO IIZUKA

1st Department of Internal Medicine, Dokkyo University School of Medicine, Tochigi, 321-02 Japan

INTRODUCTION

In this brief review the progress in the treatment of chronic heart failure is discussed from standpoint of understanding of mechanisms of heart failure.Nobody would disagree that an effective treatment must be based on thorough understanding of disease mechanisms. In reality,however,it is not the case in heart failure.We are treating heart failure without knowing its exact mechanisms.In this area,conversely,development of treatment has stimulated and accelerated studies on the mechanisms of disease.So in this article how each drug was introduced and how progress in understanding of mechanisms folloed will be presented.

Digitalis

Digitalis was introduced by empirical selection more than 200 years ago and it has long been known to have only mild inotropic effect and a definite bradycardic action and thus considered not sufficiently effective in controlling heart failure patients,especially in normal sinus rhythm.Recently,however,rather unexpectedly the efficacy of digitalis has been reconfirmed in trials for other more potent drugs.In the captril-digoxin trial in which digitalis was used as a control drug digitalis showed a definite improvement in both exercise tolerance and NYHA classification.In the study of milrinone survival for 3 months looks better for digitalis.These results prompted us to look for other mechanisms in the drug.Alteration of baroreceptor reflex has repeatedly been observed in heart failure in animals and patients. Many investigators demonstrated digitalis restores this alteration to some extent.Ferguson et al (1) clearly showed that digitalis supresses sympathetic nerve activity in heart failure patients and that this supression is not mediated by hemodynamic improvement. In addition digitalis was proved to reduce renin and aldosterone blood levels in patients with heart failure. Thus digitalis has increasingly been recognized effective in controlling chronic heart failure probably through novel mechanisms.

Diuretics

Diuretics were introduced empirically to mimic the improved state brought about by other means. Heart failure patients recovers often with marked diuresis.As a matter of fact digitalis was originally assumed to be a diuretic.Marked effects of diuretics in improving heart failure patients deepened our insight.These effects renewed our understanding of cardiac function curves. Furthermore conbination of cardiac function curve and venous return curve including a novel concept of mean systemic pressure introduced by Guyton (2) turned out quite effective in explaining effects of diuretics.It seems to me that analyses of effects of diuresis and venodilatation converted this term,mean systemic pressure,from theoretical assumption into clinical reality.However,it is well known that diuretics stimulate renin-angiotensin-aldoserone system and frequently evoke hyponatremia, a sign of poor prognosis. Thus effects of diuretics on long-term survival remain undetermined.

Vasodilators

Vasodilators are generally believed to have been introduced as a very first accomplishment of the brilliant progress in cardiac physiology indicating that cardiac performance is determined by cardiac contractile state,preload and afterload.

As for venous system and venodilators,their essential role in heart failure is accounted for as a determinant of mean systemic pressure, which was discussed in previous paragraph. My colleagues measured pressure-volume relationship in the forearms of heart failure patients by a pletysmographic method.Curves fitted by exponential functions turned out to be clearly separated according to the severity of heart failure.This increased venous stiffness was improved by treatments. But ca-antagonists and atrial natriuretic peptide were ineffective(3).

In understanding actions of arteriodilators,an epoch-making accomplishment was brought about by Sunagawa and Sagawa (4).They proposed to analyse the coupling between heart and arterial system by calculating the ratio between cardiac function Ees and arterial function Ea. Theoretical analyses gave the conclusion that ratio Ees/Ea should be 1.0 for the highest possible external work and 2.0 for the best energy economy.Many excellent clinical works were performed to confirm these conclusions.The index is distributed between 1.0 and 2.0 for normal subjects and far below for patients with heart failure. Recently,however,evidences have been accumulated indicating that effects of vasodilators can not be explained by mechanical vasodilating action alone.For example minoxidil with definite hemodynamic effects on resting hemodynamics was found without enough effect on exercise tolerance.In contrast an angiotensin converting enzyme inhibitor was found to have a significant improving effect on exercise tolerance in heart failure.In addition this effect proved to be attributed to increased leg skeletal muscle blood flow.Famous large scaled trials on the effects of vasodilators such as V-Heft,CONSENSUS and SOLVD have repeatedly disclosed that only some selected vasodilators especially angiotensin converting enzyme inhibitors have beneficial effects on long-term survival.These results have motivated investigators to search for novel actions in humoral factors and vasodilating drugs other than mechanical actions.Consequently many new actions such as direct cardiac effects,metabolic actions and influences on other factors have been proposed based on clinical and experimental studies.Now vasodilators have come to be classified in terms of both mechanical and non-mechanical actions.

Neurohumoral factors

Increasing numbers of neurohumoral factors have been proposed to be activated and to be playing important roles in the development of heart failure.

In understanding roles of these factors,investigators divided neurohumoral factors into 2 groups,beneficial group with vasodilating and diuretic actions (ANP,prostaglandins,EDRF etc) and aggravating group with vasoconstricting and water retaining actions (sympathetic nervous system,renin-angiotensin-aldosterone,vasopressin,endothelin,etc). As representing vasoconstrictor group,norepinephrine has been extensively studied.It is almost established that elevated norepinephrine blood levels are related to poor prognosis.Combined with recent abundant evidences indicating definite improving effects of ß-blocker on patients with dilated cardiomyopathy,these results have increasingly been interpreted as evidences supporting aggravating nature of sympathetic nervous system.However,its beneficial effects are still proposed and can not be denied completely.The situation is controversial and a clear-cut conclusion seems unrealistic as Packer advocates (5).
Then,how about atrial natriuretic peptide (ANP) representing vasodilator group? Blood ANP levels are also related to poor prognosis. Results of recent SOLVD trial confirmed that ANP blood levlel is the most reliable predictor of poor prognosis.Then,is ANP a truly favorable factor against progress of heart failure and promising as a drug? In the trial of short-term infusion of ANP conducted in Japan,injection of extrinsic ANP was demonstrated to be ineffective in patients with highest baseline intrinsic ANP blood level.The results may indicate saturated and inactive ANP receptors in advanced heart failure. A long-term treatment of heart failure patients with ANP has become possible by introduction of orally available inhibitors of ANP endopeptidase. A long-term trial is scheduled and we are expecting to have insights into the role played by ANP in chronic heart failure.

Inotropic agents

Opinions are controversial on the process of development and introduction of inotropic agents.Some investigators insist that the drug was developed theoretically because essential and final cause of heart failure is impaired cardiac muscle contractile state.Others are of opinion that inotropes have been selected at least so far depending solely on phenomenal mechanical effects ignoring inner mechanisms.We are all well aware of series of discouraging and disappointing results of large scaled and long-term trials of oral inotropic agents on survival without any exceptions in these several years.Since then active analyses and discussions have been made concerning mechanisms underlying aggravating effects of inotropic agents (6,7).A conclusion might be reached indicating that every inotropic agent is hazardous irrespective of its mechanisms. However,can we treat heart failure patients without inotropes? I think we still need "good inotropic agents",how small its possibility might be! Although angiotensin converting enzyme inhitors have been proved effective,their potency is still far below the level of our aspiration.Then what should we do to find this extremely limited possiblity? Studies on subcellular mechanisms in cardiac muscle should be encouraged and drugs should be selected by analyzing their effects on subcellular mechanisms.

The present state of our -nowledge on the effects of inotropic agents on cardiac subcellular mechanisms is rather poor (8). We are just at the starting point

REFERENCES

1. Ferguson DW,Berg JW,Sanders JS, Roach PJ,Kempf JS,Kienzle MG (1989) Sympathoinhibitory responses to digitalis glycosides in heart failure patients. Circulation 80:65-77
2. Guyton AC,Jones CE,Coleman TG (1973) Circulatory physiology 2nd ed.W.B.Saunders,Philadelphia
3. Ikenouchi H,Iizuka M,Sato H,Momomura S,Serizawa T,Sugimoto T (1991) Forearm venous distensibility in relation to severity of symptoms and hemodynamic data in patients with congestive heart failure. Jpn Heart J:17-34
4. Sunagawa K,Maughan WL,Sagawa K (1985) Optimal arterial resistance for the maximal stroke work studied in isolated canine left ventricle. Circ Res 56:586-595
5. Packer M (1990) Role of sympathetic nervous system in chronic heart failure. Circulation 82:suppl I 1-6
6. Katz AM (1978) A new inotropic drug:its promise and a caution. N Engl J Med 299:1409-1410
7. LeJemtel TH,Sonnenblick EH (1984) Should the failing heart be stimulated? N Engl J Med 310:1384-1385
8. Morgan JP (1990) Mechanisms of action of inotropic drugs. Update to Heart Disease ed Braunwald E, 136-144

Cardiotonic Drugs, Intracellular Calcium, and Failing Heart

TAI AKERA[1] and KYOSUKE TEMMA[2]

The National Children's Hospital Medical Research Center, Tokyo, 154 Japan, Merck Research Laboratories, West Point, PA 19486, U.S.A.[1] and Department of Veterinary Pharmacology, Kitasato University School of Veterinary Medicine and Animal Sciences, Aomori, 064 Japan[2]

KEYWORDS: intracellular calcium transients, positive inotropic agents, fura-2, pulse illumination, calcium overload of myocardial cells

INTRODUCTION

Electrical stimulation of myocardial cells causes membrane depolarization followed by a transient increase in cytoplasmic free Ca^{2+} concentration. This transient increase in Ca^{2+} concentration (Ca^{2+} transient) is an important rink in the excitation-contraction coupling mechanism [1,2]. In isolated heart muscle preparations, Ca^{2+} transient has been observed using aequorin or Ca^{2+} indicator dyes such as fura-2, indo-1 or quin-2 [3-9]. Except for few instances, signals were averaged from a number of cells making it impossible to examine the events that occur within a cell. Spatial changes in intracellular Ca^{2+} concentrations have been reported [10] in apparently Ca^{2+} overloaded myocytes. In the present study, temporal and spatial changes in intracellular Ca^{2+} concentration triggered by electrical stimulation were observed using fura 2-loaded myocytes isolated from guinea-pig heart. These myocytes responded to electrical stimulation and to inotropic agents in apparently normal manner. Positive and negative inotropic agents have unique effects on the initiation and propagation of the Ca^{2+} transient.

MATERIALS AND METHODS

Myocytes were isolated from guinea-pig heart (approximately 350 g, either sex) using collagenase during a low Ca^{2+} perfusion as described by Stemmer et al. [11]. Cells were loaded with fura-2 by incubating in the presence of 1 μM fura-2/AM (Molecular Probes, Eugene, Oregon) at 37°C for 15 min in HEPES buffer solution containing 130 mM NaCl, 5.8 mM KCl, 1 mM Na_2HPO_4, 1 mM $MgCl_2$, 1.2 mM $CaCl_2$, 10 mM glucose and 10 mM HEPES, and placed in an open chamber with a cover-glass bottom on the stage of an inverted epifluorescence microscope. Cells were superfused by a Krebs-Henseleit bicarbonate buffer solution containing 118 mM NaCl, 27.1 mM $NaHCO_3$, 4.8 mM KCl, 1 mM KH_2PO_4, 1.2 mM $MgSO_4$, 1.2 mM $CaCl_2$ and 10 mM glucose. The solution was saturated with a 95% O_2, 5% CO_2 gas mixture yielding the final pH value of 7.4. Only rod-shaped cells, which were attached to the glass bottom, were used. Cells were incubated at room temperature (27-28°C) and stimulated with an electrical field of 1 Hz with 4-msec pulses using a pair of platinum wire electrodes.

Details of fluorescence microscope and digital image analyzer system was described earlier [12]. The principle is to take a picture of a moving object using an electronic flash light and to obtain a still picture representing a given moment. By adjusting an interval between electrical stimulation and flash illumination, a fluorescence picture of a myocyte time-frozen at a given time point following

[1] Send communications to: Tai Akera, M.D., c/o MSD (Japan) Co., Ltd., 1-9-20 Akasaka, Minato-ku, Tokyo 117, Japan.

electrical stimulation was obtained. The cells were illuminated with 1.5-msec pulses of a xenon lamp with a predetermined delay (5 to 500 msec) after electrical stimulation. Resulting fluorescence image was stored on the screen of a silicone intensified target (SIT) camera until electronically scanned, and digitally stored in a computer. Even though this process takes more than 30 msec, the picture obtained represents that of the 1.5-msec period during which the cell was illuminated. This process was repeated 5-8 times for signal accumulation. Subsequently, time delay was altered and the whole process repeated to obtain images representing the entire cycle of myocyte functions.

Fluorescence pictures were taken at 500 nm with an excitation wavelength of 340 nm or 380 nm. After all pictures were obtained and digitalized, changes in free Ca^{2+} concentration were estimated using the method described by Grynkiewicz et al. [13].

RESULTS AND DISCUSSION

Stability of the Myocytes

Cardiac myocytes isolated from guinea-pig ventricular muscle maintained a striated, rod-shape appearance for several hours under the microscope. During preliminary studies, however, a gradual reduction in the cell length, representing a gradual development of contracture, was observed associated with an increase in diastolic intracellular Ca^{2+} concentrations. Under these conditions, cells started beating spontaneously after a 30 to 60-min incubation. Traveling waves of high intracellular Ca^{2+} concentrations were frequently observed as reported earlier by Takamatsu and Wier [10]. These waves were characterized by a band of an area with high Ca^{2+} concentrations that moves slowly from one end of the cell to another. When these waves were observed, cells fail to follow electrical stimulation. Subsequently, rod-shaped myocytes collapsed into rounded shape with extremely high intracellular Ca^{2+} concentrations. This sudden change in myocyte shape occurred 5-10 min after the start of spontaneous Ca^{2+} waves. Apparently, these traveling waves of high intracellular Ca^{2+} concentrations represent myocardial Ca^{2+} overload. These waves, however, do not appear to represent physiological functions of the myocyte.

The development of contracture and spontaneous Ca^{2+} waves was eliminated when the intensity of ultraviolet light was markedly reduced using a series of neutral density filters. Subsequently, a shutter was placed in the light path between the xenon lamp and the stage of an inverted microscope to reduce ultraviolet exposure. With these measures, myocytes maintained the rod shape for several hours with 1-Hz electrical stimulation. These cells were quiescent when electrical stimulator was turned off, and responded to each electrical stimulation by a transient increase in cytoplasmic Ca^{2+} concentration and a twitch contraction. Apparently slow traveling Ca^{2+} waves observed by Takamatsu and Wier [10] represents abnormal behavior of Ca^{2+} overloaded myocytes, and an excess exposure to ultraviolet light damages the cell and causes Ca^{2+} overload in isolated myocytes.

Pictures in the present study were obtained using signal accumulation technique. Changes in Ca^{2+} concentrations that are not time-locked to electrical stimulation are reduced by signal averaging whereas those triggered by electrical stimulation are enhanced into a clear picture.

Preliminary studies also indicated a slow time course for contraction and relaxation, and also a slow time course for Ca^{2+} transient. The time to peak Ca^{2+} transient was reduced as the degree of fura-2 loading was reduced by lowering fura-2/AM concentration and the reduction of incubation time with fura-2/AM. These results indicate that excessive fura-2 loading causes Ca^{2+} buffering of the cytoplasm as reported by Kim et al. [14]. The degree of fura-2 loading, therefore, was reduced until further reduction in the fura-2/AM concentration or incubation time failed to alter the time to peak Ca^{2+} transient. The reduction in the intensity of activating ultraviolet light and the reduction of fura-2 loading, however, resulted in the need for signal accumulation to obtain clear image of the intracellular Ca^{2+} distribution. The conditions described in the MATERIALS AND METHODS section are those optimized and used in the following studies.

Initiation and Propagation of Ca^{2+} Transients

Electrical field stimulation of isolated myocytes caused Ca^{2+} concentration to increase at the inner surface of the sarcolemma. Such an increase started at one fixed site within a myocyte in about 50% of the cells. In other cells, Ca^{2+} transient originated at two, three or multiple sites. The first sign of an increase in intracellular Ca^{2+} concentration was observed at 5-10 msec after electrical stimulation. Subsequently, the area of elevated Ca^{2+} concentration spread through the cell.

When a rod-shaped myocyte had a single initiating site at one end, it required about 60 msec for the Ca^{2+} transient to spread into entire volume of the cell. The length of a typical myocyte was 100 μm. The speed at which the front of the Ca^{2+} transient to advance within a myocyte is approximately 2 μm/msec. At about 25 msec after the electrical stimulation, half of area within a myocyte had high Ca^{2+} concentration whereas the other half had a low Ca^{2+} concentration of resting myocyte. The peak intracellular Ca^{2+} concentration was reached at about 80-100 msec after electrical stimulation. Subsequently, intracellular Ca^{2+} concentration decreased uniformly. During the declining phase, no difference in intracellular Ca^{2+} distribution was observed. The intracellular Ca^{2+} concentration returned to a low resting level approximately 500 msec after electrical stimulation when myocytes were stimulated at 1 Hz. These changes in intracellular Ca^{2+} concentration was closely followed by twitch shortening and relaxation of the myocyte. It was possible to observe changes in the shape of myocytes that are loosely attached to the glass bottom of the incubation chamber.

It may be noted that the time courses of Ca^{2+} transient and twitch contraction were relatively slow even when the degree of fura-2 loading was reduced. Low incubation temperature (27-28°C) is apparently responsible for slow time course of Ca^{2+} transient and also slow contraction and relaxation of isolated guinea-pig myocytes. That the reaction time for fura-2 is not the rate-limiting step was shown when similar study was performed using myocytes isolated from rat heart. Rat myocytes, which are known for short action potential duration and short twitch contraction, had shorter duration of the Ca^{2+} transient observed with the current technique. The possibility that a part of cytoplasmic Ca^{2+} is buffered by fura-2, however, cannot be excluded. Apparently, it is necessary for a part of Ca^{2+} to bind to fura-2 to cause changes in fluorescence.

In several myocytes, seemingly uniform increases in intracellular Ca^{2+} concentration responding to electrical stimulation were observed. Close examination of these cells, however, suggests that these cells have multiple foci from which Ca^{2+} transients originate.

The waves of intracellular Ca^{2+} reported by Takamatsu and Wier [10] and those observed in the present study have different characteristics. Those reported by above investigators are relatively narrow bands of high Ca^{2+} concentrations. These bands slowly move from one end of the cell to another. These waves are not time-locked to electrical stimulation. Those observed in the present study originate from one or few fixed sites within a myocyte. Instead of forming a relatively narrow band, the area of high Ca^{2+} concentration spreads from these foci to the entire cell. At the peak cytoplasmic Ca^{2+} concentration, the entire cell volume is filled with high Ca^{2+} concentration. Moreover, these Ca^{2+} transients are triggered by electrical stimulation, and apparently followed by twitch contractions.

Initiating Sites for Ca^{2+} Transients

An exposure to 0.5 μM verapamil caused 25 min later a myocyte which had two initiating foci to lose one of the sites. Apparently, one focus was eliminated by verapamil. Similar results were observed with myocytes showing multiple foci. Dose- and time-dependent extinction of the originating sites were observed. These results indicate that the initial increase in Ca^{2+} concentration at the inner surface of the sarcolemma is apparently caused by Ca^{2+} influx through the Ca^{2+} channels.

In an instance where three longitudinally connecting myocytes were isolated, electrical field stimulation caused Ca^{2+} transient to originate at one site in each cell. Punctate stimulation of one of the myocytes using a microelectrode, placed near the surface at the end opposite to the originating site observed in that cell, initiated the Ca^{2+} transient not at the site of electrode attachment but at the same site at which Ca^{2+} transient originated with electrical field stimulation. These results indicate that each myocyte has one or several sites at which membrane excitation triggers Ca^{2+} transitent more easily. It is presently unknown if Ca^{2+} channels are clustered at these sites or if there are special arrangements of intracellular organelles. These sites, however, may be inactivated by the Ca^{2+} channel blocker, verapamil.

These results are consistent with the following hypothesis. Each myocyte has one or several cytoplasmic sites at which intracellular Ca^{2+} concentration increases more easily following membrane depolarization. Such an increase in cytoplasmic Ca^{2+} concentration triggers Ca^{2+}-induced Ca^{2+}-release from the sarcoplasmic reticulum. When this occurs, cytoplasmic Ca^{2+} concentration is markedly increased at that site, and triggers Ca^{2+} release from adjacent sarcoplasmic reticulum. This process spreads into the entire cell volume.

Positive Inotropic Interventions

Ouabain (0.5 μM) enhanced the Ca^{2+} transients. The speed at which cytoplasmic Ca^{2+} concentration increases and also the Ca^{2+} concentration at the peak of the transient were markedly increased. The number of originating sites, however, was unchanged. The time course of the Ca^{2+} transient was also unchanged.

Isoproterenol (0.1 μM) also increased the Ca^{2+} concentration at the peak of the transient, and also markedly increased the speed at which cytoplasmic Ca^{2+} concentration increased. With isoproterenol, however, the time to peak Ca^{2+} transient was reduced, and the decrease in cytoplasmic Ca^{2+} concentration following the peak was rapid. Moreover, the number of originating sites were increased by isoproterenol. For example, myocytes that had only one initiating site showed several initiating sites in the presence of isoproterenol.

The effect of isoproterenol to increase the number of initiating sites was mimicked when extracellular Ca^{2+} concentration was increased. An increase in extracellular Ca^{2+} concentration, however, failed to cause a significant change in the time course of Ca^{2+} transients even though the number of originating sites was increased. An increase in extracellular Ca^{2+} concentration should increase Ca^{2+} influx. This effect seems to be responsible for the increase in the number of initiating sites. Ca^{2+} loading of the sarcoplasmic reticulum should be increased by an increase in extracellular Ca^{2+} concentration. This effect, however, was apparently unrelated to changes in the time course of the Ca^{2+} transient. Isoproterenol-induced changes in time course of the Ca^{2+} transient are likely to result from alterations in kinetics of Ca^{2+} release and Ca^{2+} uptake by the sarcoplasmic reticulum.

Theoretically, the time to peak Ca^{2+} transient should be shortened when the Ca^{2+} transient originates from multiple sites, instead of a single site especially at one end of a rod-shaped cell. The fact that this was not the case would indicate that the time to peak Ca^{2+} transient is primarily determined by the time required for Ca^{2+} to be released from the sarcoplasmic reticulum, instead of the time required for the Ca^{2+} transient to reach one end of the cell to another.

A decrease in extracellular Na^+ concentration increases Ca^{2+} loading of the sarcoplasmic reticulum via modification of the sarcolemmal Na^+/Ca^{2+} exchange reaction. When extracellular Na^+

concentration was reduced to 75 mM, changes similar to those caused by ouabain were observed. The number of initiating sites for Ca^{2+} transient was unchanged. The magnitude of the Ca^{2+} transient was markedly enhanced without changes in the time course of the Ca^{2+} transient. These results are consistent with the hypothesis that both ouabain and low extracellular Na^{+} enhance the Ca^{2+} loading of the sarcoplasmic reticulum and enhance the Ca^{2+} transient. The number of the initiating sites for Ca^{2+} transient, however, is related to Ca^{2+} influx via Ca^{2+} channels.

Failing Heart

Gwathmey et al. [15] demonstrated using aequorin that human myocardium obtained from a failing heart shows the pattern of Ca^{2+} transient typical of Ca^{2+} overloading. In isolated myocytes exposed to simulated ischemia and reperfusion, resting Ca^{2+} was elevated [16]. The magnitude of the Ca^{2+} transient was markedly reduced primarily because of an elevated resting Ca^{2+} concentration. The peak Ca^{2+} concentration *per se* was not significantly altered. During simulated reperfusion, resting Ca^{2+} concentration decreased but the magnitude of the Ca^{2+} transient was unchanged. The number of initiating sites was unchanged by simulated ischemia or reperfusion.

CONCLUSION

In fura 2-loaded myocytes, electrical stimulation initiates Ca^{2+} transient at one or few fixed sites. Agents that decrease or increase the Ca^{2+} influx may decrease or increase the number of initiating sites. Positive inotropic interventions that increase Ca^{2+} loading of the sarcoplasmic reticulum enhance Ca^{2+} transient without altering the pattern of initiation and propagation.

REFERENCES

1. Fabiato A (1983) Calcium-induced release of calcium from the cardiac sarcoplasmic reticulum. Am J Physiol 245: C1-C14
2. Blinks JR (1986) Intracellular [Ca^{2+}] measurements. In: Fozzard HA, Haber E, Jennings RB, Katz AM, Morgan HE (eds) The Heart and Cardiovascular System. Raven Press. New York
3. Allen DG, Blinks JR (1978) Calcium transients in aequorin-injected frog cardiac muscle. Nature (London) 273: 509-513
4. Wier WG (1980) Calcium transients during excitation-contraction coupling in mammalian heart: Aequorin signals of canine Purkinje fibers. Science 207: 1085-1087
5. Morgan JP, Blinks JR (1982) Intracellular Ca^{2+} transients in the cat papillary muscle. Can J Physiol Pharmacol 60: 524-528
6. Barcenas-Ruiz L, Beuckelmann DJ, Wier WG (1987) Sodium-calcium exchange in heart: membrane currents and changes in [Ca^{2+}]. Science 238: 1720-1722
7. Lee HC, Smith N, Mohabir R, Clusin WT (1987) Cytosolic calcium transients from the beating mammalian heart. Proc Natl Acad Sci USA 84: 7793-7797
8. Peeters GA, Hlady V, Bridge JHB, Barry WH (1987) Simultaneous measurement of calcium transients and motion in cultured heart cells. Am J Physiol 253: H1400-H1408
9. Thomas AP, Selak M, Williamson JR (1986) Measurement of electrically-induced Ca^{2+} transients in quin 2-loaded cardiac myocytes. J Mol Cell Cardiol 18: 541-545
10. Takamatsu T, Wier WG (1990) Calcium waves in mammalian heart: quantification of origin, magnitude, waveform and velocity. FASEB J 4: 1519-1525
11. Stemmer P, Akera T, Brody TM, Rardon DP, Watanabe AM (1989) Isolation and enrichment of Ca^{2+}-tolerant myocytes for biochemical experiments from guinea-pig heart. Life Sci 44: 1231-1237
12. Akera T, Temma K, Kondo H, Hagane K (1990) Digital imaging system for recording rapid changes in intracellular Ca concentrations triggered by electrical stimulation of cardiac

myocytes. Keio J Med 39: 168-172

13. Grynkiewicz G, Poenie M, Tsien RY (1985) A new generation of Ca^{2+} indicators with greatly improved fluorescence properties. J Biol Chem 260: 3440-3450
14. Kim D, Okada A, Smith TW (1987) Control of cytosolic calcium activity during low sodium exposure in cultured chick heart cells. Circ Res 61: 29-41
15. Gwathmey JK, Copelas L, MacKinnon R, Schoen FJ, Feldman MD, Grossman W, Morgan JP (1987) Abnormal intracellular calcium handling in myocardium with patients with end-stage heart failure. Circ Res 61: 70-76
16. Koyama T, Temma, K, Akera T (1991) Reperfusion-induced contracture develops with a decreasing $[Ca^{2+}]i$ in single heart cells. Am J Physiol 261: H1115-H1122

Myocardial Calcium Sensitivity and Energy Turnover as Modulated by Inorganic Phosphate and EMD 53998, a Novel Inotropic Agent

JOACHIM W. HERZIG, HEIDRUN DEPERSIN, and WIM J. LEIJENDEKKER

Pharmaceuticals Division, Department Research CVS, Ciba-Geigy Ltd., Basle, Switzerland

INTRODUCTION

During the last years, increasing evidence has accumulated that calcium sensitivity of the myocardium, i.e. the relationship between myocytal cytosolic free calcium and the degree of contractile activation, is not a constant but is subject to physiological and pathophysiological alterations and may also be influenced pharmacologically [1,2,3,4]. For instance, Frank-Starling's effect, i.e. the increase in contractility on the ascending limb of the myocardial pressure volume curve, appears to be based predominantly on an increase in calcium sensitivity with increasing sarcomere length [5]. On the other hand, e.g. in the hypoxic heart [6] as well as in early pump failure [7], the sensitivity of the myocardium to activator calcium is reduced. Accumulation of inorganic phosphate (Pi) under these latter conditions may lead to intracellular Pi concentrations as high as 48 mM [7], normal values being near 5 mM. In the light of this, we compared the calcium desensitizing effect of Pi with the calcium sensitizing effect of EMD 53998, a novel inotropic agent [8] (for structural formula, see Fig. 4), in skinned fibres prepared from porcine right ventricular muscle.

METHODS

Details of the methods used in the present study are described in [9]. In brief, experiments were carried out in thin bundles of porcine trabecula septo-marginalis skinned with Triton X-100. By this treatment, the membrane systems of sarcolemma and sarcoplasmic reticulum are destroyed, whereas the myofibrillar system remains functionable. The bundles were isometrically contracted in solutions containing MgATP and Ca ions buffered to distinct pCa values using EGTA. ATP consumption was determined using an NADH coupled optical assay. All experiments were carried out at room temperature.

RESULTS AND DISCUSSION

Figure 1 shows the influence of increasing inorganic phosphate (Pi) concentration on the calcium activation curve of the myocardial skinned fibres. Besides a most prominent depression of maximum calcium activation, there is also a shift of the calcium activation curve to higher calcium concentrations. This indicates that both "efficacy" and "potency" of calcium ions are reduced by Pi (cf. also [10]). The concentration range in which Pi exhibits such a calcium desensitizing action (5 to 50 mM) is the range within which inorganic phosphate has been reported to occur during early pump failure [7] of the ischaemic heart. Therefore, such calcium desensitization may be taken as a model for this particular condition of myocardial dysfunction.

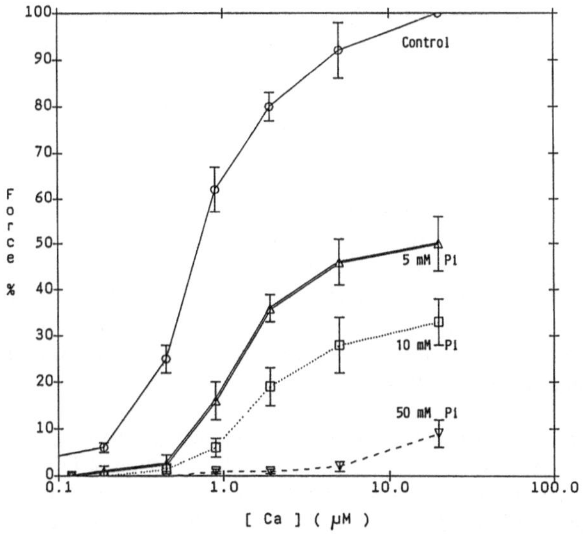

Fig. 1 Calcium dependence of force as influenced by inorganic phosphate (Pi)
Note that with increasing Pi concentration the calcium activation curve is depressed and shifted to the right to higher calcium concentrations.
Triton skinned porcine trabecula septo-marginalis, Means +/- SEM, n=6

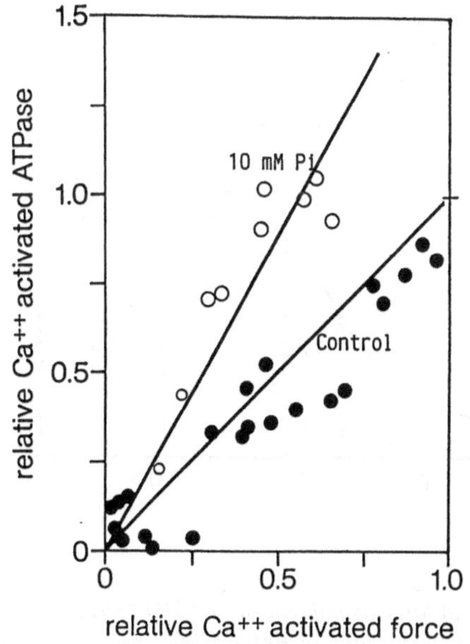

Fig.2 Influence of 10 mM inorganic phosphate (Pi) on tension cost (ATP consumed per force generated)
Note the increase in ATP consumption by Pi at any level of calcium activated force.
After [11], modified.

As already reported earlier [11], calcium desensitization with inorganic phosphate is accompanied by an increase in tension cost (see figure 2), i.e. any given active tension is, in presence of 10 mM Pi, generated at a higher actomyosin ATP turnover than in absence of Pi. Mechanical investigations suggested that this is based on an acceleration of the actomyosin crossbridge turnover, thereby reducing the time that a crossbridge dwells in the force generating state [11].

Fig. 3 shows the influence of EMD 53998, a novel calcium sensitizing inotropic agent, on the calcium activation curve of porcine myocardial skinned fibres. Roughly, the effect of this agent may be described as the opposite of the Pi effect reported above: Both "efficacy" and "potency" of calcium ions are enhanced. This leads to a prominent calcium sensitizing effect characterized by the fact that at any free calcium ion concentration between 0.01 and 48 µM, force development of the skinned fibre preparation is enhanced by EMD 53998.

Taking into account the rather opposite effects of Pi and EMD 53998 on the calcium sensitivity, we investigated whether the calcium desensitizing action of Pi (see figure 1) can be counteracted by the calcium sensitizing action of EMD 53998 (see figure 3). Fig. 4 shows that this is indeed the case. 10 µM EMD 53998 were found to be just sufficient to abolish the depression of the calcium activation curve induced by 10 mM Pi. At the same time, there is a leftward displacement of the calcium activation curve to calcium concentrations lower than under control conditions. Thus, EMD 53998 appears to counteract the depression of both calcium "efficacy" as well as calcium "potency" induced by Pi.

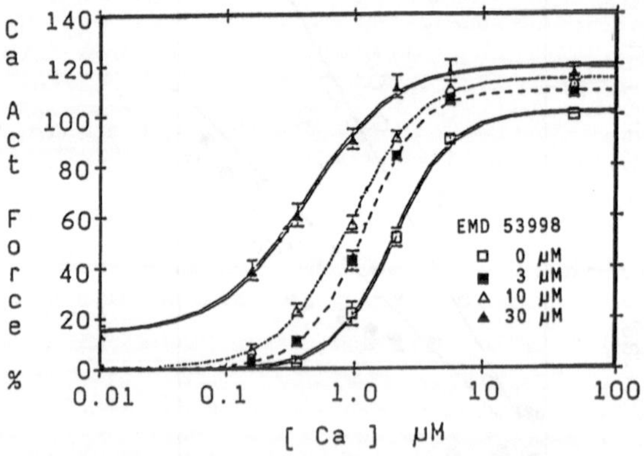

Fig.3 Calcium dependence of force as influenced by EMD 53998
Note that with increasing concentration of EMD 53998 the calcium activation curve is shifted to the left to lower calcium concentrations, and that maximum calcium activated force is potentiated.
Triton skinned porcine trabecula septo-marginalis, Means +/- SEM, n=6.

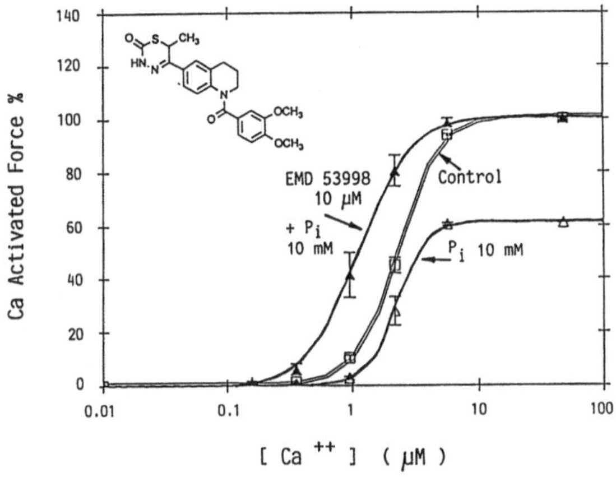

Fig.4 Influence of 10 μM EMD 53998 on the calcium activation curve suppressed by 10 mM inorganic phosphate (Pi)
Note that also in presence of 10 mM Pi, EMD 53998 leads to a leftward shift of the calcium activation curve to lower calcium concentrations, and that maximum calcium activated force is potentiated by EMD 53998, also in presence of Pi.
Triton skinned porcine trabecula septo-marginalis, Means +/- SEM, n=4.

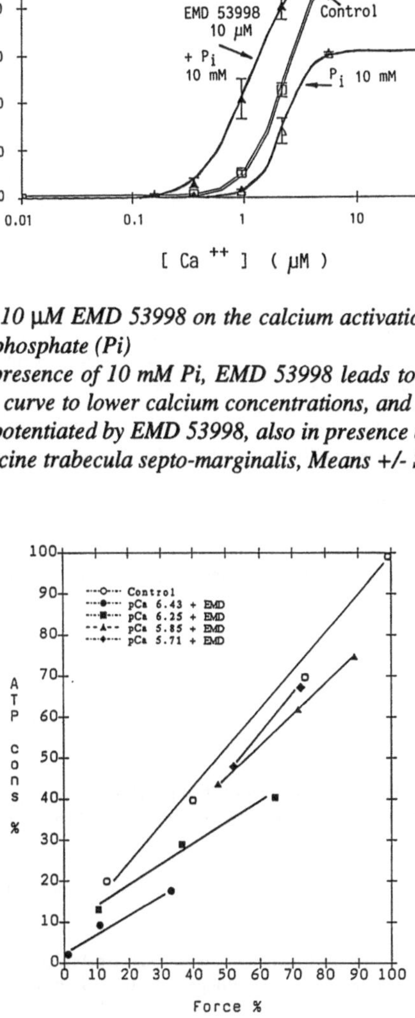

Fig. 5 Influence of EMD 53998 on tension cost (ATP consumed per force generated)
Note that only when force is increased by addition of EMD 53998, 1-30 μM, at a constant pCa of 6.25 or higher, ATP consumption is less stimulated than when similar forces are achieved by increasing the calcium concentration in absence of EMD 53998.
Triton skinned porcine trabecula septo-marginalis.

As the calcium desensitizing action of Pi is associated with an increase in tension cost (see Fig. 2), we investigated, for comparison, the effect of EMD 53998 on force and ATP consumption. Figure 5 shows that, when force is increased by addition of increasing concentrations of EMD 53998 at a constant pCa of 6.25 or higher, less ATP is split by the contractile system per force generated than under conditions when force is increased by addition of calcium ions. It is important to mention that this "economizing" effect of EMD 53998 is only observed at pCa values exceeding 6 and is abolished below pCa 6 (cf also [9]). It has been suggested that, in the range of low calcium concentrations, the crossbridge turnover rate is low [12], an effect which at normal calcium sensitivity may not be observed (due to lack of contractile response) but which is functionally unmasked by the calcium sensitizing effect of EMD 53998 (cf. [9]). This may be expected to result in a reduction of myocardial energy demand, also in the intact heart and in vivo, an effect which would be of eminent functional importance, especially in the failing heart.

REFERENCES

1. Herzig JW, Feile K, Ruegg, JC (1981) Activating effects of AR-L 115 BS on the calcium sensitive force, stiffness and unloaded shortening velocity (Vmax) in isolated contractile structures from mammalian heart muscle. Arzneim Forsch / Drug Res 31: 188

2. Solaro RJ, Ruegg JC (1982) Stimulation of calcium binding and ATPase activity of dog cardiac myofibrils by AR-L 115 BS, a novel cardiotonic agent. Circ Res 51: 290

3. Ruegg JC (1986) Effects of new inotropic agents on calcium sensitivity of contractile proteins. Circulation 73(Suppl III): 78

4. Wetzel B, Hauel N (1988) New cardiotonic agents - promising approach for treatment of heart failure. TIPS 9: 166

5. Allen DG, Kentish JC (1988) Calcium concentration in the myoplasm of skinned ferret ventricular muscle following changes in muscle length. J Physiol (Lond) 407: 489

6. Allen DG, Orchard CH (1987) Myocardial contractile function during ischaemia and hypoxia. Circ Res 60: 153

7. Kubler W, Katz AM (1977) Mechanism of early "pump" failure of the ischaemic heart: possible role of adenosine triphosphate depletion and inorganic phosphate accumulation. Am J Cardiol 40: 467

8. Lee JA, Allen DG (1990) Calcium sensitisers - a new approach to increasing the strength of the heart. Br Med J 300: 551

9. Leijendekker WJ, Herzig JW (1992) Reduction of myocardial crossbridge turnover rate in presence of EMD 53998, a novel calcium sensitizing agent. Pfluger's Arch Eur J Physiol in press

10. Kentish JC (1986) The effects of inorganic phosphate and creatine phosphate on force production in skinned muscles from rat ventricle. J Physiol (Lond) 370: 585

11. Herzig JW, Peterson JW, Ruegg JC, Solaro RJ (1981) Vanadate and phosphate ions reduce tension and increase crossbridge kinetics in chemically skinned heart muscle. Biochim Biophys Acta 672: 191

12. Herzig JW, Herzig UB (1974) Effect of calcium ions on contraction speed and force generation in glycerinated heart muscle. Symp Biol Hung 17: 85

VI: Ischemic Heart Disease

Left Ventricular Diastolic Function in Effort Angina Pectoris

AKIRA TAMURA, KAZUHIRO KATAYAMA, MASUNORI MATSUZAKI, YASUHIRO IKEDA, TAKESHI YAMAMOTO, KOHZABURO SEKI, TOSHIRO MIURA, MASAFUMI YANO, MICHIHIRO KOHNO, TAKASHI FUJII, and REIZO KUSUKAWA

The Second Department of Internal Medicine, Yamaguchi University School of Medicine, Yamaguchi, 755 Japan

KEYWORDS: effort angina pectoris, diastolic function, left ventriculography

INTRODUCTION

Diastolic function of the left ventricle is well known to be disturbed in patients with coronary artery disease [1,2]. There are few reports which analyzed left ventricular (LV) regional diastolic function using a left ventriculogram with simultaneous LV pressure. The purpose of this study was to analyze LV regional diastolic function in stable effort angina pectoris (AP) without myocardial infarction.

METHODS

Left ventriculography (biplane method:30°RAO,60°LAO) was performed using a Millar's catheter-tip micromanometer in 9 normal subjects (N) and 14 AP patients with isolated organic stenosis (≥75%) of left anterior descending (LAD) coronary artery. AP group was divided into 2 subgroups. AP1 (n=9) was defined as patients without angiographically delay. AP2 (n=5) was defined as patients with angiographically delay. There were not significant differences in mean age between 3 groups (N:51±8years,AP1:55±7,AP2:61±12). LV volume (V), regional area (S) and the first derivative of V and S (dV/dt, dS/dt) were derived from the frame-by-frame analysis of left ventriculogram. Left ventriculogram taken from a 30°RAO projection was divided into 3 regions (anterior, apex and inferior) as described before [3]. Peak filling rate (PFR) and peak atrial filling rate (PAFR) were derived from dV/dt and normalized for end-diastolic volume (nPFR, nPAFR). The ratio of filling volume to stroke volume during rapid filling, slow filling and atrial contraction phases were defined as rapid filling fraction (RFF), slow filling fraction (SFF) and atrial filling fraction (AFF). Likewise, regional PFR, PAFR, RFF, SFF and AFF were derived from S and dS/dt. We also calculated time constant of LV relaxation (T) and indexes of LV global and regional compliance at end-diastole (ED) {(dV/VdP)ed, (dS/SdP)ed} [4]. The data are presented as the mean±SD. Statistical comparison of data between 3 groups was performed by analysis of variance (ANOVA). If significant differences ($p<0.05$) were found, multiple comparison test (Fisher PLSD) was performed between 2 groups. The level of statistical significance was considered at p value less than 0.05.

RESULTS AND DISCUSSION

Time constant (T) [N:36±6msec,AP1:44±6,AP2:45±5] prolonged significantly in AP group compared with N. In AP group, nPFR significantly decreased compared with N (N:3.32±0.47 sec^{-1},AP1:2.67±0.73,AP2:2.03±0.21), however, nPAFR (N:2.72±0.89sec^{-1},AP1:2.43±0.73,

AP2:2.41±0.61) and (dV/VdP)ed [N:0.052±0.027mmHg-1,AP1:0.055±0.028,AP2:0.066±0.065] showed no significant differences between 3 groups. RFF (N:66±8%,AP1:66±4,AP2:55±6) decreased significantly in AP2 compared with other groups. SFF (N:3±3%,AP1:3±4,AP2:7±7) showed no significant differences between 3 groups. AFF (N:30±9%,AP1:31±5,AP2:38±11) tended to increase in AP2 compared with other groups.

Table 1 Regional diastolic parameters.

		N	AP1	AP2
nPFR (sec^{-1})	anterior	2.40±0.67	1.55±0.53**	1.20±0.38**
	apex	2.51±0.64	2.07±0.51	1.76±0.57*
	inferior	2.36±0.55	2.09±0.61	1.91±0.57
nPAFR (sec^{-1})	anterior	1.72±0.58	1.74±0.45	1.72±0.49
	apex	1.70±0.40	2.00±0.82	1.61±0.87
	inferior	1.17±0.53	1.00±0.36	0.88±0.32
(dS/SdP)ed ($mmHg^{-1}$)	anterior	0.038±0.017	0.044±0.022	0.056±0.057
	apex	0.032±0.020	0.042±0.022	0.048±0.067
	inferior	0.025±0.017	0.023±0.012	0.023±0.016
RFF (%)	anterior	67±5	63±8	45±9**§§
	apex	74±11	69±7	63±12
	inferior	71±13	74±7	73±10
AFF (%)	anterior	29±6	34±7	52±11**§§
	apex	22±8	29±7	31±19
	inferior	24±13	20±4	20±10

N:normal, AP1:angina pectoris group 1, AP2:angina pectoris group 2
nPFR:normalized peak filling rate, nPAFR:normalized peak atrial filling rate,
(dS/SdP)ed:normalized regional compliance at end-diastole,
RFF:rapid filling fraction, AFF:atrial filling fraction. Values are mean ± SD.
*:P<0.05 normal vs AP1 or AP2, **:P<0.01 normal vs AP1 or AP2
§:P<0.05 AP1 vs AP2, §§:P<0.01 AP1 vs AP2

End-systole (ES) of each regional area change curve (S) were almost simultaneous, and synchronicity of the LV wall motion between each region were preserved in N. However, in AP2, the time of regional ES were different between 3 regions and synchronicity of the LV wall motion was lost. Abnormal wall motions were often found during the early diastole in anterior and apex regions of AP2. As shown in Table 1, nPFR decreased significantly in anterior region of AP1 and AP2, and in apex region of AP2 compared with N. Between 3 groups of each region, nPAFR had no significant differences. (dS/SdP)ed had no significant differences between 3 groups of each region, but tended to increase in anterior and apex regions of AP group compared with N. RFF significantly decreased in anterior region of AP2 compared with other groups. SFF had no significant differences between N (anterior:4±4%, apex:4±5,inferior:5±6), AP1(anterior:4±6%,apex: 2±4,inferior:6±7) and AP2 (anterior:3±4%, apex:6±8,inferior:6±6) of each region. AFF increased significantly only in anterior region of AP2 compared with other groups. AFF had a tightest inverse correlation with RFF in anterior region (r=-0.92,p<0.001) compared with apex (r=-0.86,p<0.001) and inferior (r=-0.79, p<0.001) regions. AFF also had a significant inverse correlation with nPFR only in anterior region (r=-0.57,p<0.01). In the affected region of AP group, (dS/SdP)ed tended to increase.

Thus, LV global (T,nPFR) and regional (nPFR,RFF) early diastolic function were impaired in the affected region supplied by LAD of AP group. While the rapid filling was impaired, nPAFR was maintained and AFF was increased in the affected region supplied by LAD. Furthermore, nPFR and RFF had significant inverse correlations with AFF in anterior region. In the present study, relaxation disturbance [5], LV asynchrony [6,7] and impairment of elastic recoil [8] were considered as the major causes of LV regional early diastolic filling impairment in AP group. Moreover, LV wall of AP group seemed to be as compliant as that of N, because nPAFR was preserved almost normally and indexes of LV regional compliance at ED was not decreased in the affected region supplied by LAD of AP group compared with N. The relationships between AFF and RFF, and between AFF and nPFR suggested that the more severely LV early diastolic filling was impaired, the more greatly atrial contraction contributed to LV filling in the affected region. Although the AP group was considered to have sustained ischemia or myocardial hibernation because of chronic hypoperfusion, LV regional compliance was preserved and LV wall was stretched sufficiently at atrial contraction phase. The reason why AFF increased in the affected region supplied by LAD seemed to be the relative increase resulted from decreased RFF, without changes in SFF. In conclusion, the frame-by-frame analysis of left ventriculogram showed that left ventricular global and regional early diastolic function were simultaneously impaired at rest in patients with effort angina pectoris who had isolated organic stenosis of LAD. Although the rapid filling was impaired, the passive filling during atrial contraction was preserved in the affected region supplied by LAD of effort angina pectoris without myocardial infarction.

REFERENCES

1. Bonow RO, Bacharach SL, Green MV, Kent KM, Rosing DR, Lipson LC, Leon MB, Epstein SE (1981) Impaired left ventricular diastolic filling in patients with coronary artery disease: assessment with radionuclide angiography. Circulation 64: 315-323
2. Aroesty JM, McKay RG, Heller GV, Royal HD, Als AV, Grossman W. Simultaneous assessment of left ventricular systolic and diastolic dysfunction during pacing-induced ischemia. Circulation 1985; 71: 889-900
3. Katayama K, Matsuzaki M, Khono M, Fujii T, Ohtani N, Yatabe S, Ogawa H, Ozaki M, Matsuda Y, Kusukawa R (1990) Global and regional diastolic filling dynamics in compensated dilated cardiomyopathy. Jpn Circ J 54: 624-635
4. Gaasch WH, Battle WE, Oboler AA, Banas JS Jr, Levine HJ (1972) Left ventricular stress and compliance in man: with special reference to normalized ventricular function curves. Circulation 45: 746-762
5. Gewirtz H, Ohley W, Walsh J, Shearer D, Sullivan MJ, Most AS (1983) Ischemia-induced impairment of left ventricular relaxation: relation to reduced diastolic filling rates of the left ventricle. Am Heart J 105: 72-80
6. Yamagishi T, Ozaki M, Kumada T, Ikezono T, Shimizu T, Furutani Y, Yamaoka H, Ogawa H, Matsuzaki M, Matsuda Y, Arima A, Kusukawa R (1984) Asynchronous left ventricular diastolic filling in patients with isolated disease of the left anterior descending coronary artery: assessment with radionuclide ventriculography. Circulation 69: 933-942
7. Zile MR, Blaustein AS, Shimizu G, Gaasch WH (1987) Right ventricular pacing reduces the rate of left ventricular relaxation and filling. J Am Coll Cardiol 10: 702-709
8. Udelson JE, Bacharach SL, Cannon RO III, Bonow RO (1990) Minimum left ventricular pressure during ß-adrenergic stimulation in human subjects: evidence for elastic recoil and diastolic "suction" in the normal heart. Circulation 82: 1174-1182

The Effect of N,N,N-Trimethylsphingosine on Reperfusion Injury

KUNIHIKO IMAI[1], NOBUTUNE HIRAHARA[1], HIROSHI KAMIYAMA[1], FUMIO NAGANUMA[1], TADASHI SUZUKI[1], and SEIKI MINAMIDE[2]

Second Department of Internal Medicine, Gunma University, Gunma, 371 Japan[1] and Japan Immunoresearch Laboratories, Gunma, 370 Japan[2]

KEYWORDS: N,N,N-Trimethylsphingosine, Reperfusion Injury, Coronary Vasodilator Reserve,

INTRODUCTION

The paradoxical phenomenon of the exacerbation of myocardial injury after reintroduction of blood into the ischemic tissue of the heart is well known. It has been reported that in the relatively short time from 15 to 30 min of reperfusion, a supply of neutropenic blood reduced myocardial infarct size in ischemia-reperfusion canine models . The neutrophils play a major role in the exacerbation of myocardial injury[1][2]. N,N,N-Trimethylsphingosine(TMS) derived from sphingosine strongly inhibits oxidative burst and phagokinetic migration of neutrophils, due to its inhibitory effect on protein kinase C (Kimura S, Hakomori S, Igarashi Y, et al.,submitted). Based on this finding, the possible protective effect of TMS on reperfusion injury in dog heart was studied.

MATERIALS AND METHODS

Fourteen adult mongrel dogs(15-25 kg body weight) were divided into 2 groups of 7 dogs each, one treated with TMS and the other without TMS as control. Dogs were anesthetized with pentobarbital sodium(30 mg/kg), and ventilated by respirator. Thoracotomy was performed at the left fifth intercostal space, and the heart suspended in a pericardial cradle. A cuff occluder was set at the proximal end of the left anterior descending artery(LAD) and a point, 1.0-1.5cm distal to the occluder was cannulated in order to measure coronary artery pressure and for drug administration. Wire type tissue electrodes were set in the central portion of the ischemic and non-ischemic areas in order to measure regional myocardial blood flow by the hydrogen clearance method. To measure left ventricular end-diastolic pressure and dp/dt, a catheter was inserted into the right carotid artery through the left ventricle. The right femoral artery was cannulated to measure systemic pressure and the femoral vein was used for drug administration. After ischemia by LAD occlusion for 90 min, reperfusion by releasing occluder was maintained for 6 hrs, TMS saline solution(0.4 mg/kg) was administered by drip infusion 10 min before reperfusion and the drip infusion was continued for 60 min. Seven dogs were administered saline only as control. The systemic blood presure, heart rate, left ventricular end-diastolic pressure and dp/dt were measured before LAD occlusion as baseline and 1 hr after reperfusion. Coronary artery blood pressure and regional myocardial blood flow were measured before and during drug administration.

Abbreviation. TMS, N,N,N-Trimethylsphingosine; Ach, acetylcholine; NP, nitroprusside LAD, left anterior descending artery; RBF, regional blood flow, CVR, coronary vascular resistance.

Acetylcholine(Ach;0.1 μg/kg/min, for 4 min) and nitroprusside(NP;0.4 μg/kg/min, for 4 min) were administered into the LAD in order to estimate coronary vasodilatative reaction (Fig.1).

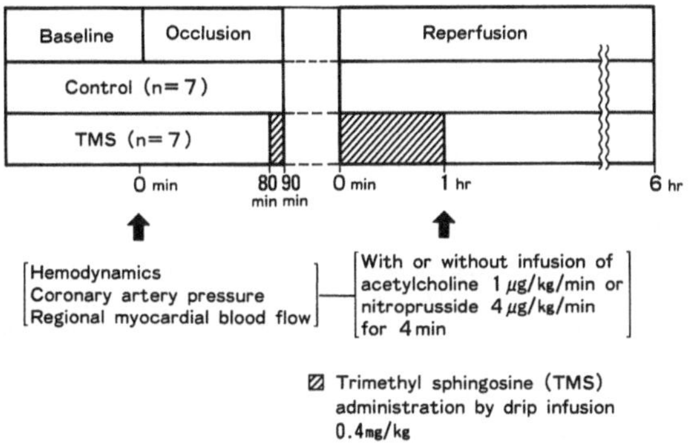

Fig.1 Experimental Protocal

After reperfusion for 6 hrs, methyleneblue(5 %, 50 ml) was administered through the left atrial appendage with ligation of LAD, and then the heart was removed after euthanasia. From a transeverse section of the heart, the ischemic area was measured using methyleneblue and the infarct size was determined using triphenyltetrazolium chlolide. Electron microscopic examination was performed on the ischemic and infarct areas. N,N,N-trimethylsphingosine(TMS, MW=342) was purchased from the Biomembrane Institute (Seattle, USA). Acetylcholine chloride, nitroprusside, triphenyltetrazolium, methyleneblue(all from Sigma), and pentobarbital sodium(Dainippon pharma.) were used in this study.

Statistics

All data were analysed by student's-test, and p<0.05 was considered statistically significant. Results were expressed as mean±SEM.

RESULTS

Regional blood flow(RBF) and coronary vascular resistance(CVR) data are summarized in Table 1. The decrease of RBF and the increase of CVR in reflow at 1 hr were noted as significant in control when compared with baseline(before occlusion) regardless Ach and NP. While the TMS treated group showed the same RBF and CVR response as control without drugs, the vasodilative vascular response to Ach and NP was satisfactorily preserved. There was no significant differences in either ischemic size nor in its ratio to left ventricular area between control and TMS treated groups(CONTROL;49.3±2.4% vs TMS;45.6± 4.9% p=NS). However, the percentage of infarct size was significantly reduced in the TMS treated group when compared to control(CONTROL;30.3±8.5% vs TMS;10.1±3.9%, p<0.05). Electron microscopic examination supported the protective effect of TMS on the reperfusion injury, namely, the appearance of vascular endothelial cells in the TMS treated dogs remained almost intact, while there were degenerative changes such as vacuolation and edema of endothelial cells and elastic lamina in control. Hemodynamic data are shown in Table 2. There were no significant differences between control and TMS treated groups. Except for mean blood pressure(both control and TMS treated groups) and end-diastolic pressure(TMS treated groups only), there were significant differences between baseline and reflow at 1 hr, and these differences may have been reflected in their influence on artificial ischemia.

Table 1 Vascular responsibility by acetylcholine and nitroprusside at baseline and reperfusion for control and TMS treated dogs

	CONTROL		TMS treated	
	Baseline	Reflow 1hr	Baseline	Reflow 1hr
RBF(ml/100g/min)				
Drug Free	89.7±5.8	51.8±2.8**	65.6±16.9	45.6±4.4*
Ach	122.6±13.3	63.4±4.2**	91.8±12.9	94.4±14.0
NP	89.6±5.7	53.4±4.2**	59.9±8.5	73.5±12.3
CVR(mmHg/ml/min)				
Drug Free	1.24±0.08	2.31±2.8**	1.44±0.09	2.36±0.26**
Ach	0.86±0.09	1.85±0.24**	1.00±0.31	1.22±0.27
NP	1.03±0.12	1.98±0.22**	1.31±0.11	1.28±0.18

Values are mean±SEM (n=7) RBF, regional blood flow; CVR, coronary vascular registance
, *, Significant difference from baseline(p<0.01, * p<0.05)

Table 2 Hemodynamic data at baseline and reperfusion for control and TMS treated dogs

		HR(bpm)	mBP(mmHg)	dp/dt(mmHg/sec)	LVEDP(mmHg)
CONTROL	Baseline	150±6	110±7	382±32	7.7±0.3
	Reflow 1hr	112±5**	120±10	241±21*	11.0±0.9*
TMS treated	Baseline	134±4	94±5	276±15	6.7±0.6
	Reflow 1hr	104±4**	105±5	204±14**	8.9±1.3

Values are mean±SEM (n=7) HR, heart rate; mBP, mean blood pressure;
dp/dt, peak positive dp/dt; LVEDP, left ventricular end-diastolic pressure
, *, Significant difference from baseline(p<0.01, * p<0.05)

DISCUSSION

The need to investigate the mechanism of reperfusion injury has increased since the discovery that the resupply of blood to ischemic tissue exacerbate damage. The reperfusion injury both myocardial and vascular dysfunction following ischemia and reperfusion has been mentioned. The neutrophils play a major role in process of myocardial injury occuring with ischemia and reperfusion[3]. These neutrophil responses are triggered by numerous stimuli, including chemotactic peptides, arachidonate and phorbol esters[4]. Due to the production of vasoreactive agents and the release of cytotoxic substances, migrated, adhered and activated neutrophils have been proposed as being toxic to endothelial cells. However, there are many successful reports on the experimental prevention of reperfusion injury by using a filter to trap neutrophils and monoclonal antibodies. We have also documented that a supply of neutropenic blood reduced reperfusion injury of canine models. As there are many limitations to clinical use, all attempts are not practically suitable for patients suffering from myocardial infarctions. TMS strongly inhibits oxidative burst and phagokinetic migration of neutrophils due to its inhibitory effect on protein kinase C indicates that it prevents exacerbation of reperfusion injury. Drug treatment for preventing reperfusion injury of heart may be possible in clincal use in the near future, and TMS and its analogues could be considered as candidates for clinical use in the prevention of heart injury.

REFERENCES

1. Imai K, Hirahara N, Kamiyama H, Naganuma F, Suzuki T, Murata K ; The role of granulocyte in reperfusion injury, in Japanese with English summary, in press, SHINKIN NO KOUZOU TO TAISYA

2. Vedder, N. B., Winn, R. K., Rice. C. L., Chi, E. Y., Arforcs, K. E., Harlan, J. M., ; Inhibition of leukocyte adherence by anti-CD18 monoclonal antibody attenuates reperfusion injury in the rabit ear, Proc. Natl. Sci. USA Vol.87, pp 2643-2646, April 1990

3. Sheridan, F. M., Dauber, I. M., Mcmurtry, I. M., Lesnefsky, E. J., Horwitz, L. D., ; Role of Leukocytes in Coronary Vascular Endothelial Injury Due to Ischemia and Reperfusion Circ Res 1991 ;69:1566-1577

4. Nishizuka, Y ., ;The role of kinase C in cell surface signal transduction and tumor promotion. Nature 308:693-698(1984)

VII: Signal Transduction

Possible Prerequisite Morphological Changes Preceeding Cell Damage During Hypoxia-Reoxygenation in Cardiac Myocytes

MITSUYOSHI NINOMIYA, YOKO HAYASAKI, and KAZUMI IWAKI

Shionogi Research Laboratories, Osaka, 553 Japan

KEYWORDS: cardiac myocyte, hypoxia-reoxygenation, cell damage, hypercontraction, BDM

INTRODUCTION

The phenomenon of reperfusion/reoxygenation injury observed in the isolated whole heart [1] is known as the oxygen paradox. It has been proposed that reperfusion/reoxygenation injury may express itself in the different forms of reperfusion/reoxygenation-induced arrhythmia, myocardial stunning and necrosis including contractile band necrosis[2, 3]. In isolated cardiac myocytes, the oxygen paradox was also reported after both brief [4] and prolonged periods of hypoxia [5] followed by reoxygenation as a marked abbreviation of the mechanical twitch and an irreversible morphological change, hypercontraction. This paper describes the morphological changes during chemical hypoxia-reoxygenation and discusses possible morphological changes during hypoxia that lead to an irreversible cell damage after reoxygenation.

MATERIALS AND METHODS

Myocyte Isolation

Adult ventricular myocytes were isolated from 2 to 3 month-old Wistar rat heart as described previously [6]. Briefly, the heart was retrogradely perfused with collagenase (Yakult) containing Ca^{2+}-free Tyrode solution. The ventricular myocytes were mechanically dissociated and suspended in a high-K^+ storage solution and kept at 4 °C. Neonatal rat myocytes were isolated from 2 to 3 day-old SD rats and cultured as described previously [7]. The cells purified by percoll density gradient centrifugation were transferred to culture dishes at a density of approx. 1 million cells/30 mm cultured dish. The cells reached confluence after 48 hours in DMEM (containing fetal bovine serum) at which point the medium was replaced with serum-free DMEM. The experiments were started 24 hours later.

Experimental Conditions

Adult ventricular myocytes were superfused at room temperature with a solution containing (mM): $CaCl_2$ (1.2), $NaCl_2$ (137), KCl (5.0), $MgSO_4$ (1.2), D-glucose (10) and N-(2-hydroxyethyl)-piperazine-N'-2-ethanesulfonic acid (HEPES, 20), pH = 7.4 (adjusted with NaOH) in an experimental chamber mounted on the stage of an inverted microscope (Nikon Diaphoto). Video images of the cells were obtained using video camera and recorded for subsequent analysis. Diastolic cell length (DCL) was measured on a video monitor. Cells were field stimulated constantly with platinum electrodes at a frequency of 0.2 Hz unless otherwise indicated. Chemical hypoxia in the adult rat myocytes was achieved by replacing glucose by 10 mM 2-deoxyglucose (2-DG) 10 min before exposure to 2 mM cyanide, and reoxygenation was performed by removing cyanide. Hypoxia was caused neonatal rat myocytes using an anaerobic jar, GasPac system (BBL microbiology system, Becton Diskinson and Co.) equipped with a GasPac hydrogen and carbon dioxide generating envelope. Cultured neonatal myocytes in glucose-free DMEM were submitted to hypoxic conditions in the anaerobic jar. Reoxygenation was performed by taking hypoxic culture plates out of the anaerobic jar, and exchanging the medium to glucose-added DMEM. Creatine phosphokinase (CPK) activity released from myocytes during hypoxia-reoxygenation was determined using CPK-test Wako (Wako Chemical Co.).

RESULTS AND DISCUSSION

Morphological Changes During Chemical Hypoxia-Reoxygenation.

In adult rat myocytes, addition of 2 mM cyanide followed by its removal from the superfusate in the presence of 2-DG caused a characteristic sequence of changes in the excitability and morphology of the cells. During the exposure to cyanide, twitch amplitude gradually decreased. The cells then became unexcitable and abruptly became shortened to a brick-like contraction state known as the ATP-depleted rigor form (R-form) [8]. The R-form occurred 13.3 $\pm$1.3 min ($n = 40$) after addition of 2 mM cyanide. DCL in the R-form decreased to 55 % of the initial length. When the cells were washed with cyanide-free solution after a period in the R-form, transient recontraction (TR) occurred immediately after cyanide removal and the cells became even shorter. DCL in TR decreased to 35 % of the initial length. Some cells then became rounded up in an irreversible hypercontracture form (H-form) with mechanical oscillation, while others partially recovered, becoming capable of stimulated twitch. Thus, irreversible cell damage after reoxygenetion occurred in an all-or-none manner. These morphological changes are similar to those reported during hypoxia-reoxygenation [5]. The incidence of the H-form (%H) increased with increasing duration from the initiation of the R-form to cyanide removal. Thus, whether H-form occurs or not depends on the duration of the R-form but not the total duration of cyanide exposure.

Effects of Experimental Conditions on Incidence of the H-form

The incidence of the H-form (%H) was determined under various experimental conditions with constant period in R-form. In the control condition (1.2 mM Ca^{2+}), 67 % of all the cells assumed to H-form when cyanide was removed at 15 min after initiation of R-formation. On the other hand, in the Ca^{2+}-free solution, %H was much lower (25 %) but R-formation and TR were only slightly affected. Similar results were also observed when the cells were exposed to cyanide in the presence of Ca^{2+} and washed out Ca^{2+}-free solution without cyanide. These indicate that H-formation is Ca^{2+}-dependent but R-formation and TR are Ca^{2+}-independent processes. The incidence of the H-form was also greatly reduced (17%) by 5 mM 2,3-butanedione monoxime (BDM) as shown in Fig. 1. A similar protective effect of BDM against irreversible cell damage was observed in the cultured neonatal rat ventricular myocytes as the reduction of CPK leakage induced by hypoxia-reoxygenation. When the cells were reoxygenated 30 min following 4 hr hypoxia, CPK leakage in the presence of 2 or 20 mM BDM was reduced to 66 % or 6 % of those in the absence of BDM, respectively. Preliminary results of this study have been presented in abstract form (9).

Relationship Between H-formation and Other Morphological Changes

BDM can prevent the oxygen paradox in the isolated whole heart [10] possibly due to an inhibitory effect [11] of BDM on the Ca^{2+}-dependent twitch. Therefore, the protective effect of BDM observed in our experiments may be induced by a decrease in the Ca^{2+}-dependent twitch amplitude during chemical hypoxia. To test this possibility, chemical hypoxia-reoxygenation was performed under the condition of non-stimulation. Under this condition, %H was reduced to 40 % but this reduction was smaller than that in the cells treated with BDM even though the cells were completely silent during the experiment and R-formation and TR were still observed. Therefore, the protective effect of BDM against reoxygenation-induced cell damage cannot be explained only by its negative inotropic effect. DCL in the R-form, TR and H-form were measured under various experimental conditions. In the cells treated with BDM, decreases of DCL in the R-form and TR were significantly small compared with that in the control (Fig. 1). Developments of R-formation and TR were slower than those in the control cells. These result suggests that Ca^{2+}-independent R-formation and TR may be prerequisite for Ca^{2+}-dependent H-formation, and the protective effect of BDM against irreversible cell damage may b partly induced by its inhibitory effect on the morphological changes that lead to the cell damage.

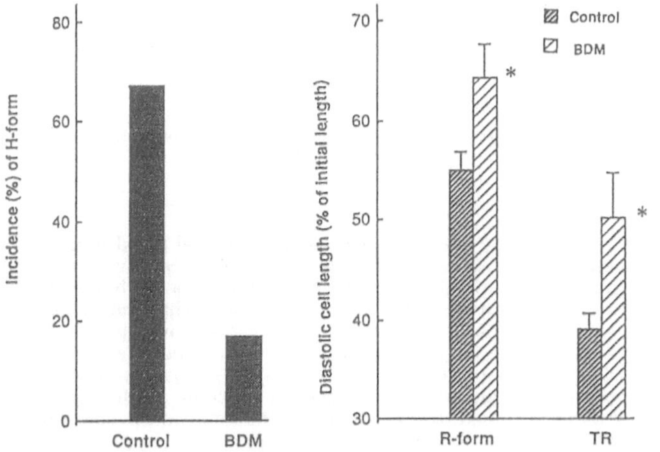

Fig. 1 Effects of BDM on incidence of H-formation (left) and on the diastolic cell length in R-form and TR in the isolated rat ventricular myocytes.

REFERENCES
1. Hearse DJ, Humphrey SM, Chain EB (1973) Abrupt reoxygenation of the anoxic potassium-arrested perfused rat heart: A study of myocardial enzyme release. J Mol Cell Cardiol 5: 395-407
2. Braunwald E, Kloner RA (1982) The stunned myocardium: prolonged, postischemic ventricular dysfunction. Circulation 86: 1146-1149
3. Kloner RA, Ganote CE, Whalen DA Jr, Jennings RB (1974) Effect of a transient period of ischemia on myocardial cells. Am J Pathol 74: 399-422
4. Silverman HS, Ninomiya M, Blank PS, Hano O, Miyata H. Spurgeon HA, Lakatta EG, Stern MD (1991) A cellular mechanism for impaired posthypoxic relaxation in isolated cardiac myocytes: Altered myofilament relaxation kinetics at reoxygenation 69: 196-208
5. Stern MD, Chien AM, Capogrossi MC, Pelto DJ, Lakatta EG (1985) Direct observation of the "oxygen paradox" in single rat ventricular myocytes. Circ Res 56: 899-903
6. Yazawa K. Kaibara M, Ohara M, Kameyama M (1990) An improved method for isolating cardiac myocytes useful for patch-clamp studies. Jpn J Physiol 40: 157-163
7. Morris AC, Hagler HK, Willerson JT, Buja LM (1989) Relationship between calcium loading and impaired energy metabolism during Na^+, K^+ pump inhibition and metabolic inhibition in cultured neonatal rat cardiac myocytes. J Clin Invest 83: 1876-1887
8. Haworth RA, Nicolaus A, Goknur AB, Berkoff HA (1988) Synchronous depletion of ATP in isolated adult rat heart cells. J Mol Cell Cardiol 20: 837-846
9. Iwaki K, Hayasaki Y (1992) Preconditioning, stunning and concepts of cardioprotection. Abstract of satellite symposium of the XIV World Congress of the ISHR. 8-9 May 1992. Sapporo Japan
10. Schluter KD, Schwartz P, Siegmund B, Piper HM (1991) Prevention of the oxygen paradox in hypoxic-reoxygenated hearts. Am J Physiol 261: H416-H423
11. Gwathmey JK, Hajjar RJ, Salaro RJ (1991) Contractile deactivation and uncoupling of crossbridges: Effects of 2, 3-butanedione monoxime on mammalian myocardium. Circ Res 69:1280-1292

Opioid Modulation of Cardiac Sympathetic Nerve Activity of Baroreceptor Reflex in Rats

MITSUHIRO YOSHIOKA, MASAHIRO TOCHIHARA, HIROKO TOGASHI, and HIDEYA SAITO

First Department of Pharmacology, Hokkaido University School of Medicine, Sapporo, 060 Japan

KEYWORDS: opioid peptides , baroreceptor reflex, cardiac sympathetic nerve activity, rats

INTRODUCTION

The baroreflex arch is the primary pathway for regulating arterial blood pressure. A number of studies have demonstrated that opioid peptide systems might be involved in this baroreflex pathway (1, 2). Morphine-like compounds are known to facilitate the baroreceptor reflex at the level of the nucleus tractus solitarii (2). It has also been reported that endogenous opioid peptides might be related to the altered baroreflex function in hypertensive animals (3,4). The opioid receptor system is recognized to have an important role in the control of autonomic functions as well (5). However, in most previous reports, the relationship between blood pressure (BP) and heart rate (HR) has been used as an index of baroreceptor function. In the present study, we used the measurements of cardiac sympathetic nerve activity to focus on the opioid modulation of the sympathetic component of the baroreceptor reflex function.

MATERIALS AND METHODS

General

Experiments were carried out on male Wistar rats weighing 200g-400g at an age of 7-12 weeks (Slc:Wistar/ST). Animals were anesthetized with 1% halothane via a precalibrated vaporizer (Fluotec Mark 3) through a tracheal cannula which was connected to a rodent respirator (Harvard apparatus , Millis, MA, model 683) during surgical preparations. Anesthesia was maintained by intravenously injected α-chloralose (50mg/kg) throughout the experiment. Halothane was withdrawn gradually. Gallamine triethiodide, a cardioselective acetylcholinergic M_2-receptor antagonist (6), was intravenously administered (10mg/kg) for the purpose of eliminating vagal components of the cardioinhibitory response to baroreceptor activation as well as for immobilization. Arterial BP was continuously recorded through a catheter inserted into the femoral artery by a pressure transducer (TP-200T, Nihon Kohden). HR was monitored from the pulse waves of BP using a tachometer (AT-601G, Nihon Kohden). Drugs were injected into the femoral vein.

Cardiac Sympathetic Nerve Activity Recordings

The inferior cardiac sympathetic nerve was isolated from the right stellate ganglion and cut near the heart under an operation microscope. Inferior cardiac nerve activity (ICNA) was recorded from the central cut end of the nerve with a platinum-iridium electrode. Nerve activity was amplified, passed through high and low cut filters and then quantified every 2 sec using a cumulative integrator (EI601G, Nihon Kohden) and a real-time data analyzer (ATAC 450, Nihon Koden).

Evaluation of Baroreceptor Reflex Function

After blood pressure was increased by a bolus injection of phenylephrine hydrochloride (0.1-64 μg), the baroreceptor reflex was evaluated from the peak responses in ICNA, HR and/or heart period (msec) defined as 60,000/HR. Baroreflex sensitivity was determined from the slope of a regression line relating ICNA or heart period change to the rise of mean BP, in accordance with the method of Weinstock and Rosin (7). Baroreflex sensitivity was determined before and 5 min after intravenous administration of a μ-opioid receptor antagonist, naltrexone (1mg/kg).

Data Analysis

Values are expressed as mean ±SEM. Data means were compared with the paired or unpaired Student's t-test. A p value less than 0.05 was accepted as the level of statistical significance.

RESULTS AND DISCUSSION

Sympathetic Component in Baroreceptor Reflex Function

The sympathetic component which might be involved in the cardioinhibitory response to activation of arterial baroreceptors was evaluated by measuring ICNA. ICNA as well as HR was reflexically reduced by increasing the BP with a pressor stimulus by a bolus injection of phenylephrine (Fig. 1). In order to clarify the contribution of a sympathetic component in the baroreflex function, HR/ heart period was determined with and without gallamine. The slope of the mean BP-heart period relationship in gallamine-pretreated rats was significantly suppressed as compared with that of non-treated rats (from 0.567 to 0.163). Gallamine is known to have a pharmacological property as a cardioselective M_2-receptor antagonist (6) . Therefore, the attenuated HR/ heart period response after gallamine treatment is thought to reflect a parasympathetic component included in the baroreflex function.

It has recently been reported that chemical sympathectomy potentiated a bradycardiac response to baroreceptor activation in conscious rats (8), indicating the possibility that the sympathetic nervous system exerts an antagonistic influence on the baroreceptor reflex as previously reported (9,10). However, the present study using ICNA recordings provides direct evidence that sympathetic components also contribute to the reflex bradycardia elicited by baroreceptor stimulation in anesthetized rats.

Effects of Naltrexone on Baroreceptor Reflex Function

Baseline BP, HR and ICNA

Mean BP, HR and ICNA were compared before and after intravenous administration of naltrexone (1mg/kg). Baseline BP tended to increase after naltrexone administration but this increase was not statistically significant. On the other hand, baseline HR and ongoing ICNA were diminished after naltrexone administration. The decrease in HR was statistically significant ($P<0.05$).

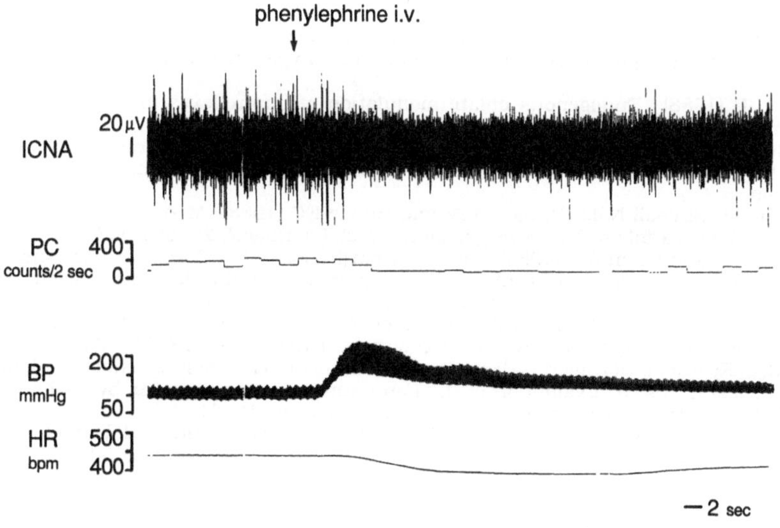

Fig. 1. Original recordings illustrate baroreflex elicited by bolus injection of phenylephrine in the anesthetized rat. Tracings from top to bottom indicate actual neurogram of ICNA, pulse counts (PC) of ICNA, arterial blood pressure (BP) and heart rate (HR).

Baroreceptor reflex sensitivity
Intravenous administration of naltrexone attenuated the reflex response of ICNA to phenylephrine in gallamine-treated rats. Thus, naltrexone significantly decreased the slope of the regression line between mean BP and ICNA from 0.494 to 0.313. Our finding indicates that the ICNA response to BP increase, a sympathetic component of the baroreceptor reflex, might be modulated via the μ-opioid receptor.

Numerous reports indicating that endogenous opioids can modulate the baroreceptor function have accumulated (1-4). However, it is likely that a species difference exists in the opioid peptide modulation of the baroreflexes; in the rabbit (1) and the rat (4), endogenous opioid peptides act to suppress baroreflex response. On the contrary, naloxone reduced the baroreceptor sensitivity in the dog,(2). In agreement with the latter, our results with anesthetized rats demonstrate that endogenous opioids are likely to stimulate the baroreflex arch via the cardiac sympathetic nerves, since the reflex decrease in ICNA was attenuated by naltrexone.

On the other hand, naltrexone did not influence the slope of the mean BP-heart period relationships, which were significantly attenuated by gallamine pretreatment. A possible explanation for the discrepancy between the effects of naltrexone on the reflex responses of ICNA and heart period is that the endogenous opioid system may be involved in the tonic control of cardiac function, since naltrexone significantly decreased baseline HR. For this reason, naltrexone might have failed to produce further cardioinhibitory effects.

Baroreceptor reflex sensitivity has previously been evaluated as a regression line between mean BP and heart period during a bolus injection of a pressor agent. Through the measurement of ICNA as a direct index, the present study clarified that the endogenous opioid system is involved in the sympathetic modulation of the baroreceptor reflex sensitivity. However, further study is needed before the precise role of the endogenous opioid peptides/receptors on the autonomic control of the baroreflex function can be assessed.

CONCLUSION

The present study demonstrated that naltrexone attenuated the reflex response of ICNA to arterial baroreceptor activation in anesthetized rats. Our findings indicate that μ-opioid receptor mechanisms might be involved in the modulation of sympathetic component of the baroreceptor reflex.

REFERENCES

1. Petty MA and Reid J (1982) The effect of opiates on arterial baroreceptor reflex function in the rabbit. Naunyn-Schmiedeberg's Arch Pharmacol 319: 206-211
2. Szilagyi JE (1987) Opioid modulation of baroreceptor reflex sensitivity in dogs. Am J Physiol 252: H733-H737
3. Ricksten SE and Thoren P (1981) Reflex control of sympathetic nerve activity and heart rate from arterial baroreceptor in conscious spontaneously hypertensive rats. Clin Sci 61:169S-172S
4. Szilagyi JE (1988) Endogenous opiate modulation of baroreflexes in normotensive and hypertensive rats. Am J Physiol 255: H987-H991
5. Arndt JO (1987) Opiate receptors in the CNS and their possible role in cardiovascular control. In: Buckley JP and Ferrario CM (eds) Brain peptides and catecholamine in cardiovascular regulation.
6. Stockton JM, Birdsall NJM, Burgen ASV and Hulme EC (1983) Modulation of the binding properties of muscarinic receptors by gallamine. Mol. Pharmacol. 23: 551-557
7. Weinstock M. and Rosin AJ. (1984) Relative contribution of vagal and cardiac sympathetic nerves to the reflex bradycardia induced by a pressor stimulus in the conscious rabbit: comparison of 'steady state' and 'ramp' methods. Clin Exp Pharmacol Physiol 11: 113-141.
8. Ferrari AU, Daffonchio A, Franzelli C and Mancia G (1991) Potentiation of the baroreceptor-heart rate reflex by sympathectomy in conscious rats. Hypertension 18: 230-235
9. Parati G, DiRienzo M, Bertinieri G, Pomidossi G, Casadei R, Groppelli A, Peddotti A, Zanchetti A and Mancia G (1988) Evaluation of the baroreceptor-heart rate reflex by 24-hour intra-arterial blood pressure monitoring in humans. Hypertension 12: 214-222
10. Mancia G, Ferrari A, Geogorini L, Parati G and Pomidossi G (1982) Effects of isometric exercise on the carotid baroreflex in hypertensive subjects. Hypertension 4: 245-250

VIII: Congestive Heart Failure

Clinical Efficacy of Flosequinan in Patients with Mild Chronic Heart Failure: a Double-Blind Placebo-Controlled Study

KATSUJI IMAI[1], MASATSUGU HORI[1], HIDEYUKI SATO[1], HITOSHI OZAKI[1], MICHITOSHI INOUE[1], MASASHI NAKA[1], MASATAKE FUKUNAMI[1], MASAKATSU FUKUSHIMA[1], KEITA KUNISADA[1], TAKENOBU KAMADA[1], and AKIRA KITABATAKE[2]
The First Department of Medicine, Osaka University School of Medicine, and Osaka Flosequinan Multicenter Trial Group, Osaka, 553 Japan[1], and Department of Cardiovascular Medicine, Hokkaido University School of Medicine, Sapporo, 060 Japan

KEYWORDS: flosequinan, mild heart failure, cardiac function, exercise capacity, subjective symptoms

INTRODUCTION

Flosequinan is a novel vasodilating agent with a mild positive inotropic effect [1]. This drug has been reported to increase exercise capacity in patients with severe heart failure [2-4]. However, its efficacy has not been studied in patients with less severe forms of heart failure. In the present study we investigated the effects of 4-week administration of flosequinan (50 mg daily) on exercise capacity, cardiac function, and subjective symptoms in patients with chronic mild heart failure in a randomized placebo-controlled double-blind clinical trial.

SUBJECTS

The criteria for patient selection were (1) underlying myocardial disease or regurgitant valvular disease, (2) cardiothoracic ratio (CTR) of greater than 55% or left ventricular fractional shortening (FS) determined by M-mode echocardiography of less than 25%, and (3) a stable New York Heart Association (NYHA) functional class of I-III for at least 2 months. Twenty-four patients who fulfilled the criteria were entered in the study. They were 16 males and 8 females, ranging in age from 37 to 76 years (mean, 58 years). The underlying disease was dilated cardiomyopathy in 16 patients, old myocardial infarction in 2, aortic regurgitation in 2, and mitral regurgitation in 4. Twenty-two patients were classified as NYHA functional class II, and the remaining two patients were class I and III. Digitalis and/or diuretics were continued throughout the study without changes in dose or regimen. Other vasodilators or inotropic agents were withdrawn 4 weeks before the study. Written or oral informed consent was obtained from all patients.

METHODS

The trial period consisted of the 2-4 weeks run-in period and the 4 weeks treatment period. Symptomatic, echocardiographic, and exercise examinations were performed two times during the run-in period and on the last day of the treatment period. A symptom-limited ramp maximal exercise test was conducted on a sitting bicycle ergometer. Gas exchange data were collected continuously during exercise. As indicators of exercise capacity, exercise time, peak oxygen uptake (peak V02) and V02 at the anaerobic threshold (AT) were obtained every 30 sec. AT was defined as the time point at which the ratio of minute ventilation to V02 begins to increase rapidly. Heart rate and blood pressure were measured at rest and every minute during exercise. The left ventricular end-diastolic dimension (LVDd) and end-systolic dimension (LVDs) were measured from M-mode echocardiograms. FS was calculated by the following equation: (LVDd - LVDs)/LVDd. The severity of heart failure was evaluated according to the NYHA classification and the new heart failure severity classification proposed by Obata and Yasuda. Within group comparison of data between the run-in period and the treatment period was performed for the flosequinan and the placebo group, using Wilcoxon's signed rank test. A comparison between the two groups was also performed, using the Mann-Whitney test. P<0.05 was regarded as statistically significant.

RESULTS

Intergroup comparison

There was no significant difference in any measurement between the two groups during the run-in and the treatment period. However, when the parameter changes from the final run-in period to the treatment period were examined, FS was increased by 2.9 ± 1.3% in the flosequinan group, but decreased by 1.3 ± 0.9% in the placebo group. This difference was statistically significant ($p<0.05$). The improvements in exercise time, AT, and the heart failure severity classification were also greater in the flosequinan group than in the placebo group, although they were not statistically significant (Table).

Table. Parameter changes from the run-in period to the treatment period

	flosequinan group	placebo group	p value
EDD (mm)	-1.7 ± 1.4	-0.9 ± 0.4	N.S.
ESD (mm)	-2.9 ± 1.4	-0.1 ± 0.5	N.S.
FS (%)	2.9 ± 1.3	-1.3 ± 0.9	p<0.05
ET (sec)	58.4 ± 17.8	30.9 ± 20.3	N.S.
peak V02 (ml/1min/kg)	0.6 ± 1.3	1.2 ± 1.0	N.S.
AT (ml/min/kg)	2.9 ± 1.0	0.8 ± 1.0	N.S.
NYHA class	-0.3 ± 0.1	-0.1 ± 0.1	N.S.
HF severity class	-0.6 ± 0.2	-0.4 ± 0.2	N.S.

Data are mean ± SE. ET; exercise time. HF; heart failure

Intragroup comparison

In the flosequinan group, 10 of the 12 patients, excluding the 2 dropouts, were studied. Moreover, AT could not be determined in three of the 10 patients, and they were excluded from analysis of AT. No significant change was observed in any measurement during the run-in period. Heart rate, systolic and diastolic blood pressure, and CTR were also not significantly altered even during the flosequinan treatment. LVDd was decreased from 64.5 ± 4.1 to 62.8 ± 4.3mm with flosequinan, and LVDs was also decreased from 55.3 ± 4.5 to 52.4 ± 5.0mm, although the changes were not significant. FS was insignificantly increased from 15.1 ± 2.1% to 18.0 ± 2.7%. The heart failure severity classification significantly improved from 2.1 ± 0.2 to 1.5 ± 0.1 ($p<0.05$), while improvement of the NYHA classification did not reach a significant level. Exercise time was also significantly prolonged ($p<0.05$) and AT significantly increased ($p<0.05$), although peak VO2 remained unchanged (Fig.). In the placebo group, no significant change was observed in any measurement during the treatment period. Severe adverse effects were not observed in both groups.

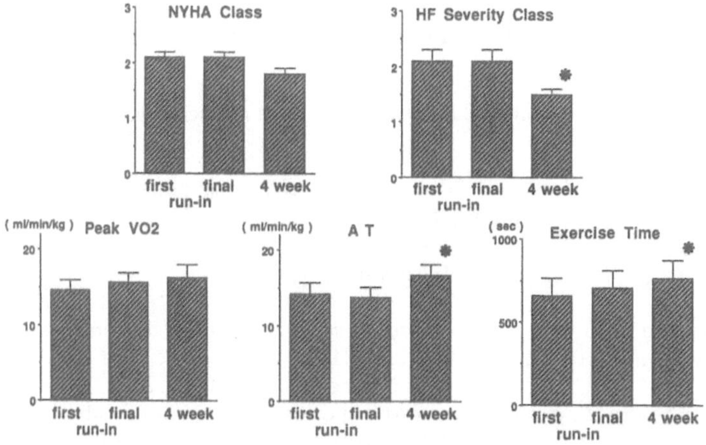

Fig. Changes in symptoms and exercise capacity in the flosequinan group (HF; heart failure. *$p<0.05$ vs final examination in the run-in period)

CONCLUSION

In the present study the effect of 4-week administration of flosequinan (50 mg daily) on exercise capacity, left ventricular function, and symptoms of heart failure were investigated in a placebo-controlled double-blind study in patients with chronic mild heart failure. Although intergroup comparison failed to demonstrate the superiority of flosequinan to placebo in improving heart failure except for FS, intragroup comparison demonstrated a significant increase in AT and prolongation of exercise time in symptom-limited maximal exercise, and improvement in the heart failure severity classification during the treatment period in the flosequinan group. These improvements were not observed in the placebo group. These results, together with favorable trends observed with intergroup comparison, suggest that this agent is promising for long-term treatment of chronic mild heart failure as well as severe heart failure.

REFERENCES

1. Yates DB (1991) Pharmacology of flosequinan. Am Heart J 121: 974-983
2. Elborn JS, Riley M, Stanford CF, Nicholls DP (1990) The effects of flosequinan on submaximal exercise in patients with chronic cardiac failure. Br J Clin Pharmacol 29: 519-524
3. Cowley AJ, Wynne RD, Stainer K, Fullwood L, Rowley JM, Hampton JR (1988) Flosequinan in heart failure: Acute hemodynamic and longer term symptomatic effects. Br Med J 297: 169-173
4. Elborn JS, Stanford CF, Nicholls DP (1989) Effect of flosequinan on exercise capacity and symptoms in severe heart failure. Br Heart J 61: 331-335

Clinical Efficacy of Pimobendan for Patients with Chronic Heart Failure — A Dose Finding Study by a Multicenter Double Blind Trial —

The UD-CG 115 BS In Chronic Heart Failure Study Group,
Toshiaki Kumada et.al.

The 3rd Division, Department of Internal Medicine, Faculty of Medicine, Kyoto University Hospital, Kyoto, 606 Japan

Key Words: pimobendan (UD-CG 115 BS), calcium sensitizer, chornic heart failure, dose finding study

INTRODUCTION

Pimobendan (UD-CG 115 BS), a benzimidazole pyridazinone derivative, is a new oral inodilator. Its positive inotropic effect is produced both by inhibition of phosphodiesterase (PDE) and by increase in sensitivity of cardiac myofilaments to Ca [1,2], and the vasodilating effect is induced by inhibition of the type III PDE. It is well absorbed after oral administration, and its effect continues for approximately 10 hours. Since it also acts as a calcium sensitizer, pimobendan has been recently spotlighted as a new type of inotropic agent. The present study was designed to investigate the effect of pimobendan and to determine the optimal dose in patients with chronic heart failure (CHF) by a multicenter placebo-controlled double-blind comparison.

SUBJECTS AND METHODS

The subjects enrolled were patients with CHF who were in New York Heart Association (NYHA) functional class IIm (moderate limitation of physical activity) or III, and whose physical findings and clinical symptoms were stable throughout the observation period. Sixteen patients had ischemic heart disease, 44 dilated cardiomyopathy, 41 valvular regurgitation, and 11 other heart diseases. Digitalis and diuretics were permitted to be used providing that their dosages were unchanged during the study period, and other cardioactive drugs were prohibited.

Patients were randomly assigned in a double-blind manner to receive either pimobendan (1.25 mg or 2.5 mg orally twice daily) or matched placebo. Following 2 weeks of the observation period, the drug (placebo or pimobendan) was administered for 4 weeks. Clinical symptoms, physical findings, NYHA functional class, physical activity indices, chest X-ray, echocardiography, 12-lead electrocardiograms (ECG), and laboratory findings were evaluated.

Physical activity indices (Index I and II) were obtained by scoring the patient's answer to a questionnaire on their daily activity. Twenty questions on a patient's physical activity were classified into 4 grades based on the metabolic equivalence (expressed as mets), with 5 questions in each grade. Index I is defined as the above described grade of the physical activity. Index II was the sum of the number of the "yes" answer to the 20 questions. Left ventricular (LV) end-diastolic and end-systolic (ESd) diameters were measured by M-mode echocardiography, and the fractional shortening (%FS) was calculated. At the end of treatment period, the physician assessed the degree of global improvement in his patients based on the extent of improvement of his or her clinical symptoms and physical findings, and then determined the utility of the drug based on the degree of the global improvement and on the safety. Before starting this trial, a written or oral informed consent was taken from each patient.

Data are presented as means± standard error. The base-line characteristics of the three groups were compared by the Kruskal-Wallis test or the chi-square test. Treatment effects for nonparametric results were evaluated with Kruskal-Wallis test, Dunn multiple-comparison test, or signed rank test. Statistical analysis of parametric data was performed with Student's t-test or Dunn multiple-comparison test.

RESULTS

Sixty-three men and 49 women with milde to moderately severe CHF, aged from 28 to 92 years old, were enrolled in this study. Thirty seven patients received 1.25 mg of pimobendan b.i.d. (the 1.25 mg group), 38 had 2.5 mg of pimobendan b.i.d. (the 2.5 mg group), and 37 had the placebo b.i.d. (the placebo group). There were no differences in the baseline patients' characteristics among the 3 groups. Three patients were excluded from the analysis of the clinical efficacy because they were below NYHA class IIm.

Clinical symptoms and physical findings improved most significantly during treatment in the 2.5 mg group. Improvement rates of the physical activity indices I and II, and the NYHA functional class were also higher in the 2.5 mg group compared to those in the placebo group. Similarly, CTR as well as LVESd were reduced and %FS was increased in the 2.5 mg group alone. Then, the global improvement rate in the evaluation by the physician in charge was 58.8 % in the 2.5 mg group, which was significantly higher than in the placebo group (Fig. 1). The incidence of side effects was 10.8% in the 1.25 mg group, 10.5% in the 2.5 mg group and 0% in the placebo group, but no serious symptoms were observed. In addition, there were no problematic abnormalities in laboratory examinations and ECG. The utility rate was 57.1 % in the 2.5 mg group, highest among the 3 groups (Fig. 2).

Fig. 1 Global improvement rate

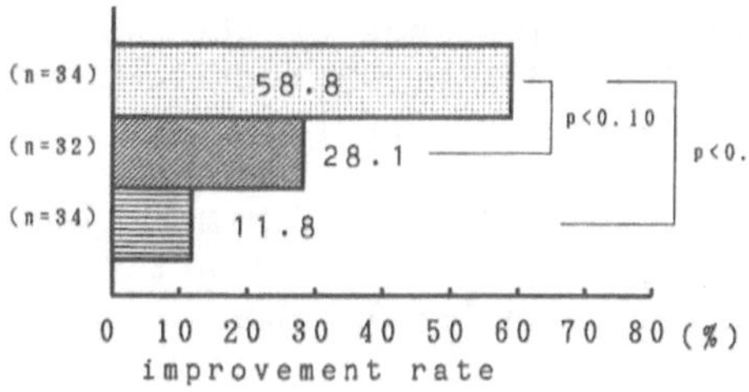

Fig. 2 Utility rate

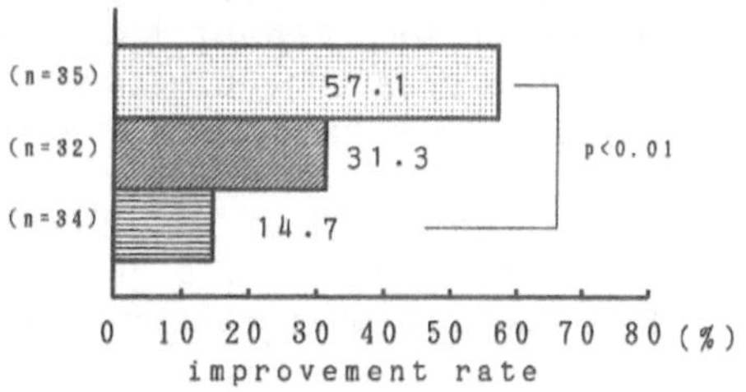

:Pimobendan2.5 ▩ :Pimobendan1.25 ▤ :Placebo (Dunn multiple-comparison)

Compared to the 1.25 mg and the placebo groups, the global improvement rate and the utility rate were highest in the 2.5 mg group, and the difference was significant between the 2.5 mg and the placebo group ($p<0.01$).

DISCUSSION

PDE inhibitors increase intracellular Ca to exert the positive inotropic property. However, because of its arrhythmogenic effects or aggravation of myocardial function resulting from increased myocardial oxygen consumption [4], the risk of sudden death may increase. A placebo-controlled comparison study on milrinone demonstrated that the rate of arrhythmia aggravation was 4% in the placebo group and as high as 18% in the milrinone group. Pimobendan improves the utility efficacy of ATPase without a significant increase in myocardial oxygen consumption and is expected to be a promising drug with lesser risk of increasing mortality. A clinical study [5] conducted in the United State showed that the mortality rate was 6% in the placebo group and 5% in the pimobendan group in which 1.25 mg, 2.5 mg or 5.0 mg of pimobendan was given twice a day.

In this study, the improvement rate of clinical symptoms, physical findings, NYHA functional class, and physical activity index were all significantly higher in the 2.5 mg group compared to in the placebo and 1.25 mg groups. The global improvement rate and utility rate were 58.8 % and 57.1 % in the 2.5 mg group, highest among the three groups. In addition, there were no serious side effects in any of the 3 groups. One patient in the 1.25 mg group died suddenly during the treatment period, but the causal relation to pimobendan was denied.

It is concluded that pimobendan is a useful and safe inodilator in the treatment of patients with milde to moderately severe CHF, and the optimal dose is 2.5 mg twice a day.

REFERENCES

1. Scheld HH, JCA van Meel et al (1989) Pimobendan increases calcium sensitivity of skinned human papillary muscle fibers. J Clin Pharmacol 29 : 360-365
2. Fujino K, Solaro RJ et al (1988) Sensitization of dog and guinea pig heart myofilaments to Ca^{++} -activation and the inotropic efect of pimobendan: comparison with milrinone. Circulation Res 63 : 911-922
3. Packer M (1988) Do positive inotropic agents adversely effect the survival of patients with chronic congestive heart failure? Ⅱ. Protagonist's viewpoint. J Am Coll Cardiol 12 : 562-569
4. Holubarsch CH, Alpert NR et al (1989) Influence of the positive inotropic substance pimobendan (UD-CG 115 BS) on contractile economy of guinea pig papillary muscles. J Cardiovasc Pharmacol 14 (Suppl. Ⅱ) : S13
5. Kubo MS, Gollub S et al (1992) Benificial effects of pimobendan on exercise tolerance and quality life in patients with heart failure -Results of a multicenter trial. Circulation 85: 942-949

Effect of Lisinopril on Hemodynamics and Cardiac Hypertrophy in Rats with Aortocaval Fistula

TAMIKO OKA, HIKARU NISHIMURA, MASAKUNI UEYAMA, JIRO KUBOTA, and KEISHIRO KAWAMURA

The Third Department of Internal Medicine, Osaka Medical College, Osaka, 569 Japan

KEYWORDS: Wistar rats, volume-overload heart failure, thermodilution, laser-Doppler flowmetry, neurohumoral factors

INTRODUCTION

Angiotensin converting enzyme (ACE) inhibitors such as captopril and enalapril are effective in relieving signs and symptoms of patients with congestive heart failure [1-3]. Enalapril reduced the mortality of patients with mild to severe heart failure, and decreased the number of hospitalizations [2-3]. However, it is not known whether the other ACE inhibitors are equally effective in heart failure. We therefore evaluated the effects of lisinopril on hemodynamics, cardiac hypertrophy, and neurohumoral factors in rats with high-output failure induced by aortocaval fistula. Unlike enalapril, lisinopril is not a prodrug, though otherwise lisinopril possesses many features common to enalapril.

MATERIALS AND METHODS

Animals and Surgical Procedures

Ten-week-old male Wistar rats (n=45) were randomly divided into 3 groups: an aortocaval fistula group (n=15), a fistula group with lisinopril (n=15), and a sham-operation group (n=15). Under anesthesia with ether, aortocaval fistula (1 mm) was created between the infra-renal abdominal aorta and inferior vena cava. A sham operation was performed in the same way except for the fistula creation. Lisinopril (1mg/kg/day) was given in drinking water to rats with fistula (n=15) for 4 weeks.

Hemodynamic and Echocardiographic Determinations

Conscious blood pressure was determined using the tail-cuff method before and every week after fistula operation. Under pentobarbital anesthesia, left ventricular (LV) function was determined using a 2F catheter-tip micromanometer: aortic pressure, LV pressure, mean aortic pressure (MAP), pulse pressure, LV end-diastolic pressure (LVEDP) and dp/dt_{max} were recorded. A venous catheter (PE 50) was inserted to the right atrium (RA). Cardiac output (CO) was measured by the thermodilution method. Stroke volume (SV) and total peripheral resistance (TPR) were calculated as follows: SV = CO/heart rate × 1,000, TPR = MAP/CO. Renal blood flow (RBF) was assessed with laser-Doppler flowmetry. Echocardiograms were taken using a 7.5 MHz transducer directed upward to the anterior chest. Under the guidance of 2 dimensional echocardiogram, LV end-diastolic internal diameter (Dd), end-systolic internal diameter (Ds), and end-diastolic external diameter (ED) were measured on M-mode recordings, as illustrated in Fig. 1.

Blood Sampling and Organ Weights

Plasma renin activity (PRA) was determined by radioimmunoassay and norepinephrine (NE) levels by high-performance liquid chromatography. Blood urea nitrogen (BUN) and creatinine levels were measured by an autoanalyser. Finally, weights of LV, right ventricle (RV), and kidney were measured.

RESULTS

Body, Heart and Kidney Weights

Body weight was similar in the 3 groups. The untreated rats with fistula exhibited greater heart weight than the sham-operated rats due both to LV (18%) and RV (33%) hypertrophy. Lisinopril significantly decreased heart weight by reducing only LV mass ($p<0.05$). Kidney weight was similarly decreased in both fistula groups ($p<0.05$). Lisinopril decreased the mortality rate (20% vs 33%, $p<0.05$).

Hemodynamic and Echocardiographic Data

At 1 week after the operation, conscious blood pressure was significantly lower in the fistula groups but then it returned toward control values. Rats with fistula possessed higher CO than control rats, due to an increase in SV (both $p<0.05$) because heart rate was similar between the fistula and sham-operated groups. In the untreated rats with fistula, LVEDP, RA and pulse pressures were significantly higher, whereas aortic diastolic pressure, TPR and RBF were lower than in control rats (all $p<0.05$). Lisinopril did not affect heart rate, MAP, dp/dt_{max}, CO, SV, and TPR. Echocardiograms taken at the time of catheterization (Fig. 1) showed significantly increased LV internal (Dd and Ds) and external (ED) dimensions in the untreated rats with fistula than in the sham-operated rats (all $p<0.05$). Lisinopril did not alter the LV dimensions.

Neurohumoral Data and Renal Function

While plasma NE levels were significantly elevated in the untreated rats with fistula than in the sham-operated rats ($p<0.05$), PRA was significantly increased only in the lisinopril-treated rats ($p<0.05$). Serum creatinine and BUN levels were significantly higher and RBF was lower in the treated and untreated rats with fistula compared with the sham-operated rats (all $p<0.05$).

CONCLUSION

The untreated rats with fistula had biventricular hypertrophy, signs of volume-overload heart failure, impaired renal function, and higher mortality. Lisinopril reduced LV mass without compromising cardiac and renal hemodynamics, and decreased the mortality rate. Regression of LV hypertrophy with lisinopril occurred without significant decreases in LV pre- and afterload, suggesting factors other than the hemodynamic variables play a role in the regression. Neurohumoral factors such as angiotensin II (ANG II) [4] and NE [5] can cause myocardial hypertrophy independent of blood pressure. In this study, PRA in the treated rats was significantly elevated, indicating the adequate blockade of the renin-angiotensin system. Because the renin-angiotensin system is also present in the heart [6], lisinopril might have blocked directly the local effects of ANG II. Further, lisinopril attenuated the increase in plasma NE levels. This may also contribute to the reduction of LV mass by the ACE inhibitor. On the other hand, RV hypertrophy was not reversed by the treatment. This is probably because volume overload to the RV was much greater than to the LV, as evidenced by more prominent RV hypertrophy, offsetting the beneficial effects of lisinopril. In summary, lisinopril regressed LV hypertrophy in rats with high-output failure in a dose that did not significantly decrease arterial or venous pressures. The blockade of the renin-angiotensin system and the attenuation of the enhanced sympathetic nervous system may play a role in the regression of LV hypertrophy.

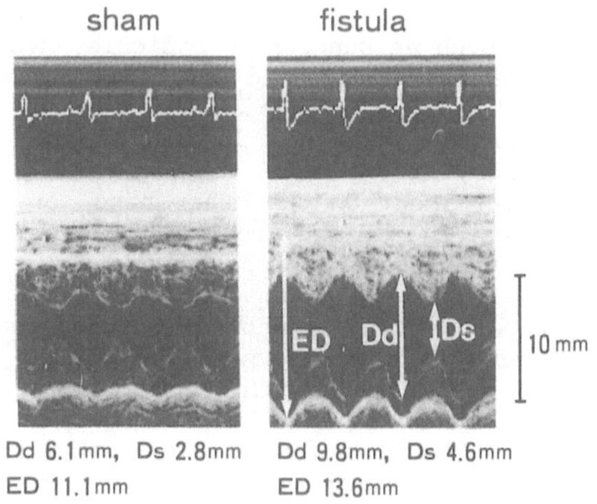

Fig. 1 Representative M-mode echocardiograms of the fistula and sham-operated rats, showing a significant cardiomegaly in a fistula rat.

REFERENCES

1. The Captopril-Digoxin Multicenter Research Group (1988) Comparative effects of therapy with captopril and digoxin in patients with mild to moderate heart failure. JAMA 259:539-544
2. The CONSENSUS Trial Study Group (1987) Effects of enalapril on mortality in severe congestive heart failure: results of the Cooperative North Scandinavian Enalapril Survival Study (CONSENSUS). N Engl J Med 316:1429-1435
3. The SOLVD Investigators (1991) Effect of enalapril on survival in patients with reduced left ventricular ejections and congestive heart failure. N Engl J Med 325:293-302
4. Simpson P, McGrath A (1983) Norepinephrine-stimulated hypertrophy of cultured rat myocardial cells is an $alpha_1$ adrenergic response. J Clin Invest 72:732-738
5. Robertson AL Jr, Khairallah PA (1971) Angiotensin II: rapid localization in nuclei of smooth and cardiac muscle. Science 172:1138-1139
6. Unger T, Gohlke P, Ganten D, Lang RE (1989) Converting enzyme inhibitors and their effects on the renin-angiotensin system of the blood vessel wall. J Cardiovasc Pharmac 13 (suppl 3):S8-S16

Increased Plasma Lipid Peroxide in Patients with Congestive Heart Failure

KIMINORI KAJIYAMA, YOSHINORI KOGA, YUKARI TSUJI, GENSHO IWAMI, TSUTOMU OTSUKI, and HIRONORI TOSHIMA

The Third Department of Internal Medicine, Kurume University, School of Medicine, Fukuoka, 830 Japan

KEY WORDS: lipid peroxide, free radical, heart failure, norepinephrine

INTRODUCTION

Oxygen free radicals such as superoxide radicals, hydrogen peroxide or hydroxyl radicals have been suggested to play an important role in ischemia-reperfusion injury, catecholamine injury or adriamycin cardiomyopathy[1)-3)]. However, the half life of these free radicals is a matter of microseconds, too short a period for their clinical significance to be determined. On the other hand, oxygen free radicals react with membrane phospholipid and produce lipid peroxide which can be reliably measured by thiobarbituric acid test[4)]. Several invesitigators [5)-7)] have reported increases in plasma lipid peroxide in animal models of adriamycin cardiomyopathy, alcoholic cardiomyopathy or genetic cardiomyopathy. However, few reports have investigated the alteration of plasma lipid peroxide in patients with chronic heart failure, and the clinical significance of lipid peroxide is largely unknown. Therefore, we measured plasma lipid peroxide in patients with dilated cardiomyopathy (DCM), hypertrophic cardiomyopathy (HCM), ischemic heart disease (IHD) and mitral valve disease (MVD) to determine the clinical significance of lipid peroxide in the pathophysiology of congestive heart failure.

PATIENTS AND METHODS

We studied 167 patients with heart diseases, 112 males and 55 females, ranging in age from 16 to 74 years (average 53 ± 13 years). They included 25 patients with DCM, 30 patients with HCM, 52 patients with IHD and 20 patients with MVD. Of these, 145 patients were treated for heart failure with agents including diuretics, digitalis, angiotensin converting enzyme (ACE) inhibitors, calcium antagonists and antiarrythmic agents. Twenty healthy volunteers, 16 males and 4 females ranging in age from 27 to 65 (average 45 ± 10) served as controls. In the fasting and resting state, a blood sample was drawn from the cubital vein. Plasma lipid peroxides were measured by thiobarbituric acid test which detected malondialdehyde (MDA) products of peroxidised lipid and carbohydrates. As we found that storing samples in the freezer significantly decreased measurements, the assay was performed by using plasma immediately after sampling. Plasma norepinephrine (NE) was determined by high pressure liquid chromatography, plasma cyclic AMP by radioimmunoassay, plasma natriuretic peptide (ANP) by radioimmunoassay. The plasma superoxide dismutase (SOD) was measured using Xanthine-Xanthine oxidase method as the radical scavenger. As for clinical and hemodynamic variables, we measured left ventricular ejection fraction (EF) by echocardiogram, cardio thoracic ratio (CTR) in chest X-ray and left ventricular enddiastric pressure (LVEDP) or pulmonary capillary wedge pressure (PCWP) by cardiac catheterization. The statistical comparisons of group means were performed by ANOVA, with Scheffes's multiple comparison test. Peason's product moment was used to determine correlation coefficients.

RESULTS

The average plasma lipid peroxide level (nmol/ml; MDA) was 2.61 ± 0.7 in controls, 4.63 ± 2.0 in DCM, 3.16 ± 1.1 in HCM, 2.76 ± 1.0 in IHD and 3.53 ± 1.3 in MVD (Fig 1). The patients with DCM had significantly higher plasma lipid peroxide than controls ($p<0.001$). No significant differences were observed among the other groups.

Figure 2 shows the relation between severity of heart failure (by NYHA classification) and the plasma lipid peroxide level. The average plasma lipid peroxide level was 2.5 ± 0.6 in NYHA II, 3.9 ± 0.8 in NYHA III and 5.8 ± 1.7 in NYHA IV. The plasma lipid peroxide values increased with the severity of the NYHA classification.

Figure 1 Plasma lipid peroxide in patients with underlying cardiac diseases

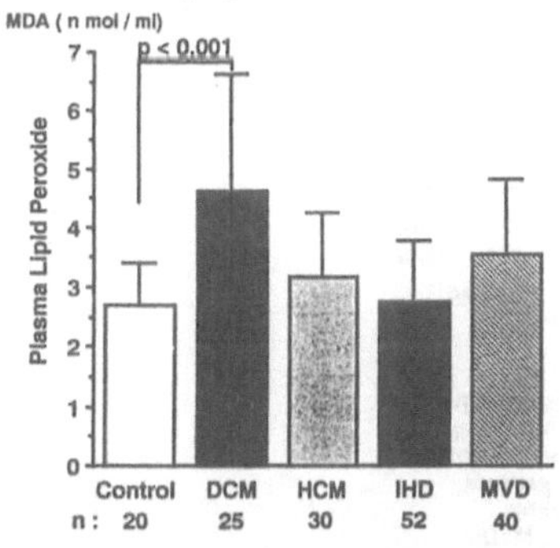

Values are mean ± SD. N means numbers of patients. DCM: dilated cardiomyopathy, HCM:hypertrophic cardiomyopathy, IHD: ischemic heart disease, MVD: mitral valve disease, MDA:malondialdehyde

Figure 2 Plasma lipid peroxide vs NYHA clssification

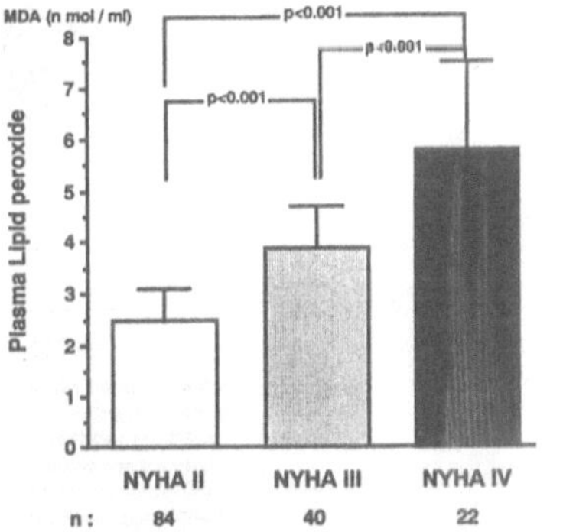

Values are mean ± SD. N means numbers of patients. MDA:malondialdehyde

Table 1 Correlation coefficienct between plasma lipid peroxide and various neurohormonal variables and hemodynamic parameters

		ANP	NE	cAMP	SOD	EF	LVDd	CTR	EDP	PCWP
All heart diseases	r =	0.39	0.50	0.08	0.10	- 0.41	0.30	0.35	0.10	0.30
	p =	0.001	0.001	NS	NS	0.001	0.003	0.001	NS	0.024
DCM	r =	0.57	0.60	0.06	0.11	- 0.54	0.30	0.59	0.31	0.34
	p =	0.005	0.002	NS	NS	0.005	NS	0.003	NS	NS

r: correlation coefficient, p: p values, NS means no significance.
ANP: plasma natriuretic peptide, NE: norepinephrine, cAMP: cyclic AMP, SOD: superoxide desmutase, EF: left ventricular ejection fraction, LVDd: left ventricular dyastric dimension, CTR: cardiac thoracic ratio, EDP left ventricular end-dyastric pressure, PCWP: pulmonary capillary wedge pressure, DCM: dilated cardiomyopathy

The plasma lipid peroxides showed significantly correlations between plasma ANP (r=0.47, p=0.001) and plasma NE (r=0.50, p=0.001) in the analysis of all the study patients as a whole. The correlations attained higher coefficients in the analysis using patients with DCM alone (ANP; r=0.57, p=0.005, NE; r=0.60, p=0.002). However there was no significant correlation between plasma lipid peroxide levels and SOD activity. The plasma lipid peroxide levels also showed a significant correlation with EF (r=0.41, p=0.001) ,CTR (r=0.35, P=0.001) or PCWP (r=0.30, p=0.024). The correlation coefficients with EF (r=-0.54, p=0.005) and CTR (r=0.59, p=0.003) were again higher in patients with DCM alone (Table 1).

The decrease in plasma lipid peroxide level was associated with an improvement of heart failure after treatment with diuretics, ACE inhibitors, digitalis, antiarrythmic agents and antioxidant (Vitamin E and Vitamin C), etc (5.4 ± 1.0 to 2.7 ± 0.9 in Fig 6).

Figure 3 The alteration of plasma lipid peroxide in patients with CHF after treatment

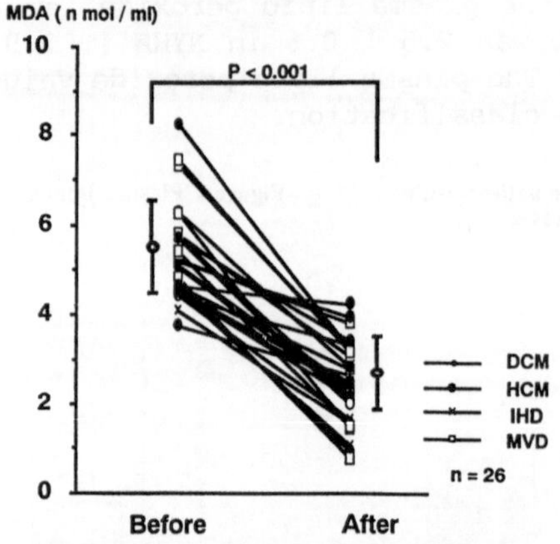

Mean levels before or after treatment of congestive heart failure by diuretics, digitalis, angiotensine converting enzyme inhibitors, antiarrythmic agents or antioxidants. Values are mean ± SD. N means number of patients. DCM:dilated cardiomyopathy, HCM:hypertrophic cardiomyopathy, IHD:ischemic heart disease, MVD: mitral valve disease, MDA:malondialdehyde

DISCUSSION

In the present study, we observed an increase in plasma lipid peroxide level in patients with heart failure, especially in those with dilated cardiomyopathy (DCM). Detailed analyses revealed that plasma lipid peroxide was significantly elevated in association with left ventricular ejection fraction, plasma NE or ANP. These correlations were higher in the analyses using patients with DCM alone than in the analyses using all of study patients as a whole. This observation indicated that plasma lipid peroxide was elevated in correlation with increasing severity of heart failure, rather than in association with underlying mechanisms of heart failure.

It is of interest that the highest correlation coefficient observed was between plasma lipid peroxide and NE. Catecholamines are known to produce free radicals by autooxidation[8]. Thomas et al[9] demonstrated that free radicals such as superoxide anions react with lipid hydroperoxides to form alkoxy radicals in phospholipid membranes. The product, lipid peroxides, are incorporated into polyunsaturated side chains of cell membranes and can then decompose cell membranes producing alkoxy and peroxy radicals in the presence of transition metals such as iron and copper. The enhanced sympathetic nerve function and elevated plasma catecholamines levels in patients with congestive heart failure thus could lead to an increased generation of lipid peroxide in the cell membrane, since iron and copper are present in sufficiently amount in plasma or cell membranes. It is therefore likely that an elevation of plasma lipid peroxide can be attributed to activated peroxidation of cell membrane lipid possibly due to autoxidation of catecholamines. The sympathetic activation in congestive heart failure, which has long been considered to be a compensatory and adaptive response, could instead damage cellular membrane function in various tissues, including myocardium.

In summary, we showed that plasma lipid peroxide was increased in patients with heart failure, especially those with dilated cardiomyopathy. The close correlation of plasma lipid peroxide with parameters of left ventricular function and plasma norepinephrine suggested that enhanced sympathetic activity due to heart failure could induce plasma lipid peroxide production which could in turn induce further myocardial injury. These observations was provide a further rationale for the use of beta-blockades in patients with heart failure.

Reference

1. McCord JM. (1985) Oxygen-derived free radicals in post ischemic tissue injury N Engl J Med 312: 159-63
2. Singal PK, Kapur N, Dhillon KS, Beamish RE, Dhalla NS (1982) Role of free radicals in catecholamine-induced cardiomyopathy Can J Physiol Pharmacol 60: 1390-1397
3. Kajiyama K, Sugiyama M, Iwahashi H, Hidaka T, Entman ML, Shimada I, Ogura R (1987) Electron Spin Resonance Studies on the spin label of rat cardiac mitochondria treated with driamycin Kurume Med J 34: 59-64
4. Ohkawa h, Ohishi S, Yagi K (1979) Assay for lipid peroxides in animal tissues by thiobarbituric acid reaction Anal Biochem 95: 351-358
5. Goodman J, Hochstein PL, (1977) Generation of free radicals and lipid peroxidation by redox cycling of adriamycin and daunomycin Biochem Biophysic Res Commun 77: 797-803
6. Garucia-Bunuel L, (1984) Lipid peroxidation in alcoholic myopathy and cardiomyopathy Medical Hypotheses 13: 217-231
7. Sakanashi T, Sako S, Nozuhara A, Adachi K, Okamoto T, Koga Y, Toshima H (1991) Biochem Biophysic Res Commun 181: 145-150
8. Belch JJF, Bridges AB, Scott N, Chopra M (1991) Oxgen free radicals and congestive heart failure Br Heart J 65: 245-248
9. Thompson JA Hess ML (1986) The oxgen free radical system: A fundamental mechanism in the production of myocardial necrosis Progress cardiovascular Diseases 28: 449-462
10. Thomas MJ, Mehl KS, Pryor WA (1978) The role of superoxide anion in the Xanthine-oxidase induced autooxidation of linoleic acid Biochem Biophisic Res Commun 83: 927-932

Dopamine Sulfate and the Cardiovascular System

TOMOMI KAWAGUCHI[1], KAYOKO TAKENAKA[1], TORU ENDO[1], MASARU MINAMI[1], KOSEI OHNO[2], SATOSHI TAKEO[3], KOICHIRO HAGIHARA[4], KAZUHIKO YAMADA[4], and YOSHIKUNI SUZUKI[4]

Department of Pharmacology[1], Synthetic and Pharmaceutical Chemistry[2], Faculty of Pharmaceutical Science, Higashi-Nippon-Gakuen University, Tobetsu, 061-02 Japan and Department of Pharmacology, Tokyo College of Pharmacy, Tokyo, 192-03 Japan[3] and Pharmaceutical Research Center, Nisshin Flour Milling Co., Ltd., Saitama, 354 Japan[4]

KEYWORDS: DA-4-O-sulfate, DA-3-O-sulfate, Positive inotropic effect, Rabbit papillary muscle, cAMP

INTRODUCTION

Approximately 80% of the total NE and Ep and 90% of the total DA in circulation consists of conjugated catecholamines (1-3). Kuchel et al (4) reported that increased plasma concentrations of DA-S were observed in patients with essential hypertension. In a recent study (5), we found that the levels of DA-S in the plasma of patients with CHF were 3-fold higher than control values. We also reported that DA-4-S has a positive inotropic effect on isolated rabbit papillary muscles (6). However, the source and physiological role of the sulfate catecholamines remain unknown. In order to investigate the site and the mechanism of action of DA-S, we have synthesized DA-4-S and DA-3-S (Fig.1). The present study was undertaken to determine the affinity for the receptor related to the positive inotropic effect. An attempt was also made to determine the role of sulfate in the conversion of DA-S into free DA and cAMP in various tissues of the rabbit.

MATERIALS AND METHODS

Isolated cardiac muscle preparation

Papillary muscle preparations were obtained from the right ventricle of male white rabbits (approximately 3 kg). They were driven by electrical stimulation (rectangular wave, 5 ms duration, 1 Hz) (Nihon Kohden, Japan, MSE-3R). Each preparation was suspended in an organ bath containing Locke Ringer solution. The bath temperature was maintained at 37 °C and the solution was continuously aerated with a mixture of 95% O_2 and 5% CO_2. The isometric tension was recorded by a strain gauge transducer (Shinkoh, Japan, U-gage U-L).

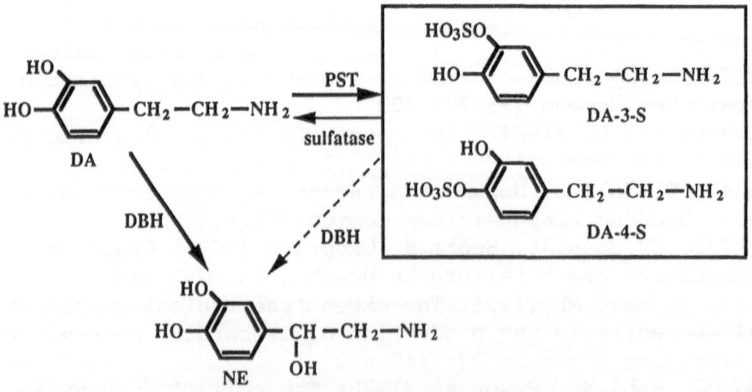

Fig.1 Biochemical pathway of catecholamine

[1]Abbreviation. DA, dopamine; DA-S, dopamine-sulfate; DA-4-S, dopamine-4-O-sulfate; DA-3-S, dopamine-3-O-sulfate; cAMP, cyclic adenosine monophosphate; NE, norepinephrine; Ep, epinephrine; CHF, congestive heart failure; RV, right ventricle; RA, right atrium; LV, left ventricle; LA, Left atrium.

Biochemical assays

Sulfatase assay was based on the simplified method described by Roy (7). Receptor binding assay was performed using the rat brain (8). Using beating atrial preparations of the rat, we measured their myocardial cAMP contents by the method of Honma et al. (9). Protein determinations were carried out by the method of Lowry et al. (10).

Statistical analysis

Statistically significant differences were determined by Student's t-test. Values are expressed as mean ± SE.

RESULTS AND DISCUSSION

Effect on rabbit papillary muscle

As shown in Fig. 2, DA-4-S increased contractile force in a concentration dependent manner in rabbit papillary muscle. The 20% increase in isometric tension represents the inotropic effect of DA-4-S. This positive inotropic effect was not inhibited by propranolol (10^{-5}M), haloperidol (10^{-6}M) or domperidone (10^{-6}M). Prazosin (10^{-6}M) and phentolamine (2.6×10^{-5}M) also did not inhibit this inotropism. Amosulalol (10^{-5}M), α and β blocker, failed to inhibit the positive inotropic effect of DA-4-S. Endoh et al. (11) reporter that the positive inotropic effect of DA was antagonized by amosulalol. Dopaminergic receptor antagonists also failed to alter the effect of DA on rabbit papillary muscle (12). These reports support the possibility that free DA is not responsible for the positive inotropic action of DA-4-S. Furthermore, the synthesized DA-3-S did not have any significant effect on the guinea pig atria. As sulfatase is a nonspecific enzyme, both DA-4-S and DA-3-S could be converted to free DA by sulfatase. Free DA is not responsible for this positive inotropism.

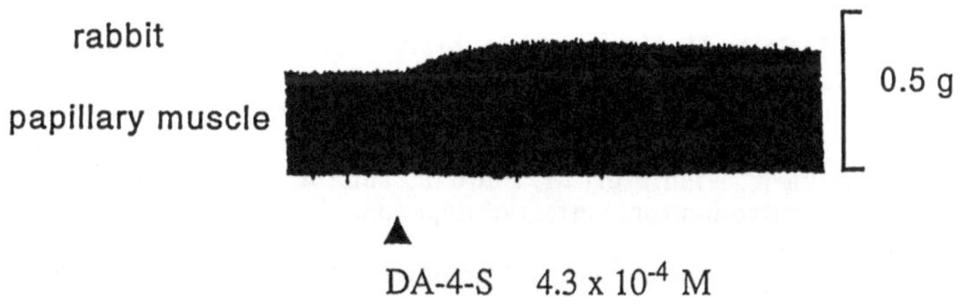

Fig. 2 Positive inotropic effect of DA-4-S on the isolated rabbit papillary muscle.

Sulfatase activity

Free DA was detected in the organ bath containing DA-4-S treated guinea pig atria. Increased sulfatase activity was observed in the atrial tissue of the guinea pig and rabbit.

Receptor binding assay

As shown in Table 1, the receptor binding assay demonstrated that DA-4-S had no affinity with adrenergic or dopaminergic receptors.

cAMP assay

In the beating rat heart muscle, myocardial cAMP content increased significantly after administration of DA-4-S (4.3×10^{-4} M)(vehicle n=5, 3.18 ± 0.51 vs DA-4-S n=5, 6.31 ± 0.69 pmol/mg protein).

Table 1. Affinity of DA-4-S with adrenergic and dopaminergic receptors

Receptor	Ligand	% Inhibition of 10^{-5} M
α_1–adrenergic	^{3}H-Prazosin	-5
α_2–adrenergic	^{3}H-Rauwolscin	15
β–adrenergic	^{3}H-DHA	-2
Dopamine D_1	^{3}H-SCH23390	-2
Dopamine D_2	^{3}H-Raclopride	23

In summary, DA-4-S had a positive inotropic effect on the isolated heart muscle of guinea pigs and rabbits. Furthermore, DA-4-S caused a significant increase of myocardial cAMP. These findings suggest that DA-4-S might be appropriate for the clinical diagnosis and treatment of CHF.

REFERENCES

1. Kuchel O, Buu NT, Fontaine A, Hamet P, Beroniade V, Larochelle P, Genest, J (1980) Free and conjugated plasma catecholamines in hypertensive patients with and without pheochromocytoma. Hypertension 2: 177-186
2. Johnson GA, Baker CA., Smith RT (1980) Radioenzymatic assay of sulfate conjugates of catecholamines and dopa in plasma. Life Sci 26: 1591-1598
3. Joyce DA, Beilin LJ, Vandongen R, Davidson L (1982) Plasama free and sulfate conjugated catecholamine levels during acute physiological stimulation in man. Life Sci 30: 447-454
4. Kuchel O, Buu NT, Hamet P, Larochelle P, Bourque M, Genest J. (1984) Catecholamine sulfates and platelet phenolsulfotransferase activity in essential hypertension. J Lab Clin Med 104: 238-244
5. Endo T, Minami M, Saito H, Yamazaki N, Matsumoto M, Takeo S, Parvez SH. (1989) Significance of sulfate conjugated dopamine, epinephrine and norepinephrine in patients with congestive heart failure and chronic hemodialysis: In vitro correlations. Biogenic Amines 6: 571-580
6. Minami M, Takenaka K, Nishikiori M, Endo T, Tanabe T, Saito H, Yasuda H, Takeo S, Parvez SH. (1991) Positive inotropic effect of dopamine-4-O-sulfate; A preliminary study. Asia Pacific J Pharmacol 6: 165-170
7. Roy AB. (1960) The sulphate of ox liver. 7. The intracellular distribution of sulphatases A and B. Biochem J 77: 380-386
8. Greengrass P, Bremner R (1979) Binding characteristics of ^{3}H-prazosin to rat brain α-adrenergic receptors. Eur J Pharmacol 55: 323-326
9. Honma M, Satoh T, Takezawa J, Ui M. (1977) An ultrasensitive method for the simultaneous determination of cyclic AMP and cyclic GMP in small-volume samples from blood and tissue. Biochem Med 18: 257-273
10. Lowry OH, Rosebrough NJ, Farr AL, Randall RJ. (1951) Protein measurements with the folin phenol reagent. J Biol Chem 193: 265-275
11. Endoh M, Schümann HJ, Krappitz N, Hillen B (1976) α-Adrenoceptors mediating positive inotropic effects on the ventricular myocardium: Some aspects of structure-activity relationship of sympathomimetic amines. Jap J Pharmacol 26: 179-190
12. Motomura S, Broddle OE, Schümann HJ (1978) No evidence for involvement of dopaminergic receptors in the positive inotropic action of dopamine on the isolated rabbit papillary muscle. Jap J Pharmacol 28: 145-153

Systemic Study of the Hemodynamic Effects of Nitroglycerin in Conscious Dogs: New Aspect of Mechanism of its Antianginal Action

KAZUKO NONAKA and AKIRA UENO

Department of Pharmacology and Experimental Therapeutics, Nagasaki University School of Medicine, Nagasaki, 852 Japan

KEYWORDS: nitroglycerin, conductance-resistance-capacitance arteries, unanesthetized dog

INTRODUCTION

Nitroglycerin (GTN) has been widely used as an antianginal agent for more than a century. However, the exact mechanism of the effect of GTN is still uncertain and, in some aspect, controversial. A majority believes that GTN reduces myocardial wall tension by lowering preload and afterload due to dilation of capacitance vessels and this improves the the transmural distribution of the blood flow to the subendocardial layer of the myocardium [1, 2]. Brown et al.[3] clearly showed by angiography that GTN increases the luminal area in both normal and diseased portions of epicardial large coronary arteries, and concluded that vasodilation of epicardial coronary stenosis is usually a major component of the beneficial response to GTN. But they have not ruled out the role of venodilation.
The purpose of this communication was to provide information on the large and small arterio-venous and cardiac effects of GTN in unanesthetized and unrestrained normal dogs with special reference to the susceptibility of conductance, resistance and capacitance vessels to GTN, and on the mode of action of its anti-anginal activity.

MATERIALS AND METHODS

Mongrel dogs, aged over 5 y, either sexes, 8.5 to 17 kg in body weight and in total 17 were participated in the experiment 1-3 months. The parameter examined included coronary blood flow (CBF), diameter of LCX (CD), internal diameter of the left ventricle (LVID) blood flow in the aorta (CO) and vena cava (vcBF), diameters of the aorta, carotid, mesenteric, iliac internal thoracic and pulmonary arteries and vena cava, pressure in the left ventricle, abdominal aorta and pulmonary arteries, organ thickness of the spleen, liver and sartorius muscle, and rate of rise in arterial pressure pulses at the abdominal aorta (Adp/dt). The recordings were made with aid of electromagnetic blood flow meter (Transflow 601, Skalar Med., Delft, Holland) and ultrasonic sonomicrometer (UDM 5C, Mecc, Fukuoka, Japan). Sublingual administration of GTN tablet was carried out by holding the dog's jaw for 1 min after placing the corrected dose tablet under the tongue.

1) Based on Nonaka K, Ueno A (1991) Systemic Study of the Hemodynamic Effects of Sublingual Nitroglycerin in Unanesthetized Dogs. Arch int Pharmacodyn 312: 5-26, with permission.

RESULTS AND DISCUSSION

The effects of GTN, administered sublingually (s.l.) and intravenously (i.v.) at doses of 5, 10, 15 and 25 micro-grams/kg, were investigated. GTN, at dose of 5-15 micro-grams/kg, s.l., produced a slight but persistent fall in systolic pressure (sBP) and no definite changes in diastolic pressure (dBP), heart rate (HR), CO and vcBF in about 1/3 of the cases. The remainder of the dogs responded to GTN by showing an increased HR, a slight fall in mean blood pressure and slight increase of CO and vcBF, but these changes were transient, lasting for 10 to 60 sec. As the s.l. dose increased, the changes became more apparent and longer lasting. GTN, at dose of 5-15 micro-grams/kg, s.l., essentially produced no effect on CBF in most cases, although there was a slight transient increase in CBF with a concomitant HR increase in response to systolic pressure fall, followed by a slight but persistent decrease in coronary blood flow. These responses in CBF, responses of coronary resistance vessels, could be attributable to increased and decreased oxygen demands of the myocardium. On the other hand, GTN, s.l., i.v., consistently and efficiently dilated epicardial large coronary arteries. This action was apparent not only in the coronary artery but also in all systemic arteries tested.
It is, therefore, proposed that this action of GTN could be called "selective conductance arterial dilation".

GTN s.l., had no effect on LVEDP, LVID, pressure and diameter of pulmonary artery. There was no reduction in preload in unanesthetized dogs, as far as changes in HR and CO were concerned. Reduction of preload, decrease of LVID with reduction of LVEDP, were noted only in case where GTN, in a large dose, elicited a definite fall in mBP with concomitant marked increases in HR, LVdp/dt and CO. Therefore, the reduction of preload by GTN appeared to be a phenomenon induced secondary by cardio-acceleration in response to hypotension.
GTN i.v., always produced transient fall in BP and transient increases in HR, CO and LVdp/dt and reductions in LVEDP and LVID and sustained increase in CD, indicating participation of dilation of resistance vessels when exposed to a high concentration of GTN.

GTN, s.l., 5 micro-gram/kg, essentially had no effect on mBP. GTN, i.v., caused a transient fall in mBP. However, in both situations, a slight but persistent decrease in sBP was observed in most cases. Adp/dt, first derivative of the pressure at the caudal portion of abdominal aorta, was reduced persistently throughout the period of lowered sBP and both LVdp/dt and CO remained unchanged or were increased. Thus, GTN-produced systemic conductance arterial dilation increased the Windkessel volume, and which is responsible for the fall in sBP, and could be an important factor in reducing cardiac work load.

Although GTN has long been believed to cause both arteriolar and venous dilation, with venodilation being predominant, in the present study it was found that the diameter of the vena cava and the thickness of the spleen, liver and sartorius muscle, which reflect changes in vascular capacity, mainly in the venules in each organ, never increases by GTN, s.l. and i.v., and that vcBF and CO responded with either no change or with an increase, and that GTN s.l., without effect on LVEDP and LVID. The results in unanesthetized dogs indicate that the

veins, at least, in the splanchnic and hind limb areas do not respond to GTN with an effective venodilation.
The present results clearly indicate that the primary vascular action of a therapeutic s.l. dose of GTN is solely conductance arterial dilation. Other actions, such as reduction of LVID and LVEDP, increase in HR, LVdp/dt and CO, are secondary effects due to the baroreceptor reflex triggered by the fall in BP.
It is well documented that, during an anginal attack, LVEDP, pulmonary wedge pressure and central venous pressure are markedly elevated, and that the use of GTN reduces the elevated pressures dramatically.

From the present results, this effect of GTN can be explained as follows: most of the pathologic narrowings in the coronary arteries manifested epicardial large arteries [5, 6], and coronary conductance arterial dilation by GTN acts directly on diseased portion to dilate, and improves blood flow into the ischemic part of the myocardium. Therefore, the heart regains its ventricular function and pumps stagnant blood from heart, lungs and veins to arterial side, resulting in a reduction of elevated preload to normal levels in anginal patients.

It is concluded that the therapeutic significance of s.l. administered GTN lies in a novel selective conductance arterial dilation which occurs in both the coronary and systemic arteries. The effect of the former would be directly on stenotic lesions in the epicardial large coronary artery, improving blood flow to the ischemic part of the myocardium, whereas the latter might be beneficial for reducing cardiac work and lowering sBP by increasing the Windkessel volume. And the present study rule out the therapeutic role of venodilation. A recently published paper [4] on the role of nitroglycerin in angina pectoris is available for more comprehensive discussion.

REFERENCES

1. Burggraff GW, Parker JO (1974) Left ventricular volume changes after amyl nitrate and nitroglycerin in man as measured by ultrasound. Circulation 49: 136-143
2. Swain JL, Parker JP, McHale PA, Greefield JC Jr (1978) Effect of nitroglycerin and propranolol on the distribution of transmural myocardial blood flow during ischemia in the absence of hemodynamic changes in the dog. J clin Invest 64: 947-953
3. Brown BG, Bolson EL, Petersen RB, Pierce CD, Dodge HT (1981) The mechanism of nitroglycerin action: Stenosis vasodilation as a major component of the drug response. Circulation 64: 1089-1097
4. Nonaka K, Ueno A (1991) Systemic study of the hemodynamic effects of sublingual nitroglycerin in unanesthetized dogs. Arch int Pharmacodyn 312: 5-26
5. White NK, Edwards JE, Dry TJ (1950) The relationship of degree of coronary atherosclerosis with age, in men. Circulation 1: 645-654
6. Yasue H (1983) Electrocardiographic, hemodynamic, and angiographic consequences. In: Chahine RA (ed) Coronary artery spasm. Futura. Mount Kisco, New York. pp85-118

Load Dependence of Systolic and Diastolic LV Function — On-line Recorded in the Isolated Perfused Guinea Pig Heart. Effects of Ouabain, Caffeine, Gallopamil and $[Mg^{++}]_o$

JOACHIM DÖRING[1], VOLKER HILLER[1], and PAISAN BUNSIRICOMCHAI[2]

Physiological Institute, University of Freiburg, D-7800 Freiburg/Germany[1] and Research Fellow of the Faculty of Medicine, Siriraj Hospital, Mahidol University, Bangkok, Thailand[2]

KEYWORDS: load-dependence of $-dp/dt_{max}$, ouabain, caffeine, gallopamil, magnesium

INTRODUCTION

For about 20 years the diastolic part of the cardiac cycle was increasingly taken into consideration [1, 9, 2] especially with respect to ischemic heart disease [6, 7]. Particularly the load-dependence of relaxation - the analogue of the FRANK-STARLING LV function curves - occupied high interest. Using the four tools ouabain, caffeine, gallopamil and Mg^{++} the following studies should contribute to elucidate the interaction between myocardial intra-/extracellular Ca status and load dependence of $-dp/dt_{max}$ (as a measure of diastolic relaxation).

MATERIALS AND METHODS

Hearts from guinea pigs (280 - 350 g) were perfused at constant pressure (50 mmHg) with modified KREBS-HENSELEIT solution and stimulated electrically (270/min). The following parameters were measured or calculated: 1. left ventricular isovolumetric pressure by means of an intraventricular balloon catheter connected to a Statham P23 Db transducer; 2. $p_s - p_d$ (dLVP), 3. $+dp/dt_{max}$, 4. $-dp/dt_{max}$, 5. the ratio $-dp/dt_{max} : +dp/dt_{max}$ (termed "Q"), coronary flow above the aortic cannula using an electromagnetic flowmeter (Biotronex BM 402), 6. perfusion pressure (PP) with a Statham P23 Db transducer. Using an electronic perfusion pressure control unit PP was increases stepwise to load the hearts repetitively. All data were fed into a PC which controlled the experimental protocol by specially developed software. By means of quantitative evaluation of the experiments the following function curves were obtained:

1. FRANK-STARLING function curves from dLVP, $+dp/dt_{max}$ and $-dp/dt_{max}$ (see paper by Bunsiricomchai et al., this book).
2. The ratio "Q" vs. PP.

The LANGENDORFF set-up by Hugo Sachs Elektronik, D-7806 March/Germany was used. For details of the method see [3, 4, 5,].

RESULTS AND DISCUSSION

Our studies on the ratio of LV -dp/dt_{max} and +dp/dt_{max} (= Q) in guinea pig hearts have revealed three different types of cardiac relaxation/contraction ratios:

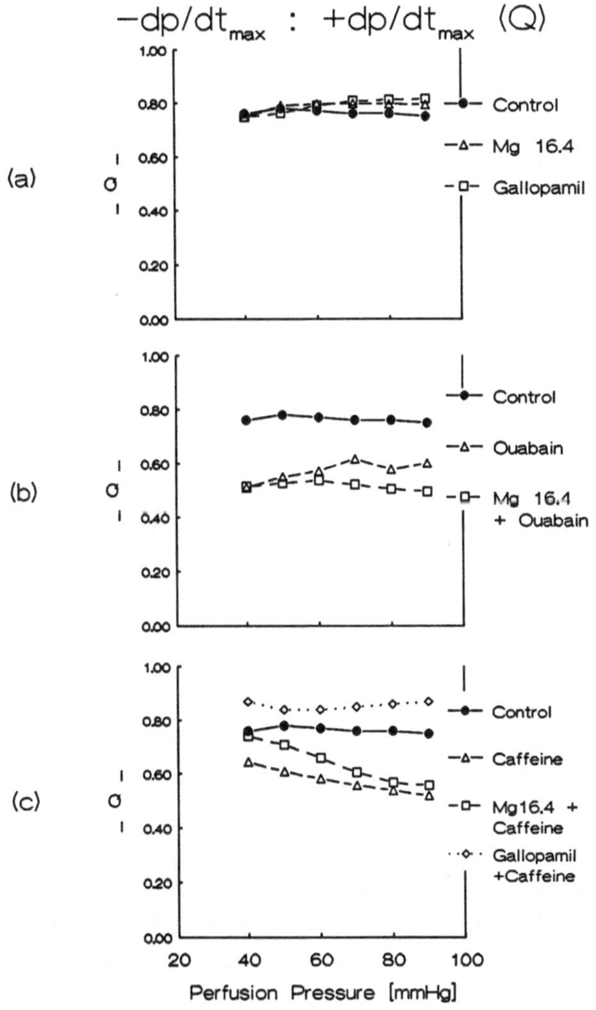

Fig.1 Load-dependence of -dp/dt_{max} : +dp/dt_{max} (= Q) of guinea pig left ventricle.
(a) In control hearts, with various Mg^{++} concentrations (here only 16.4 mmol/l shown) or the Ca antagonist gallopamil "Q" amounts to about 0.8, independently of perfusion pressure load.
(b) Ouabain (1.4 × 10^{-6} mol/l) depressed "Q" to 0.5 to 0.6 due to an increase of +dp/dt_{max} without a concomitant increase in -dp/dt_{max}. Mg^{++} exerts no influence.
(c) Caffeine (12 mmol/l) depressed "Q" PP-dependently due to PP-dependent decrease in -dp/dt_{max}. Gallopamil but not Mg^{++} abolished the influence of caffeine.

Normal type

During perfusion with normal solution or various $MgSO_4$ concentrations (0 to 16,4 mmol/l) or gallopamil (10^{-8} mol/l) "Q" remained constant at 0.8 to 0.9 independent of PP-load, though contractile force varied in a wide range (Fig.1a). This means that -dp/dt_{max} is slightly lower than +dp/dt_{max} and its load dependence shows a similar course than +dp/dt_{max}.

Ouabain type

Ouabain (1.4×10^{-6} mol/l), which is known to inhibit relaxation, depressed "Q" to values of 0.5 to 0.6 independently of PP (Fig.1b). The combination with 4 different Mg concentrations (0, 1.64, 3.28, 16.4 mmol/l) did not influence "Q".

Caffeine type

With Caffeine (12 mmol/l) "Q" took a downsloping course with the increase of PP (Fig.1c). This is due to the development of myocardial contracture. Various Mg^{++} concentrations (0, 8.2 and 16.4 mmol/l) exhibit no influence on the PP-dependent course of "Q". Gallopamil, however, restored the caffeine-induced, load-sensitive depression of "Q".

The reason might be a stretch-induced inhibition of the Ca storage capacity of the sarcoplasmic reticulum which might be enhanced under the influence of caffeine and which preferably results in a decrease in $-dp/dt_{max}$.

REFERENCES

1. Brutsaert DL, Sonnenblick, EH (1971) The early onset of maximum velocity of shortening in heart muscle of the cat. Pflügers Arch 324: 91-99
2. Cohn PF,. Liedtke AJ, Serur J, Sonnenblick EH, Uschel CW (1972) Maximal rate of pressure fall (peak negative dp/dt) during ventricular relaxation. Cardiovascular Res 6:263-267
3. Döring HJ, Dehnert H (1988) The isolated perfused heart according to LANGENDORFF. Biomesstechnik-Verlag March GmbH, March/ Germany
4. Döring HJ (1989) Differentiation of various cardiovascular drugs by means of specific myocardial and vascular load tests. Experiments at the isolated perfused heart. Arzneim Forsch (Drug Res) 39: 1535-1542
5. Döring HJ, Schlicht I, Hiller V, Jiang X-R (1989) Myogenic autoregulation of coronary vessels and heterometric autoregulation of the myocardium. Korean J Physiol 23: 225-235
6. Kumada T, Karlinger JS, Pouleur H, Gallagher KP, Shirato K, Ross J (1979) Effects of coronary occlusion on early ventricular diastolic events in conscious dogs. Am Heart J 237: H542-H549
7. Mann T, Goldberg S, Mudge GH, Grossman W (1979) Factors contributing to altered left ventricular diastolic properties during angina pectoris. Circulation 59: 14-20
8. Mason DT (1969) Usefulness and limitations of the rate of rise of intraventricular pressure (dp/dt) in the evaluation of myocardial contractility in man. Am J Cardiol 23: 516- ???
9. Strauer BE (1971) Evidence for a positive inotropic effect of nitroglycerol on isolated human ventricular myocardium. Pharmacol Res Comm 3: 377-383

Different Load Dependence of $-dp/dt_{max}$ in Rat and Guinea Pig Hearts and the Influence of Ouabain and Caffeine

PAISAN BUNSIRICOMCHAI[1], JOACHIM DÖRING[2], and VOLKER HILLER[2]

Research Fellow of the Faculty of Medicine, Siriraj Hospital, Mahidol University, Bangkok, Thailand[1] and Physiological Institute, University of Freiburg, D-7800 Freiburg/Germany[2]

KEYWORDS: load-dependence of $-dp/dt_{max}$, diastolic function, caffeine, ouabain.

INTRODUCTION

Isovolumic rate of LV pressure decrease ($-dp/dt_{max}$) depends on fibre prestretch similar to $+dp/dt_{max}$; its stretch-induced increase, however, is less pronounced. The rate of both values ($-dp/dt_{max}$: $+dp/dt_{max}$) is influenced by various interventions [1].
The following experiments were performed to investigate load dependence of $-dp/dt_{max}$ in guinea pig and rat hearts implementing two tools: ouabain and caffeine.

MATERIALS AND METHODS

Hearts of guinea pigs (280 - 350 g) and Wistar rats (280 - 350 g) were perfused according to LANGENDORFF with a modified KREBS-HENSELEIT solution. LV isovolumic pressure, coronary flow, and perfusion pressure (PP) were measured; $+dp/dt_{max}$, $-dp/dt_{max}$, and the ratio $-dp/dt_{max}$: $+dp/dt_{max}$ (Q) were calculated. Myocardial load was changed by increases of perfusion pressure (PP) in the range of 40 - 150 mmHg (for details of method see [1] and [2]).

RESULTS AND DISCUSSION

Influence of Steady-state Contractile Force

Rat hearts are generally more resistant to load than guinea pig hearts. This is demonstrated in the upper right diagram of the figure in which a LV function curve from rat hearts is drawn from $+dp/dt_{max}$ vs PP: The ascending branch of this curve reaches from 70 to 150 mmHg with

$+dp/dt_{max}$ values ranging from 3500 to 6100 mmHg/s (= +74%). In contrast, the increase of the $-dp/dt_{max}$ curve peaks already at a PP of 130 mmHg with a maximum value of 3290 mmHg/s (31% increase). Thus "Q" takes a descending course if PP increases (lower right diagram).
On the other hand maximum PP-tolerance of guinea pig hearts amounts to about 100 mmHg. In the range of 40 - 90 mmHg $+dp/dt_{max}$ rises from about 1150 mmHg/s to 1860 mmHg/s (+62%) (upper left diagram). Simultaneously, $-dp/dt_{max}$ increases with about the same rate (57%) from 870 to 1360 mmHg/s. Thus, "Q" shows only a minor load-dependence (lower left diagram), (see also [3]).

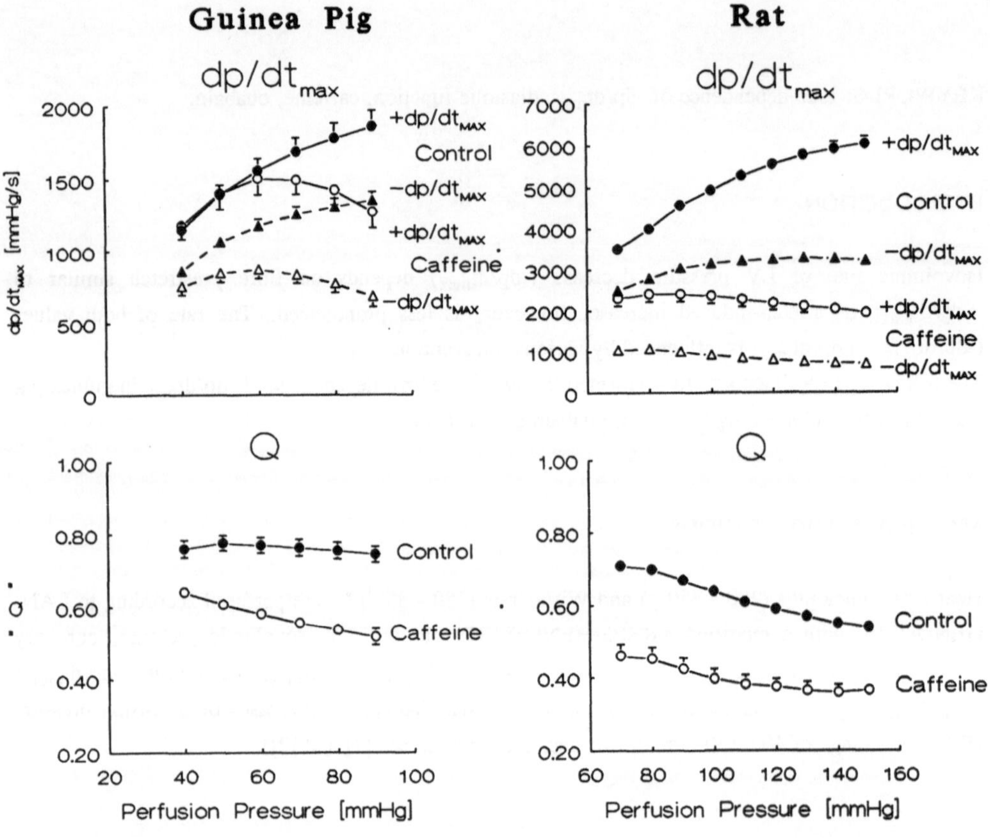

Fig.1 Load-dependence of $-dp/dt_{max}$ and $+dp/dt_{max}$ (upper diagrams) and the ratio (Q) of both (lower diagrams) in guinea pig and rat hearts.

Following a more exact analysis of the data it became apparent that in guinea pig hearts with a high level of $+dp/dt_{max}$ (1895 mmHg/s) "Q" shows a decreasing (-11%) load-dependence whereas in those with a low level of $+dp/dt_{max}$ (1170 mmHg/s) it even shows an increasing (+11%) load-dependence. The reason for this different behavior obviously is that the load-dependent inotropic effect is more marked and more variable than the lusitropic effect; one might speculate that in some types of cardiac failure the ratio of systolic and diastolic function is shifted in favour of diastole. Thus, "Q" may increase, be constant or may decrease during PP load depending on the initial contractile force of the heart.

Changes in cellular calcium status

Two substances, ouabain and caffeine, are known to induce alterations in contractile function, particularly with regard to the rates of systolic and diastolic LV pressure changes.
In guinea pig hearts, after 1.4×10^{-6} mol/l ouabain "Q" was depressed by 40% and remained constant at this level during load. This is due to a specific inhibition of the load-dependent increase of $-dp/dt_{max}$. After 12 mmol/l caffeine "Q" was depressed by 20%, but, in addition, took a downsloping course during load similar to normal rat ventricles (upper and lower left diagrams). This functional change may be related to a disturbance in the Ca-sequestration of the sarcoplasmic reticulum. In rat hearts, after 12 mmol/l caffeine, no change in the slope of "Q" was observed when compared with control rats but the curve was shifted parallel to even lower levels (upper and lower right diagrams). (The influence of ouabain was not investigated.)

CONCLUSION

Load dependence of "Q" is related to the steady-state contractile force of the heart but on the other hand it may reflect the functional integrity of the sarcoplasmic reticulum.

REFERENCES

1. Döring HJ, Dehnert H (1988) The isolated perfused heart according to LANGENDORFF. Biomesstechnik-Verlag March GmbH, March/ Germany
2. Döring HJ (1989) Differentiation of various cardiovascular drugs by means of specific myocardial and vascular load tests. Experiments at the isolated perfused heart. Arzneim Forsch (Drug Res) 39: 1535-1542
3. Döring HJ, Hiller V, Bunsiricomchai P (1992) Load dependence and diastolic LV function - on-line recorded in the isolated perfused guinea pig heart. Effects of ouabain, caffeine, gallopamil and Mg^{++}. This book.

Depressed Endothelium-Dependent Vesodilator Response in the Hindquarter Resistance Vessels in Heart Failure Dogs

MASAHIRO UENO, SEINOSUKE KAWASHIMA, MASATO MORITA, SADAYA TSUMOTO, TOMOHIRO KONDO, and TADAAKI IWASAKI

The First Department of Internal Medicine, Hyogo College of Medicine, Hyogo, 663 Japan

KEYWORDS : congestive heart failure, EDRF, resistance vessels

【INTRODUCTION】

Congestive heart failure (CHF) is a clinical syndrome characterized by the inability of the heart to provide adequate nutrient supply to the metabolically active tisse. Abnormalities in vasomoter tone are well-known in this condition.

This study was undertaken to examine whether endothelium-dependent vasodilator response in the hindquarter resistance vessels is altered in congestive heart failure.

【METHODS】

〈Model of experimental heart failure〉

CHF was produced in eleven mongrel dogs (10-30 kg) by rapid ventricular pacing. Briefly, a pacemaker generator was inserted into a cervical pocket, and a unipolar pacemaker lead was positioned in the right ventricular free wall under general anesthea. After dogs were recovered from anesthea, pacemakers were programmed to pace at 250 beats/min. Dogs were then returned to a chronic-care facility where they recieved a standard diet and free access to water over the following 2 weeks.

〈experimental protocol〉

After 2 weeks, under anesthemic condition, blood from the left carotid artery was pumped into a reservoir situated above the dog and, then, perfused into the left femoral artery at constant pressure equivalent to mean aortic pressure. A Swan-Ganz catheter was inserted into the femoral vein and advanced to the pulmonary artery. A small polyethylene catheter was inserted into to the right femoral artery and advanced to thratic desending aorta for monitor arterial blood pressure. (Fig 1)

(protocol 1)

After stabilization of hemodynamic variables, changes in femoral blood flow to vasodilator substances were observed. Acetylcholine (ACh), Adenosine 5'-Diphosphate Disodium Salt (ADP) and Nitroglycerin (NTG) were administered into the perfusion line. The order of the administration of the three drugs were randomized.

(protocol 2)

In another group of five dogs without CHF, vascular responses to various doses of ACh was examined before and after intravenous administration of aspirin (25 mg/kg).

(protocol 3)

In five dogs with CHF, changes in femoral blood flow in response to L-N^{G}-monomethyl L-arginine (LNMMA), No synthesis inhibitor was observed. LNMMA (1.0 mg/kg/min) was infused into the perfusion line.

	MAP(mmHg)	H.R(/min)	LVEDP(mmHg)	C.I(ml/min/kg)	%FS	
Control group (n=7)	113±15	145±38	9.3±1.9	108±21.9	46.6±9.6	mean±SE *:p<0.05
CHF group (n=6)	110±10	150±8	34.0±12.2**	79.6±19.6*	18.3±9.8**	**:p<0.01

Table 1. Cardiac and Hemodynamic Variables in Dogs with Heart failure and Control Dogs.
Values are mean±SE. MAP;mean aortic pressure, H.R;heart rate
LVEDP;left ventricular end-diastolic pressure, C.I;cardiac index, %FS;%fractional shortening
* : p<0.05, vs Control. ** : p<0.01, vs Control.

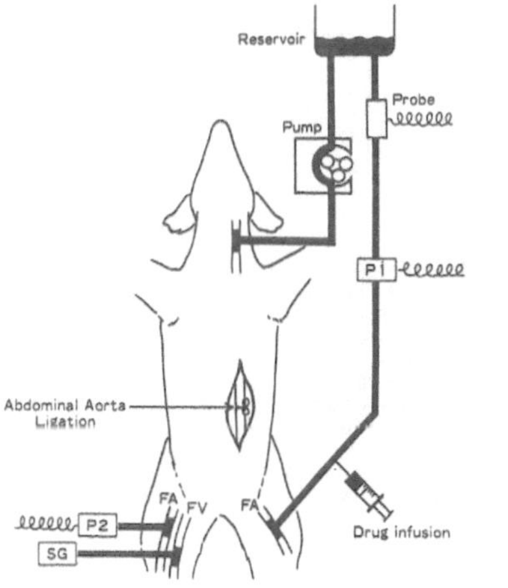

P1 : Perfusion pressure P2 : Aortic pressure
SG : Swan-Ganz catheter

Fig 1. Under anesthemic condition ,blood from the left carotid artery was pumped into a reservoir situated above the dog and, then, perfused into the left femoral artery at constant pressure equivalent to mean aortic pressure.
A Swan-Ganz catheter was inserted into the femoral vein and advanced to the pulmonary artery. A small polyethylene catheter was inserted into to the right femoral artery and advanced to thoratic desending aorta for monitor arterial blood pressure.

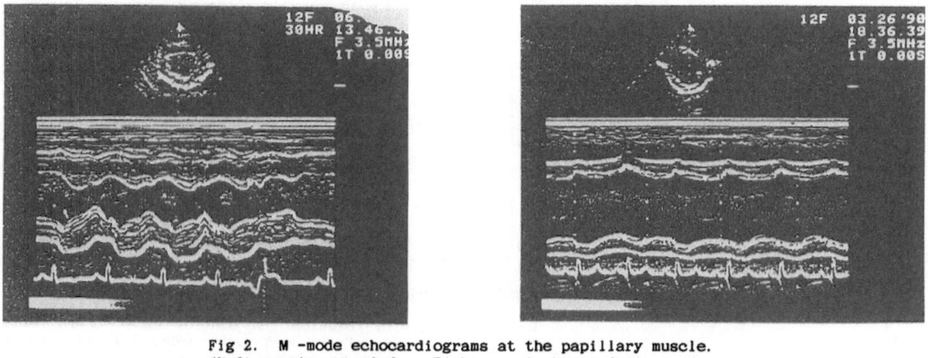

Fig 2. M -mode echocardiograms at the papillary muscle.
(Left panel: cotrol dog, Right panel: heart failrure dog.)
In heart failure dog, left ventricular end-diastolic dimension is markedly dilated, left ventricular thickness is thin and left ventricular contraction is diminished.

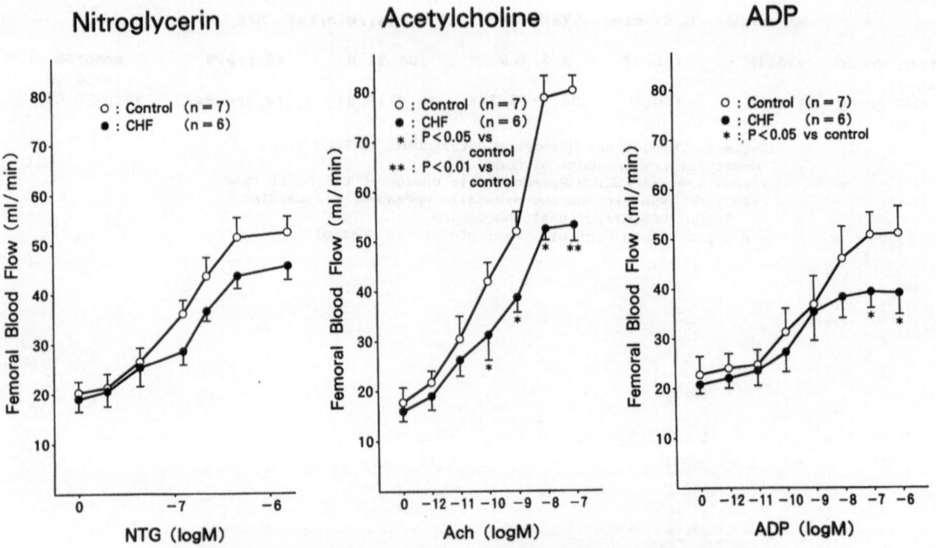

Fig 3. Left panel: Cumulative Nitroglycerin(NTG) dose-response relationships in control (○;n=7) and heart failure (●;n=6) dogs. No significant difference existed between heart failure dogs and control dogs at all concentrations. Middle panel: Cumulative Acetylcholine(Ach) dose-response relationships in control (○;n=7) and heart failure (●;n=6) dogs. In heart failure dogs, vasodilator response to Ach is significantly depressed at the doses higher than 1×10^{-9} mol. Right panel: Cumulative ADP dose-response relationships in control (○;n=7) and heart failure (●;n=6) dogs. In heart failure dogs, vasodilator response to ADP is significantly depressed at the doses higher than 1×10^{-7} mol. Values are mean±SE. * : $p<0.05$, vs Control. ** : $p<0.01$, vs Control.

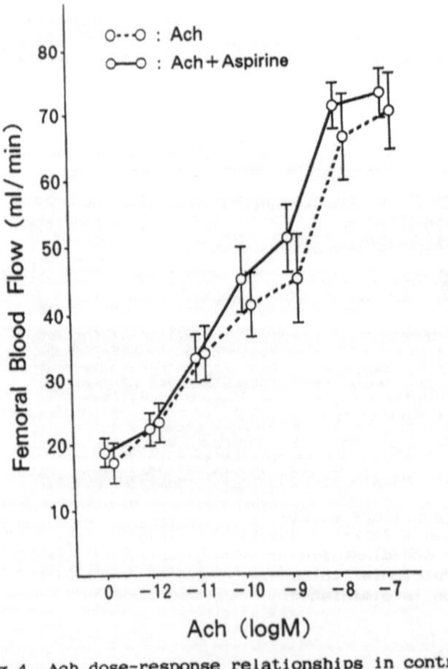

Fig 4. Ach dose-response relationships in control dogs before (○—○) and after (○···○) aspirin preteatment (n=5). Aspirin did not significantly alter Ach-induced vasodilation. Values are mean±SE.

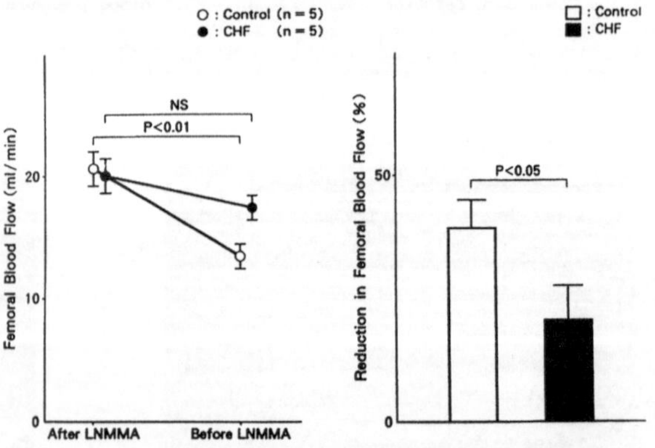

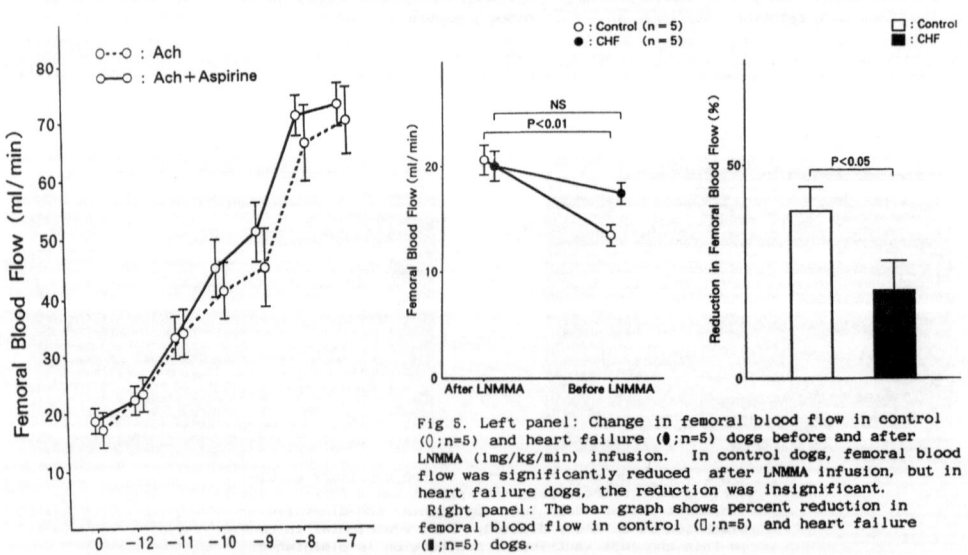

Fig 5. Left panel: Change in femoral blood flow in control (○;n=5) and heart failure (●;n=5) dogs before and after LNMMA (1mg/kg/min) infusion. In control dogs, femoral blood flow was significantly reduced after LNMMA infusion, but in heart failure dogs, the reduction was insignificant. Right panel: The bar graph shows percent reduction in femoral blood flow in control (□;n=5) and heart failure (■;n=5) dogs.

[RESULT]

Basal cardiac and hemodynamic variables in control and those with CHF are shown in table 1. There were no differences in heart rate or mean aortic pressure between the two groups of the dog. Left ventricular end-diastolic pressure (LVEDP) was significantly elevated, and % fractional shortening (% FS) was decreased in dogs with CHF (Fig 2). The vasodilator responses to NTG tended to be attenuated was in dogs with CHF, but no significant differences existed in any doses of NTG between the two groups (Fig 3 left panel). The vasodilator responses to ACh, however, was significantly attenuated in dogs with CHF compared to control dogs at the doses of higher than 1×10^{-9} mol (Fig 3 middle panel). Furthermore, the vasodilator responses to ADP was decreased at the doses higher than 1×10^{-7} mol (Fig 3 right panel). In control dogs, the pretreatment with aspirin did not affect the vasodilator responses of the femoral artery to ACh (Fig 4). LNMMA induced reduction in femoral blood flow in both group. The reduction in femoral blood flow by LNMMA was smaller in CHF dogs than in control dogs (-39.8 ± 10 % vs -20.4 ± 13 %) (Fig 5).

[DISCUSSION]

This study demonstrates that the endothelium-dependent vasodilation is depressed in the femoral resistance vessels of dogs with pacing-induced heart fairure. The attenuation of endothelial NO synthesis is probably related depressed vasodilator responses. The enhanced peripheral resistance seen in heart failure is shown to be resulted mainly from augmented sympathetic tone and increased circulating vasoconstrictive substances such as cathecholamine and angiotensin (1, 2). The vasodilator responses to ischemia and exercise is also shown to be attenuated in congestive heart failure (3). As the mechanism of the attenuated vasodilator response, fluid retention in the vascular wall has been suggested (4). The attenuated vasodilator response found in the present study may be partly related to such mechanisms. The vasodilator actions of ACh and ADP are shown to be endothelium-dependent, wheres that of NTG endothelium-independent. The vasodilator actions of ACh is shown to be mediated partly by prostaglandins in certain vasuclar beds. The participation of prostaglandins is, however, unlikely in the present preparation, because pretreatment with aspirin did not modify vasodilator response to ACh. Since the vasodilator response to both ACh and ADP were selectively depressed, our study indicated that endothelium-dependent vasodilation in the femoral resistance vessels in dogs with CHF. Our study consistent with the study of Kaiser et al, who have reported that endothelium-dependent vasodilator respose in the femoral conductance vessel depressed in dogs with pacing-induced heart failure (5). Endothelium-dependent vascular relaxation is mediated by EDRF, which is recently revealed NO (6). We examined the effect of LNMMA, which is NO synthesis inhibitor, on femoral blood flow. In control dogs as well as CHF dogs showed vasoconstrictor responses to LNMMA. This findings imply the importance of EDRF as a modulator of vascular tone in the femoral resistance vessels in dogs. The extent of the reduction in femoral blood flow after LNMMA administration was attenuated in dogs with CHF. It is suggested, therefore, that NO synthesis in the vascular endothelium is depressed in dogs with CHF. The mechanism of the attenuation of NO synthesis is unclear. The attenuation of endothelium-dependent vascular relaxation has been shown in various conditions such as atherosclerosis and hypertension (7, 8). The depressed endothelium-dependent vasodilator response may contributed to the pathophysiologic condition of CHF.

(reference)

1. Zelis R. et al : Cardiocirculatory dynamics in the normal and failing heart.
   Ann Rev Physiol 1981 ; 43 : 455 – 476
2. Zelis R. et al : A comparison of regional blood flow and oxygen utilization during dynamic forearm exercise in normal subjects and patient with congestive heart failure.
   Circulation 1974 ; 50 : 137 – 143
3. Epstein SE. et al : Characterization of the circulatory response to maximal upright exercise in normal subjects and patient with heart disease.
   Circulation 1967 ; 35 : 1049 – 1062

4. Zeli R. et al : A comparison of the effect of vasodilator stimuli on peripheral resistance vessels in normal subjects and in patients with congestive heart failure.
J Clin Invest 1968 ; 47 : 960 – 970

5. Kaiser L. et al : Heart failure depresses endothelium-dependent responses in canine femoral artery.
Am J Physiol 1989 ; 25 : H 962 – H 967

6. Moncada S. et al : Nitric Oxide : physiology, pathophysiology, and pharmacology.
Pharmacol Rev 1991 ; 43 : 109 – 142

7. Freiman PC. et al : Aterosclerosis impares endothelium-dependent vascular relaxation to acetylcholine and thrombin inprimates.
Circ Res 1986 ; 58 : 783 – 789

8. Tesfamariam B. and Halpern W. : Endothelium-dependent and endothelium-independent vasodilation in resistance arteries from hypertensive rats.
Hypertension 1988 ; 11 : 440 – 444

Effects of Calcitonin Gene-Related Peptide on Systemic and Regional Hemodynamics in Dogs with Congestive Heart Failure

SADAYA TSUMOTO, SEINOSUKE KAWASHIMA, MASAHIRO UENO, MASATO MORITA, TOMOHIRO KONDO, and TADAAKI IWASAKI

First Department of Internal Medicine, Hyogo College of Medicine, Hyogo, 663 Japan

KEYWORDS: calcitonin gene-related peptide, congestive heart failure, regional blood flow

INTRODUCTION

Calcitonin gene-related peptide (CGRP) is a novel 37 amino acid peptide that is localized in the nervous, vascular and endocrine systems (1). In the heart and peripheral arteries, specific CGRP binding sites linked to the stimulation of adenylate cyclase activity have also been recognized (2). Probably through the interaction with these receptors CGRP exterts potent cardiovascular effects that include positive chronotropic and inotropic actions on the heart, hypotension, and vasodilation (3). These findings suggest that endogenous CGRP may play a role in the regulation of cardiovascular control. In this study, we investigated the effects of CGRP on systemic and regional hemodynamics in dogs with congestive heart failure, and the effects were compared with those by sodium nitroprusside (SNP).

MATERIALS AND METHODS

-Surgical preparation of animals-

Material mongrel dogs (n=7, weight 17.2 ± 1.7kg)

Method Congestive heart failure was produced by rapid right ventricular pacing method (4).

Pacemaker generator (Model 5984, Medtronic Inc., USA)

Pacing rate 250 ppm, for 2 weeks

-Experimental preparations and protocol-

These animals were anesthetized with a low dose of sodium pentobarbital (10~15 mg/kg, iv), intubated and mechanically ventilated. The experiment was carried out after the pacing was stopped. Under fluoroscopic guidance, catheters were inserted into the abdominal aorta and left ventricle to measure aortic pressure and left ventricular pressure. A Swan-Ganz catheter was inserted into the right ventricle. Heart rate was monitored by ECG and left ventricular wall motion was assessed by echocardiography. Regional blood flow was measured by a nonradioactive colored microsphere technique (5). The microsphere (diameter: 15 ± 2 μm) were obtained from E-Z Trac Inc., California, USA.

Protocol:

At random manner, either CGRP (80 pmol/kg/min) or sodium nitroprusside (SNP: 10 μ g/kg/min) was infused itravenously for 5 min. Hemodynamic measurements and blood sampling for regional blood flow measurements were carried out at baseline and at the end of the infusion period.

RESULTS AND DISCUSSION

Animals underwent rapid ventricular pacing over 2 weeks showed prominent signs of congestive heart failure with prominent ascitis, elevated left ventricular end-diastolic pressure and decreased cardiac output at the time of the experiments.

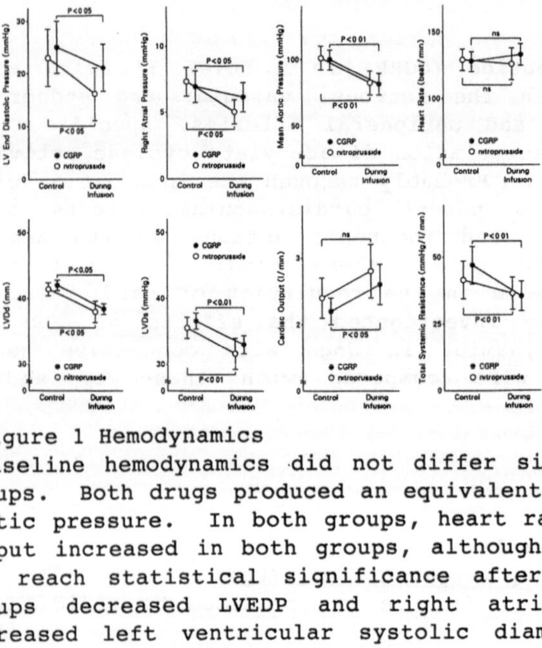

Figure 1 Hemodynamics

Baseline hemodynamics did not differ significantly between the two groups. Both drugs produced an equivalent degree of reduction in mean aortic pressure. In both groups, heart rate did not change. Cardiac output increased in both groups, although the extent of increase did not reach statistical significance after SNP administration. Both groups decreased LVEDP and right atrial pressure. Both drugs decreased left ventricular systolic diameter as well as diastolic diameter.

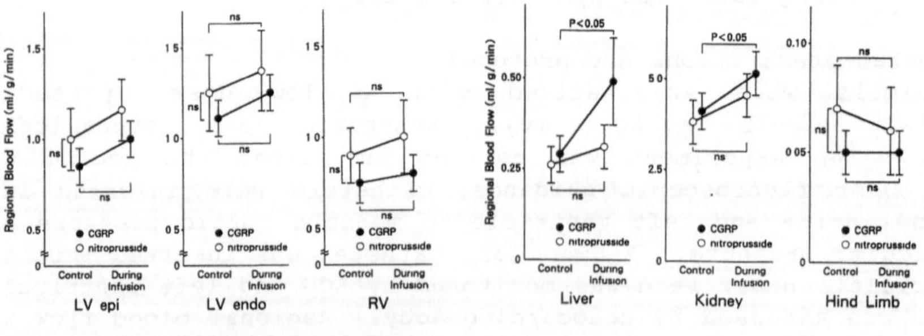

Figure 2 Regional blood flow

CGRP increased blood flow in the kidney and liver with a concomitant reduction in vascular resistance in these organs. Blood flows in these organs showed only marginal increases after SNP. Blood flow did not change in the hindlimb muscle after administration of either drugs.

CGRP and SNP decreased aortic pressure and increased cardiac output to similar extents. The reduction in LVEDP and right atrial pressure tended to be smaller in CGRP than in SNP, although the difference were insignificant. Our data shows that CGRP, like SNP, dilates venous vessels as well as artery but the venodilator action is relatively week compared to SNP. In addition to its vasodilator effect, CGRP might increase cardiac output by its inotropic action on the heart (3). On the other hand, most experimental studies have shown a direct positive inotropic effect of CGRP in the atrium (6). In our study, therefore, increased contraction in the atrium itself might improve ventricular filling and result in an increase in cardiac output. Heart rate did not change by either CGRP or SNP administration. In the similar experimental preparation performed on normal dogs without congestive heart failure, we have observed an increase in heart rate to the equivalent reduction in aortic pressure. The impaired baroreflex system, which have been documented in congestive heart failure, is probably responsible for the unchanged heart rate (7). The absence of tachycardia appears an important character of a drug as the strategy of treating heart failure. CGRP caused a rather selective vasodilation in the regional circulation compared to SNP, CGRP produced prominent increase in blood flows in the kidney and liver. The different vasodilator effects of CGRP on various organs is probably related to the distribution of its specific receptor in the body.

CGRP can be used as a possible strategy for the treatment of heart failure complicated with renal and/or hepatic dysfunction.

REFERENCES

1. Amara SG, Jonas J, Rosenfeld MG, Ong ES, Evans RM.(1982) Alternative RNA processing in calcitonin gene expression generates mRNAs encoding different polypeptide products. Nature 298:240-244

2. Edwards RM, Stack EJ, Trizna W. (1991) Calcitonin gene-related peptide stimulates adenylate cyclase and relaxes intracerebral arterioles. J Pharmacol, Exp. Ther 257: 1020-1024

3. Gennari C and Fischer JA. (1985) Cardiovascular action of calcitonin gene-relatede peptide in humans. Calcif Tissue Int 37: 581-584

4. Dibner-Dunlap ME and Thames MD. (1990) A simplified technique for the production of heart failure in the dog by rapid ventricular pacing. Am J Med. 300:0288-290

5. Hale SL, Alker KJ, Kloner RA. (1988) Evaluation of nonradioactive, colored microspheres for measurement of regional myocardial blood flow in dogs. Circulation 78: 428-434

6. Franco-Cereceda A, Gennari C, Nami R, Agnusdei D, Pernow J, Lundberg JM, Fischer JA. (1987) Circ Res 60:0393-397

7. Ellenbagen KA, Mohanty PK, Szentpetery S, Thomas MD. (1989) Arterial baroreflex abnormalities in heart failure: reversal after orthotopic cardiac transplantation. Circulation 79: 217-222

Remarkable Improvement in Congestive Heart Failure in Ventricular Septal Rupture by Dopexamine Infusion

YASURO ISHIKAWA, MASAHIRO KUDOH, MASATO OHMURA, TOMOHIDE SATO, and HIDEO MIYASHITA

Second Department of Internal Medicine, Teikyo University, Tokyo, 173 Japan

KEYWORDS:dopexamine, congestive heart failure, ventricular septal rupture, myocardial infarction

INTRODUCTION

Recently a new β_2 stimulant "Dopexamine" has been developed and is expected to be effective in the treatment of congestive heart failure (CHF). We used it in a case of severe CHF in ventricular septal rupture due to anterior myocardial infarction and saw excellent improvement. The usefulness of this drug in severely reduced cardiac function is discussed in this paper.

PRESENTATION OF CASE

The patient was a 73-year-old woman. She had firstly chest oppression on climbing stairs in January, 1989. She awoke at midnight with severe chest pain and was hospitalized in another institution with acute anterior myocardial infarction on March 22, 1990. She was discharged on July 2, 1990 but was subsequently admitted to the same institution several times due to CHF. She was transferred to our hospital in order to have recurrent CHF treated on September 11, 1990.

On physical examination the pulse was 92/min and blood pressure was 132/88mmHg;her height was 143 cm and body weight was 47.5 kg. She had neither cyanosis nor jugular vein dilatation, but had moist rales in the bilateral lower lungs. A third heart sound and holosystolic ejection murmur at the apex (Levine V/VI) were heard and slight hepatomegaly and slight leg edema were found.

The chest X-ray on admission revealed remarkable cardiomegly and pulmonary congestion. An electrocardiogram demonstrated broad anterior myocardial infarction. A cardiac ultrasonograhpic study on October 3 showed that both the right ventricle (RV) and the left ventricle (LV) were dilated and the contraction of the anterior wall in LV was severely reduced with aneurysmal change at the apex. A shunt jet from LV to RV was observed at the paillary muscle level by color-flow Doppler mapping. Laboratory data showed slight anemia, but renal and liver functions were almost within the normal range. In right heart catheterization elevated pulmonary arterial pressure, the high pulmonary capillary wedge pressure (PCW), and a significant step-up at RV in oxygen saturation were found. Therefore, we diagnosed that she had ventricular septal rupture (VSR) after myocardial infarction. Despite conventional therapy such as the use of diuretics and usual vasodilators, the condition did not improve. Finally we decided to use a dopexamine drip infusion at a rate of 0.5 γ /kg/min initially and maximally up to 4 γ /kg/min. The hemodynamic data markedly improved (Fig.1); mean PCW decreased from 25 to 9 mmHg, cardiac output (C.O.) increased from 3.2 to 10.3 l/min, and Qp/Qs decreased from 2.7 to 1.5;TSR and PVR markedly decreased, but heart rate (H.R.) slightly increased from 98 to 111 beats/min.

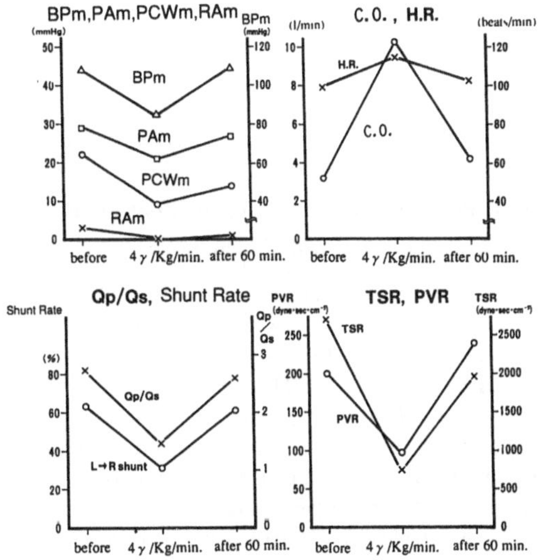

Fig.1 Hemodynamic changes after dopexamine infusion.

After using this drug the heart failure was compensated day by day by the additional combination therapy of diureics, nitrate, ACE inhibitor, and digitalis. On the 10th of October the surgical closure of VSR and aneurysmectomy of LV were performed successfully. She could leave our hospital on foot on December 20, 1990.

DISCUSSION

This case demonstrated the usefulness of dopexamine in congestive heart failure caused by ventricular septal rupture after myocardial infarction. The rupture of the venturicular septum was suspected to have occurred during hospitalization in the previous hospital because CHF did not clearly improve at that institution.

Dopexamine hydrochroride was recently developed as a new catecholamine for short-term intravenous administration in the treatment of low cardiac output states. The chemical structure resembles dobutamine more than dopamine. In the clinical profile it has both cardiac and renal performance. Its major pharmacological actions are listed in table 1. The vasodilator effects are based on strong β_2-adrenergic stimulation, with additional renal vasodilation caused by selective dopamine (DA1)receptor stimulation [1]. Its has a positive inotropic effect via three major actions such as the indirect stimulation of myocardial β_1-adrenoceptors resulting from inhibition of neuronal uptake of catecholamines (uptake-1), the stimulation of myocardial β_2-adrenoceptors, and baroreceptor reflex mechanisms[2]. It possesses only very weak and clinically insignificant direct β_1-adrenoceptor agonist activity. There is no α-adrenergic agonist activity nor vasoconstrictive action.

Actions	Pharmacological activites(Dopamine:1)
β1-stimulant	0.17
β2-stimulant	60
α-stimulant	0
DA1-stimulant	0.34
DA2-stimulant	0.17 ~ 0.23
Uptake-1 blocking	10
Thyramine-like	0
Provocating arrythmia	0

Table 1 Pharmacological actions of dopexamine (as compared with dopamine)

In our patient systemic blood pressure (BP), PCW, mean right atrial pressure (RA), TSR, and PVR fell because of vasodilative actions. However, heart rate slightly increased. The overall effects finally reduced the shunt rate and Qp/Qs and therefore the condition improved. In England this drug is usually used in clinical cases in acute exacerbations of heart failure and in hemodynamic support of cardiac surgery patients [3, 4]. However, its usefulness has not yet been demonstrated in many other patients of CHF until now. Our experience showed the possibility of its use in VSR. In VSR, intra-aortic balloon pulsation is currently thought to be one of the most effective treatments for improving hemodynamics. This drug has the potential to replace this method in the treatment of VSR with CHF. This drug needs to be considered further.

SUMMARY

1) Dopexamine acted as a β_2-stimulant and in VSR due to myocardial infarction, BP, RA, and PCW decreased. 2) It increased cardiac output and decreased L-R shunt and Qp/Qs. 3)It is effective for CHF in VSR due to myocardial infarction. 4) Dopexamine is expected to become a new treatment in congestive heart failure.

REFRENCES

1. Smith GW, Hall JC, Farmer JB (1987) The cardiovascular actions of dopexamine hydrochloride, an agonist at dopamine receptors and β_2-adrenoceptors in the dog. J Pharm Pharmacol 39:636-641.
2. Brown RA, Dixon J, Farmer JB (1985) Dopexamine: a novel agonist at peripheral dopamine receptors and β_2-adrenoceptors. Br J Pharmacol 85:599-608.
3. Dawson JR, Thompson DS, Signy FS (1985) Acute heamodynamic and metabolic effects of dopexamine, a new dopaminergic receptor agonist, in patients with chronic heart failure. Br Heart J 54:313-320.
4. Hakim M, Foulds H, Latimer RD, English TAM (1988) Dopexamine hydrochroride, a β_2-adrenergic and dopaminergic agonist;heamodynamic effects following cardiac surgery. Eur Heart J 9:853-858.

Direct Prevention Against Progressive 201TL Perfusion Defects by Captopril Treatment in Patients with Mild to Moderate Heart Failure

MAKOTO SUZUKI, MAREOMI HAMADA, MICHIHITO SEKIYA, TAKUMI SUMIMOTO, and KUNIO HIWADA

Second Department of Internal Medicine, Ehime University, Ehime, 791-02 Japan

KEYWORDS: heart failure, captopril, thallium-201 scintigraphy, renin-angiotensin system

INTRODUCTION

Angiotensin-converting enzyme inhibitors are effective for the treatment of patients with severe congestive heart failure and have been shown to alleviate symptoms and improve prognosis (1,2). Furthermore, in the stable, compensated phase of heart failure, the circulatory renin-angiotensin system is not activated (3), but angiotensin converting enzyme inhibitor improves cardiac function and normalizes regional blood flow. On the other hand, thallium-201 (201TL) myocardial imaging has become an accepted diagnostic tool to detect and assess the extent of myocardial damage in cardiology. The aim of this study is to evaluate the effect of captopril on 201TL perfusion defects in patients with mild to moderate heart failure (NYHA class II or III).

PATIENTS AND METHODS

Patient Population and M-mode Echocardiography

Twenty patients with NYHA class II or III heart failure were studied. Of the 20 patients, 12 were received captopril (Group 1: 10 men and 2 women, mean age 54±10 years) in addition to conventional treatment for heart filure and 8 were received only conventional treatment (Group 2: 8 men, mean age 59±10 years). There were no significant differences between the two groups with regard to follow-up periods (3.1±1.7 vs. 1.8±1.7 months; NS) and the presumptive causes of heart failure. A mean dose of 27 mg of captopril a day (range 12.5 to 37.5 mg) was given to patients with Group 1. M-mode echocardiogram were performed by standard technique in all patients. Mean velocity of circumferential fiber shortening was calculated according to the standard formula. Furthermore, peak and end systolic meridional wall stress was calculated using the equation of Wilson et al (4).

Single Photon Emission Computed Tomography and Heart/Lung Ratio of 201TL Activity

On the day of the radionuclide study, 20 patients were instructed to have no breakfast, but all medications were continued. Approximately 111 MBq of 201TL was injected into an antecubital vein and the single photon emission computed tomographic imaging (SPECT) (General Electric U.S.A., STARCAM 400 AC/T) was started 15 minute thereafter. In order to quantify the abnormality of 201TL SPECT, we got extent score from the extent polar map according to the methods of Garcia et al (5). The mean value and standard deviation of circumferential profiles were established from the pooled data of 20 age-matched normal subjects. For profiles, normal limits were determined as the curves representing 2 standard deviations below the mean and were used as the threshold for detection.

In the unprocessed anterior projection image, the heart/lung ratio of 201TL activity was measured using a region of interest (ROI) method. Separate square ROIs of 10 x 10 pixels (4.7 x 4.7 cm) were defined for areas of the right upper lung and left ventricular myocardium. The heart/lung ratio was determined as the mean counts/pixel in the heart ROI divided by that in the lung ROI. The heart/lung ratio in 20 normal subjects was 2.19±0.55.

Statistical Analysis

All data are expressed as mean±1SD. Data between two groups were compared by the unpaired t test, and data between the initial and repeated study were compared by the paired t test. A value of $p<0.05$ was considered statistically significant.

RESULTS

Clinical and Echocardiographic Data (Table 1)

Table 1. Clinical and echocardiographic data of the two groups

	NYHA	HR (beats/min)	SBP (mmHg)	DBP (mmHg)	LVEDD (cm)	LVESD (cm)	meanVcf (circ / sec)
Initial Study							
Group 1	2.8 ± 0.5	70 ± 5	109 ± 19	72 ± 15	7.5 ± 0.9	6.5 ± 1.0	0.61 ± 0.20
Group 2	2.5 ± 0.5	68 ± 14	113 ± 10	75 ± 7	6.3 ± 1.0 *	5.2 ± 1.1 *	0.81 ± 0.37
Repeated Study							
Group 1	2.8 ± 0.5	70 ± 9	106 ± 13	72 ± 8	7.2 ± 1.1	6.1 ± 1.4	0.71 ± 0.30
Group 2	2.4 ± 0.4	63 ± 7	109 ± 8	69 ± 8	6.2 ± 1.0	5.0 ± 1.1	0.79 ± 0.35

***P < 0.05 vs. Group 1. NYHA = New York Heart Association functional class ; HR = heart rate ; SBP = systolic blood pressure ; DBP = diastolic blood pressure ; LVEDD = left ventricular end-diastolic diameter ; LVESD = left ventricular end-systolic diameter ; mean Vcf = mean velocity of circumferential fiber shortening.**

No differences were observed between the two groups with regard to clinical and echocardiographic data except for left ventricular dimensions in the initial study. Furthermore, these variables showed no significant differences between the initial and the repeated study in both groups.

Peak-systolic and End-systolic Meridional Wall Stress (Fig. 1)

In both groups, peak systolic wall stress was significantly decreased, but end systolic wall stress was significantly decreased in only Group 1.

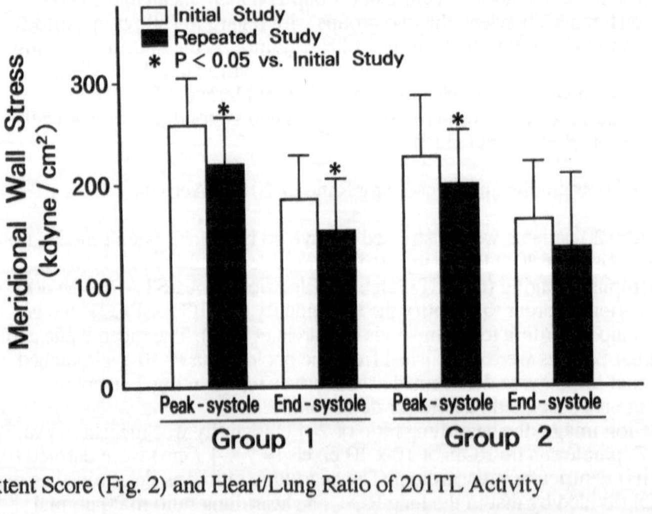

Fig. 1 Peak and end systolic meridional wall stress of the two groups.

Extent Score (Fig. 2) and Heart/Lung Ratio of 201TL Activity

In the repeated study, the extent score of Group 1 was significantly decreased (48±16 vs. 38±16%, $p<0.05$), but that of Group 2 was not changed (42±24 vs. 44±16%, NS). There was no significant difference in the heart/lung ratio between the initial and repeated study in both Groups 1 (2.10±0.64 vs. 2.31±0.61, NS) and 2 (2.06±0.48 vs. 1.87± 0.24, NS). Furthermore, the ratios in the two groups were not significantly different from that in normal subjects.

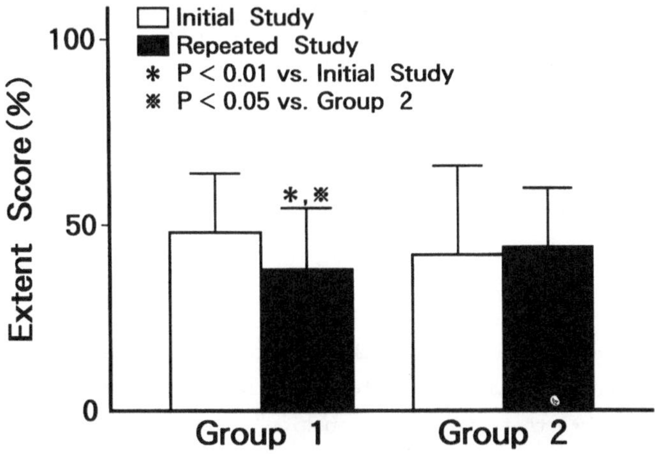

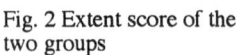

Fig. 2 Extent score of the two groups

DISCUSSION

The present study demonstrates that the treatment with captopril improves 201TL myocardial perfusion defects in patients with mild to moderate heart failure. In failing heart, 201TL myocardial SPECT is affected by two factors, which are pulmonary thallium uptake and the condition of failing heart itself. Previous studies (6,7) indicated that pulmonary uptake was high in patients with severely depressed left ventricular function, and an decreased heart/lung ratio was observed in patients with a low left ventricular ejection fraction and a high left ventricular end-diastolic pressure.However, the heart/lung ratio in both groups was in normal range.This result suggested that transduation of fluid into the lungs was under control at rest in both groups.From the point of view that approximately 60% of 201TL influx is dependent on membrane Na-K ATPase (8), the extent score seems to reflect the energy starvation state of myocardium to a certain degree. In this study, meridional wall stress, which is an index of afterload, improved in both groups, but the extent score improved in only Group 1. These findings suggested that the beneficial effect of angiotensin converting enzyme inhibitor could not be simply explained by the reduction of afterload. Recent data suggest that tissue renin-angiotensin systems may be important in the regulation of local tissue function (9,10). Therefore, the direct effects of angiotensin converting enzyme inhibitor on the cardiac renin-angiotensin system may play an important role in the prevention of progressive 201TL myocardial perfusion defects.

CONCLUSION

Captopril could prevent the progression of 201TL perfusion defects irrespective of lung 201TL uptake or loading condition in patients with mild to moderate heart failure.

REFERENCES

1. The CONSENSUS trial study group. (1987) Effects of enalapril on mortality in severe congestive heart failure. results of the cooperative north scandinavian enalapril survial study (CONSENSUS). N Engl J Med 316:1429-1435.
2. The SOLVD investigators. (1991) Effect of enalapril on survial in patients with reduced left ventricular ejection fractions and congestive heart failure. N Engl J Med 325:293-302.
3. Dzau VJ, Colucci WS, Hollenberg NK, Williams GH. (1981) Relation of the renin-angiotensin-aldosterone system to clinical state in congestive heart failure. Circulation 63:645-651.
4. Wilson JR, Reichek N, Hirshfeld J, Keller CA. (1980) Noninvasive assessment of load reduction in patients with asymptomatic aortic regurgitation. Am J Med 68:664-674.
5. Garcia EV, Train KV, Maddahi J et al. (1985) Quantification of rotational thallium-201 myocardial tomography. J Nucl Med 26:17-26.
6. Gill JB, Ruddy TD, Newell JB, Finkelstein DM, Strauss HW, Boucher CA. (1987) Prognostic importance of thallium uptake by the lungs during exercise in coronary artery disease. N Engl J Med 317:1485-1489.
7. Mannting F. (1990) Pulmonary thallium uptake: correlation with systolic and diastolic thallium-201 uptake during exercise. Am Heart J 119:1137-1146.
8. McCall D, Zimmer LJ, Katz AM. (1985) Kinetics of thallium exchange in cultured rat myocardial cells. Circ Res 56:370-376.
9.Dzau VJ .(1988) Cardiac renin-angiotensin system. molecular and functional aspects. Am J Med 84 (suppl 3A):22-27.
10.Hirsh AT, Talsness CE, Schunkert H, Paul M, Dzau VJ. (1991) Tissue-specific activation of cardiac angiotensin converting enzyme in experimental heart failure. Circ Res 69:475-482.

An Optimal Control Strategy for Regulation of Cardiovascular System

H. HIRAYAMA[1] and K. ONO[2]

Department of Public Health Asahikawa Medical College, Asahikawa, 078 Japan[1] and Department of Information Science, Muroran Institute of Technology, Muroran, 050 Japan[2]

PREFACE

Biological system always seek to operate in an equailibrium state. In such circum stances, usual explanation is tentative optimal state or stable state Although there are many works that afford "explanation", there scaserly find what is the "optimal state" or how a given system will behave if the system is controlled under optimal st rategy. In the present study, an optimal control theory was applied to cardiovascular system to disclose what is the control strategy or regulatory policy of cardiovascula system.

MATHEMATICAL THEORY.

Cardiovascular system was expressed by simple Wind Kessel model as

$$Ia(t) = Pa(t)/Ra + Ca\, dPa(t)/dt \quad \text{-------- (1)}$$

$$P(t) = Ia(t)\, r + Pa(t) \quad \text{------- (2)}$$

$$V(t) = Vo - \int_0^{Te} Ia(t)\, dt \quad \text{------- (3)}$$

where Ia(t); aortic flow rate. Pa(t) ; arterial blood pressure. P(t) ; ventricula pre ssure. V(t) ; ventricular volume, Vo ; end diastolic volume. Ra ; flow resistance. Ca ; aortic compliance.r ;aortic valvular resistance. Te; durarion of ejectin period.

Since flow rate its self have its own upper limitation following integral constra int was imposed as control variable

$$Vs = \int_0^{Te} Ia(t)\, dt \quad \text{-------- (4).}$$

Since flow rate is zero at beggining and end ejection time,

$$Ia(0) = Ia(te) = 0. \quad \text{---------(5)}$$

Relation of arterial blood pressure during diastolic phase is determined by passive properties of artreial system as

$$Pa(0) = K\, Pa(te) \quad ; \quad K = \exp(-Td/(Ra\, Ca)) \quad \text{------ (6)}$$

Then equ(1) to equ(6) describes the instantaneous behaviour of srteial system. Next the performance function that minimize reasonable physiological demand must be pres cribe exactly. In present work we used following criterion function

$$J = \int_{0}^{TE} \left[\text{beta} [P(t)] + q [Pa(t)] + \text{alpha}\ P(t)\ Ia(t) \right] dt + \text{gamma}\ P(te)$$

This function menalze the time dependent fluctuation of ventricular ejection press ure P(t) and arterial blood pressure Pa(t) and also minimize ventricular external wo rk P(t) Ia(t) which have linear relation between oxygen consumption of ventricule. Term out side of integral correlates with potential energy of ventricule if it does not eject out blood. Consequently sum of third and fourth terms is parallel to press ure volume area of given cardiac cycle. The coefficients beta , q, alpha and gamma indicate relative contribution of each terms to minimization of performance function.

It is convenient to utilyze Hamiltonian to associate these complex syste and also convert variable from ordinal to state variables and control variables. Here we set X1(t)=Pa(t), X2(t)= V(t), X3(t)=Ia(t) and Ia(t)=U(t) as optimal control variable. T The co-state variables (adjoint variables) are set as p1(t), P2(t). P3(t) then hamiltonian is

$$H[X(t), U(t), P(t)] - \text{dif}\ J(t)/dt + p1(t) \left(-X1(t)/(RaCa) + X3(t)/Ca\ 0 - p2\ X3(t) \right. \\ + p3(t)\ u(t)$$

Then optimal control uopt can be obtained by d H/d u =0. , The differential equatio for state variable and co-state variable are obtained as

$$\dot{p}1(t) = - d\ H/d\ X1, \qquad \dot{p}2(t) = - d\ H/dX2, \qquad \dot{p}3(t) = - d\ H/dx3.$$

Integral coefficients were obtained by boundary conditions expressed in equ(4,5,6)

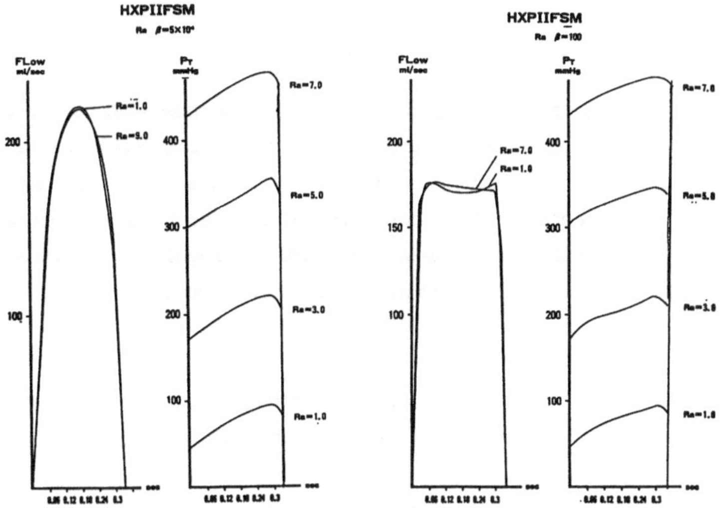

Fig 1.

RESULTS

Fig 1 show aortic flow curves and ventricular pressure curves by changes in Ra. There was little changes in flow curves by Ra howver marked depression occureed for smaller beta (= 100). The ventricular pressure increased almost parallelly with Ra there was no definite differences of pressure curves by changes in beta.

Fig 2 show effects of changes in Ca. For smaller Ca maximum flow rate depressed and peak flow had been postphoned while for larger Ca, peak flow time was shortened and maximum flow rate increased. However for smaller beta, those characteristic feau tres of flow curves were depressed and flow curve became flatt. The ventricular pre

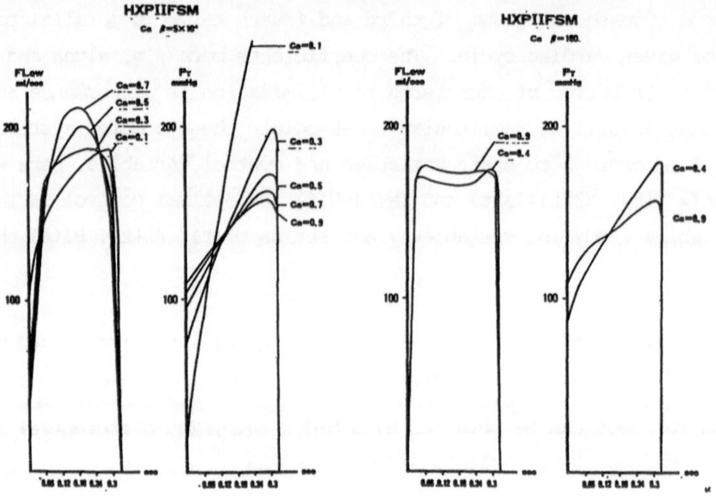

Fig 2.

increase very rapidly with smaller Ca and diastolic pressure was decreased. On the other hand for larger Ca, diastolic pressure increased while peak pressure was depre ssed and pressure curve became totally flatt.

DISCUSSION.

Although it is not possible to compare flow curves or with pressure curves between present study, typical charateristic feautres of these variables could be reconstruc ted. Because some parametric coefficients such as beta or q are not availabe in bio logical experiments the effects of these terms in relative contribution are difficult to evaluate, some harmonic mutual interdependency between regulation of these quanti ties seems to be important to produce normal physiological pressure and flow pattern.

CONCLUSION.

. Minimization of ventriclar and arterial pressure oscullation and pressure volume area is important to produce physiological pressure and flow curves.

Reference.

1. Hirayama.H., Yasuda,H. IEICE. MBE. 90.22. 91-98,1990.

Myocardial Protection with Ryanodine and CoQ_{10} Against Post-ischemic Reperfusion Injury of Rabbit Heart

MASAFUMI MORITA[1], YOSHIHIDE SAWADA[1], SEIICHIRO MINOHARA[1], YONEZO HIKITA[1], SHINJIRO SASAKI[1], ATSURO TAKEUCHI[1], IKUKO NAKAGAKI[2], and SADAO SASAKI[2]

Departments of Thoracic Surgery[1] and Physiology[2], Osaka Medical College, Osaka, 569 Japan

Key words: Ryanodine, CoQ_{10}, Reperfusion Injury, X-ray Microanalysis

ABSTRACT

The effect of Ryanodine and CoQ_{10} on intracellular electrolyte alterations of rabbit heart was investigated. Electrolyte concentrations in the contractile element (A band) of the myocardial cells (ventricular cells) were measured by X-ray microanalysis employing thin sections of freshly freeze-dried myocardium.
These data suggest that intracellular Ca accumulation may occur during reperfusion and the accumulation may be prevented by the administration of Ryanodine and CoQ_{10}.
The possible mechanism of the effects of Ryanodine and CoQ_{10} on the electrolyte alterations of myocardium are discussed.

INTRODUCTION

There remains the question as to whether there is a "Ca paradox" or not in the case of cardiac surgery performed under hypothermic global ischemia (1). Analysis of the intracellular electrolyte alterations is very important, although there remains methodological problems regarding quantification of intracellular elements.
X-ray microanalysis is a method that can be the direct quantitative estimation of the elemental composition with a simultaneous observation of the fine structure of the cells (2-3). In this study, alterations of Ca, Mg, K, Na and Cl in the contractile element of the myocardial cells were measured, and the effects of Ryanodine and CoQ_{10} on dynamic changes of the intracellular electrolytes were studied.

MATERIALS AND METHODS

Twenty-four rabbits (body weight 2.5 kg) for the isolated working heart model were divided into four groups according to the administration and concentration of Ryanodine [control group (no Ryanodine), 10^{-9} M, 10^{-8} M, 10^{-7} M Ryanodine groups]. Ryanodine was added to GIK cardioplegic solution. The basic cardioplegic solution contained: 5% glucose 1,000 ml, KCl 20 mEq, insulin 20 u, $NaHCO_3$ 14 mEq, β-methasone 1 mg/kg.
In addition, six rabbits subjected to combined administration of CoQ_{10} and Ryanodine (10^{-7} M) were studied. CoQ_{10} (5 mg/kg) was injected intravenously one hour before experiment.

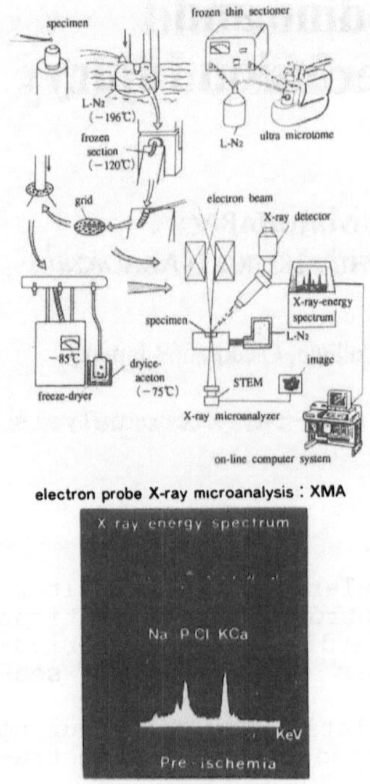

Fig. 1 X-ray microanalysis (XMA) method and X-ray energy spectrum of the cytoplasm from a frozen dried thin section of a rabbit ventricular myocardium

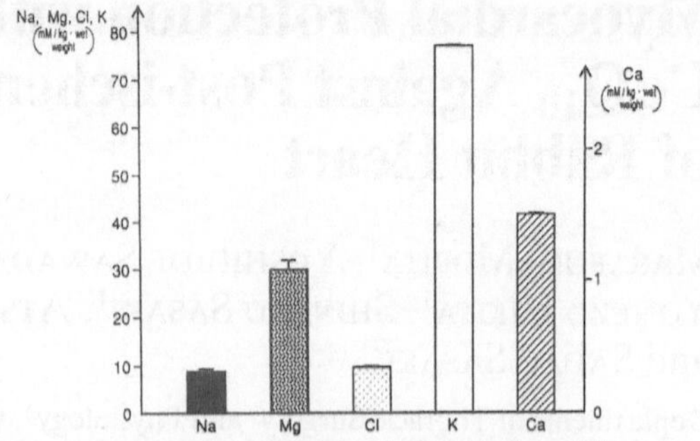

Fig. 2 Elemental concentrations in the sarcoplasm of the ventricular myocardium during preischemia

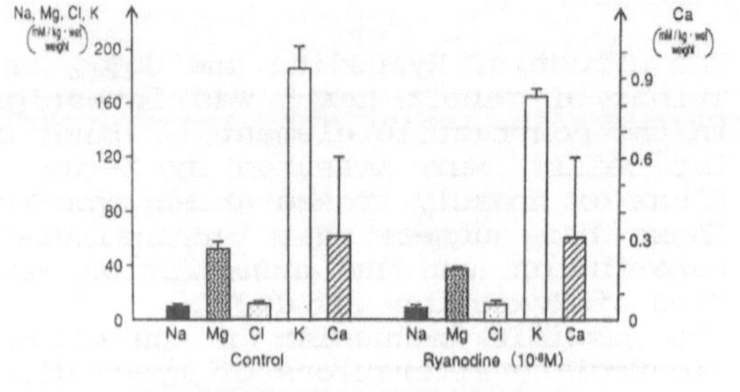

Fig. 3 Elemental concentrations during (90 mins) ischemia in Ryanodine 10^{-8}M group

Experiment

After isolation of the heart, 30 mins' non-working perfusion (Langendorff) and 15 mins' preischemic working perfusion were performed. Cardiac arrest of 90 min was induced with cold (4 °C) GIK cardioplegic solution (40 ml). During cardiac arrest, injection of the solution (20 ml) was repeated every 30 min and the myocardial temperature was kept at 15 °C. After aortic declamping (29 °C), 30 min' non-working perfusion (Langendorff) and 30 min' post-ischemic working perfusion were performed.

Specimens and Technique of X-Ray Microanalysis: (Fig.1)

Myocardial biopsy specimens were obtained at the endocardial side of left ventricular wall before ischemia (preischemia), just before aortic declamping (ischemia), 3 min and 60 min after aortic declamping (reperfusion). The specimens were presented for X-ray microanalysis study. Details of the procedure have been reported (2).

RESULTS

The X-ray spectra over bands of contractile elements (A band) of myocardium obtained during preischemia showed high peaks for K and low peaks for Ca, Mg, Na and Cl (Fig.2). Those obtained during ischemia showed higher peaks for K than preischemia, and lower peaks for Ca, Mg, Na and Cl than during preischemia in control and Ryanodine groups.

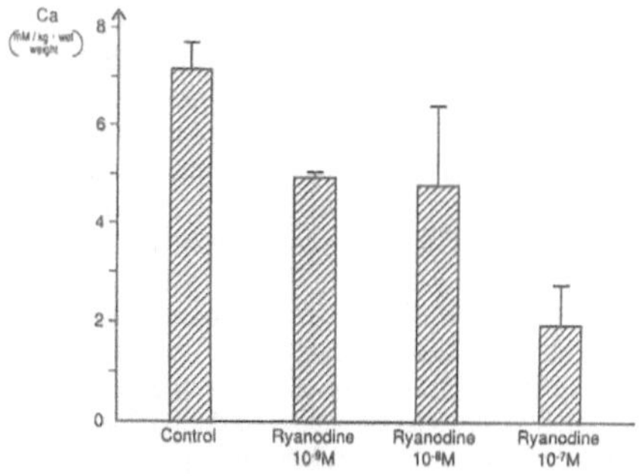

Fig. 4 Ca concentrations 3 mins after reperfusion in each Ryanodine group

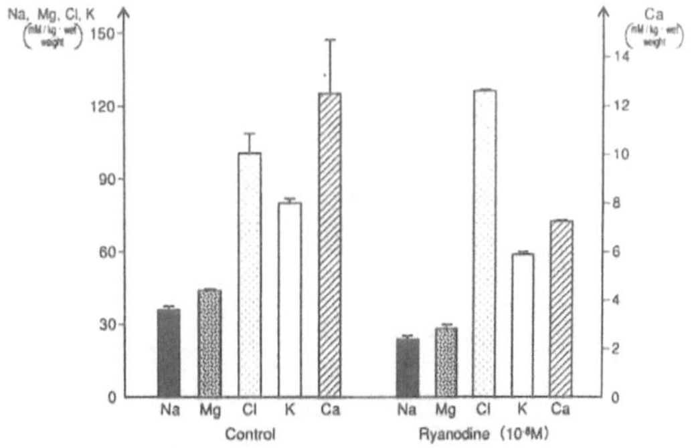

Fig. 5 Elemental concentrations during (60 mins) reperfusion in Ryanodine 10^{-8}M group

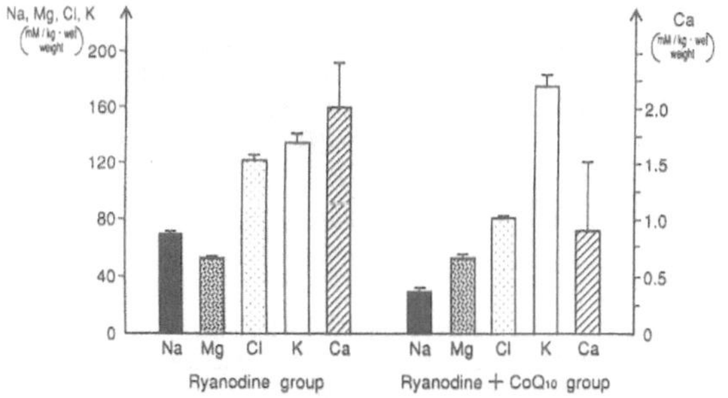

Fig. 6 Elemental concentrations during (60 mins) reperfusion in Ryanodine, and Ryanodine + CoQ_{10} groups

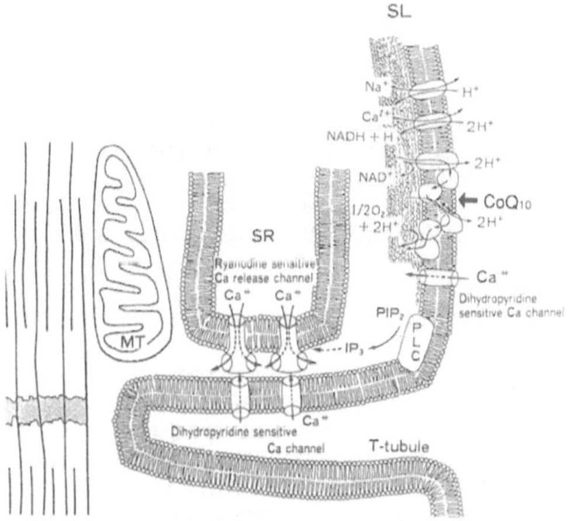

Fig. 7 A hypothetical schema of Ca chamels and effect of CoQ_{10}

There were no remarkable differences among all the groups during ischemia (Fig.3). Representatively, changes of Ca are indicated in Fig. 4. In control group, intracellular Ca significantly increased during reperfusion (3 min), and in Ryanodine groups were lower and were suppressed dose-dependently. The X-ray spectra obtained during reperfusion (60 min) showed higher peaks for all electrolytes (particularly Cl) than preischemia. In Ryanodine groups, those showed lower peaks than in control groups, and had returned to the level of preischemic state (Fig.5).
In Ryanodine $+CoQ_{10}$ group, those showed lower peaks for Ca, Na and Cl, and higher peaks for K than Ryanodine alone groups (Fig.6).

DISCUSSION (Fig.7)

Reliable measurements of electrolytes are often difficult with conventional methods: they destroy the distribution of elements in vivo, and disrupt the cell structure. With these methods, it is impossible to keep the integrity of intracellular organelles or narrow extracellular spaces. X-ray microanalysis is a method that allows such precise measurement per unit mass of the microvolume within the specimen, such as small area of A band of contractile element of myocardium in a

non-destructive fashion as Gupta and Hall (3) described.
It has been reported that the increase in intracellular and intramitochondrial Ca during reperfusion period compromise the cellular energy system and ultrastructure. The Ca overload may lead to a deleterious effect in all function of the myocardium, and this may be the irreversible step leading to cell death (4-6). To obtain favorable cardiac function after surgery, prevention of intracellular Ca accumulation is of great importance.
In this study, it was showed that Ca concentration during ischemia was lower than during preischemia, because a Ca-free cardioplegia solution (GIK) was perfused during ischemia, and during reperfusion intracellular Ca accumulation was suppressed with Ryanodine dose-dependently. Increase in intracellular Ca during reperfusion may result from the inflow of the sarcolemma or the release of an intracellular Ca store (sarcoplasmic reticulum: SR). Recently, it has been regarded that an intracellular store of Ca is important and that the release mechanism of Ca is "Ca induced Ca release" (CICR) (7-8). Ryanodine combines selectively with the Ca release channel of SR and fixes it open (9-11). Therefore, Ryanodine seems to keep Ca concentration in SR low during ischemia and contrarily to keep intracellular Ca accumulation low during reperfusion because of the recovery of positive action to store the Ca in SR. With a results to be suppressed the Ca release of SR by Ryanodine, the function of CoQ_{10} is considered. Combined use of CoQ_{10} and Ryanodine maintained intracellular Ca level lower compared with the use of Ryanodine alone. Therefore, it is suspected that CoQ_{10} would have an effect of intracellular carcium through sarcolemma or SR membrane to pump intracellular Ca out.

REFERENCES

1) Rebeika IM, Axford-Gatly RA, Bush BD, del NIdo PJ, Mickle DAG, Remaschin AD, Wilson GR: Calcium paradox in an in vivo model of multidose cardioplegia and moderate hypothermia. Prevention with diltiazem or trace calcium levels. J. Thorac Cardiovasc Surg 1990; 99: 475-483.
2) Sasaki S, Nakagaki I, Mori H, Imai Y: Intracellular calcium store and transport of elements in acinar cells of the salivery gland determined by electron probe X-ray microanalysis. Jpn J Physiol 1983; 33: 69-83.
3) Gupta BL, Hall TA: Electron microprobe X-ray analysis of calcium. Annals New York Academy of Sciences 1978; 307: 28-51.
4) Donovan PJ, Douglas AP: Calcium and its role in cardiac arrest: understanding the controversy. J Emerg Med 1985; 3: 105-116.
5) Murphy JG, Marsh JD, Smith TW: The role of calcium in ischemic myocardial injury. Circulation 1987; 75 (suppl V), V-15 - V-24.
6) Marban E, Koretsune Y, Corretti M, Chacko VP, Kusuoka H: Calcium and its role in myocardial cell injury during ischemia and reperfusion. Circulation 1989; 80 (suppl IV), IV-17 - IV-22.
7) Morad M, Goldman Y: Prog. Biophys. Mol. Biol. 27, 257 (1973)
8) Mitchell MR, Powell T, Terrar DA, Twist VW: Br. J. Pharmacol. 81, 13 (1984)
9) Fleischer S, Ogunbunmi EA, Dixon MC, Flee EAM: Proc. Natl. Acad. Sci. U.S.A. 82, 7256 (1985)
10) Inui M, Saito A, Fleischer S: J. Biol. Chem. 262, 15637 (1987)
11) Anderson K, Lai FA, Lui QY, Rousseau E, Erickson HP, Meissner G: J. Biol. Chem. 264, 1329 (1989)

Angiotensin II Potentiates Collagen Synthesis in the Hypertrophied Heart

Hitoshi Sano, Hitoshi Okada, Yoshihito Sakata, Hiroshi Okamoto, Hideaki Kawaguchi, Hisakazu Yasuda, and Akira Kitabatake

Department of Cardiovascular Medicine, Hokkaido University School of Medicine, Sapporo, 060 Japan

KEYWORDS: angiotensin II, collagen, cardiac fibroblasts, cardiac hypertrophy

INTRODUCTION

In cardiac hypertrophy, collagen accumulation in the myocardial interstitium is associated with hypertrophy of cardiomyocytes [1]. Collagen remodeling causes impaired ventricular compliance, abnormal electrical conduction and impaired oxygenation of the cardiomyocytes [2]. At present, factors that regulate cardiac collagen metabolism are not elucidated. Eghbali et al [3] found that cardiac fibroblasts are mainly responsible for the synthesis of fibrillar type I and III collagen. Recent studies have demonstrated that angiotensin II (A II), in addition to its inotropic and chronotropic actions, may exert effects by acting as a growth factor in the cardiovascular system and that there may be local autocrine or paracrine renin-angiotensin system in several tissues [4]. There are no data concerning the effects of A II on cardiac nonmyocytes. In this study we examined the effects of A II on collagen synthesis by cardiac fibroblasts in normotensive and hypertensive rats.

MATERIALS AND METHODS

<u>Cell culture</u> Cardiac fibroblasts were obtained by enzymatic digestion of the myocardial tissue of ten-week old spontaneously hypertensive rats (SHR) and Wistar-Kyoto rats (WKY) [3]. They were maintained in Dulbecco's modified Eagle's medium (DME) supplemented with 10% fetal bovine serum (FBS), penicillin (100 units/ml) and streptomycin (100 μg/ml). For all studies, we used cells from passages 4-12.

<u>Collagen synthesis</u> In preparation for experiments, the cells were grown to confluence in DME containing 10% FBS and were then made quiescent by placing them in a serum-free medium containing 0.1 mM ascorbic acid for 24 hours. A II was then added in the culture. After indicated periods, the cells were labeled with 74kBq/ml L-[2,3-^{3}H] proline and the cells were incubated for 12 hours. Collagen synthesis in the medium and the cell layer was determined by the bacterial collagen digestion [5]. The proteins in the medium and the cell layer were dialyzed against 0.05 M acetic acid containing 25 mM EDTA, 10 mM N-ethylmaleimide and 1 mM phenylmethylsulfonyl fluoride, and then lyophylized. Radioactivity in collagenase-sensitive protein was regarded as collagen synthesis and radioactivity in collagenase-insensitive protein was regarded as non-collagen synthesis.

Data are expressed as mean±SEM. Differences between groups were assessed by analysis of variance with subsequent Scfeffe's test.

RESULTS

The number of cells remained unchaged for 64 hours after A II treatmemt. Figure 1 depicts the time course of collagen synthesis in cardiac fibroblasts with A II treatment. 8 hours after addition of A II, collagen synthesis was elevated, peaked in 48 hours, and persisted for 64 hours. Basal collagen synthesis in SHR cells was 1.5-fold greater ($p<0.01$) than in WKY cells (Fig. 2). A II stimulated collagen synthesis in a dose-dependent manner. 24 hours after adding 1 μM A II, collagen synthesis increased by 230±18% in SHR cells and 204±19% in WKY cells (Fig. 2). To determine whether increased collagen synthesis was mediated by A II receptor, we examined the effect of the specific competitive inhibitor saralasin on A II-induced collagen synthesis. Saralasin blocked the A II-stimulated increase in collagen synthesis (Fig. 3).

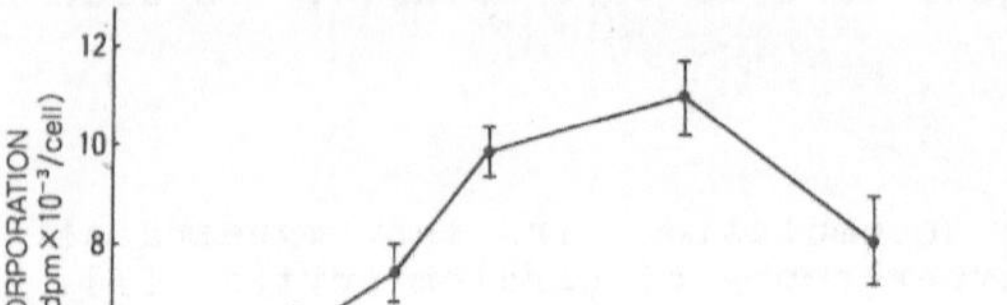

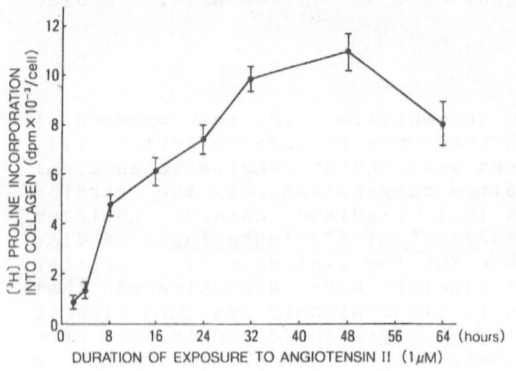

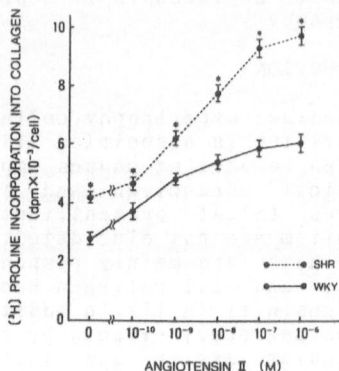

Fig. 1 Time course of collagen synthesis by WKY cariac fibroblasts after treatment with A II.

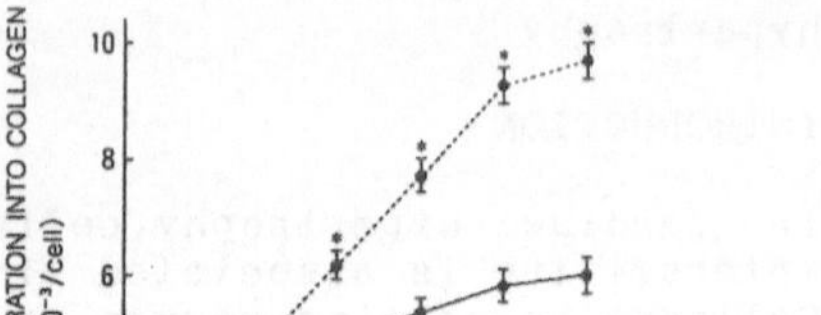

Fig. 2 Effect of A II on collagen synthesis by SHR and WKY cardiac fibroblasts. *$p<0.01$ vs. WKY

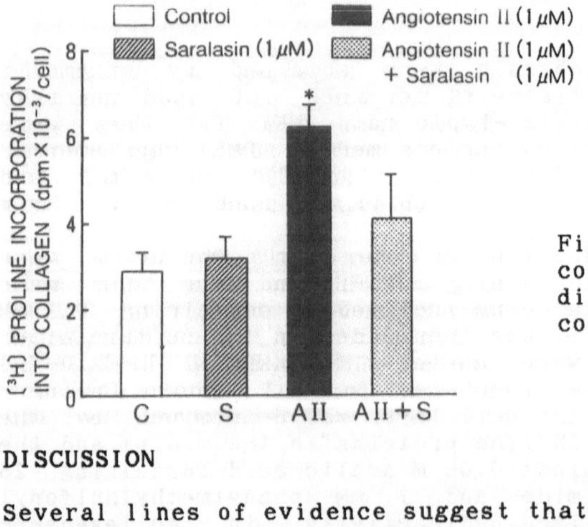

Fig. 3 Effect of saralasin on collagen synthesis by WKY cardiac fibroblasts. * $p<0.01$ vs. control

DISCUSSION

Several lines of evidence suggest that renin-angiotensin system is involved in an accumulation of fibrillar collagen in cardiac interstitium accompanied by cardiac hypertrophy. Brilla et al demonstrated that treatment with lisinopril in SHR with established left ventricular hypertrophy reversed interstitial collagen accumulation [6]. However, direct regulatory actions of A II on cardiac collagen biosynthesis have not been reported. Our results have demonstrated that A II does stimulate collagen synthesis by cardiac fibroblasts <u>in vitro</u>. This effect is dose-dependent and receptor-specific because it can be abolished by the competitive A

II inhibitor saralasin.

In vascular smooth muscle cells, A II stimulates protein synthesis and causes hypertrophy, not hyperplasia [7].Kato et al showed that A II stimulated collagen synthesis in vascular smooth muscle cells [8].These findings imply that A II provokes pathological vascular hypertrophy.Previous studies illustrated that A II activates phosphoinositide turnover,increases intracellular calcium and induces expressions of platelet-derived growth factor and the proto-oncogenes in vascular smooth muscle cells [9].Indeed,it may be the case in cardiac fibroblasts that A II induces collagen synthesis by the same mechanisms.Alternatively,it has been argued that other vasoactive substances and growth factors participate in this process.Transforming growth factor β1 is one candidate.This peptide stimulates collagen synthesis in vitro and in vivo [10].It is possible that A II indues transforming growth factor β1 gene expression and stimulates collagen synthesis in cardiac fibroblasts.

In summary,A II stimulated collagen synthesis in cardiac fibroblasts.Cardiac fibroblasts from SHR showed enhanced basal collagen synthesis and an increased response to A II.Thus,A II may play an important role in cardiac collagen accumulation in cardiac hypertrophy.

REFERENCES

1. Weber KT,Brilla CG (1991) Pathological hypertrophy and cardiac interstitium: Fibrosis and renin-angiotensin-aldosterone system. Circulation 83:1849-1865
2. Salzmann J-L,Labopin M,Belichard P,Camilleri J-P,Michel JB (1990) Collagen remodelling in cardiac hypertrophy. In: Swynghedauw B(ed) Research in Cardiac hypertrophy and failure.INSERM/John Libbey Eurotext.London Paris.pp293-309
3. Eghbali M,Czaja MJ,Zeydel M,Weiner FR,Zern MA,Seifter S,Blumenfeld OO (1988) Collagen chain mRNAs in isolated heart cells from young and adult rats.J Mol Cell Cardiol 20:267-276
4. Lindpaintner K, Ganten D (1991) The cardiac renin-angiotensin system: An appraisal of present experimental and clinical evidence. Circ Res 68:905-921
5. Peterkofsky B,Diegelmann R (1971) Use of a mixture of proteinase-free collagenases for the specific assay of radioactive collagen in the presence of other proteins.Biochemistry 10:988-994
6. Brilla CG,Janicki JS,Weber KT (1991) Cardioreparative effects of lisinopril in rats with genetic hypertension and left ventricular hypertrophy. Circulation 83:1771-1779
7. Geisterfer AAT,Peach MJ,Owens GK (1988) Angiotensin II induces hypertrophy, not hyperplasia, of cultured rat aortic smooth muscle cells.Circ Res 62:749-756
8. Kato H,Suzuki H,Tajima S,Ogata Y,Tominaga T,Sato A,Saruta T (1991) Angiotensin II stimulates collagen synthesis in cultured vascular smooth muscle cells. J Hypertens 9:17-22
9. Naftilan AJ,Pratt RE,Dzau VJ (1989) Induction of platelet-derived growth factor A-chain and c-myc gene expressions by angiotensin II in cultured rat vascular smooth muscle cells. J Clin Invest 83:1419-1424
10. Roberts AB,Sporn MB,Assoian RK,Smith JM,Roche NS,Wakefield LM,Heine UI,Liotta LA,Falanga V,Kehrl JH,Fauci AS (1986) Transforming growth factor type β: Rapid induction of fibrosis and angiogenesis in vivo and stimulation of collagen formation in vitro. Proc Natl Acad Sci USA 83:4167-4171

Polyphosphoinositide Metabolism in Hypertrophic Rat Heart

MIKAKO SHOKI, HIDEAKI KAWAGUCHI, HIROSHI OKAMOTO, HITOSHI SANO, HISAKAZU YASUDA, and AKIRA KITABATAKE

Department of Cardiovascular Medicine, Hokkaido University, School of Medicine, Sapporo, 060 Japan

KEYWORDS : Phosphatidylinositol, Phospholipase C, Cardiac Hypertrophy

INTRODUCTION

The metabolism of phosphatidylinositol-4,5-bisphosphate(PIP_2) has been studied extensively in the heart(1). The hydrolysis of PIP_2 generates two second messengers, inositol-1,4,5-trisphosphate(IP_3) and sn-1,2-diacylglycerol(DAG)(2). It is known that IP_3 mobilizes intracellular Ca^{2+}. DAG stimulates membrane-bound phospholipid-dependent, Ca^{2+}-dependent protein kinase C(PKC)(3). IP_3 may have an important role in controling Ca^{2+} levels after hormonal stimulation, but it remains to be proved that this phenomenon exists in cardiac cells. It has been reported that catecholamines, especialy α_1-adrenergic stimulation may cause myocardial hypertrophy, using neonatal rat heart cell cultures(4). However, its role in adult cardiac myocyte hypertrophy is not yet clear. We consider that this phospha-tidylinositol(PI)-turnover pathway has quite an important role in inducing cardiac myocyte hypertrophy, even in adult rat myocytes. The purpose of this experiment was to study the polyphosphoinositide metabolism in the hypertrophic adult rat heart.

MATERIALS AND METHODS

Animals: We used male spontaneously hypertensive rat (SHR) as hypertrophic rats aged 5,10 20,30 and 40 weeks old and age-matched male Wistar Kyoto rat (WKY) as normal controls.

Subcellular fractions: The left ventricule was minced and homogenized. The homogenate was centrifuged at 10,5000g for 60min. The resultant supernatant was used for each assay as the cytosolic fraction(5).

PI-PLC activity: The cytosolic fraction was incubated with [^{14}C]arachidonic acid-labeled phospholipids in 0.1 M Tris-HCl pH 7.0, 5 mM $CaCl_2$ for 2 min at 37 ℃(6). DAG and free AA were analysed by thin-layer chromatography(7).

PIP_2-PLC actibity: The cytosolic fraction was incubated with 50 μM of [^3H]PIP_2 in 50 mM Tris-HCl pH 6.5, 10 μM Ca^{2+} for 2 min at 37℃ and terminated by adding $CHCl_3$/MeOH(2:1,v/v) The radioactivity in the aqueous phase was counted.

IP_3 Kinase activity and IP_4 Phosphatase activity: Cytosolic fraction was incubated with 1 μM of [^3H]IP_3 in 50mM Tris-malate pH 7.0, 10 mM ATP, 20 mM $MgCl_2$, 5 mM 2,3-dephosphoglycerate and 10 μM Ca^{2+} for 20 min at 37℃(8). IP_3 and IP_4 were separated by AG-1 X8 columns with a gradient of ammonium formate(0.2-1.2M)(9). About the IP_4 phosphatase activity, the incubation mixture was the same as that of the IP_3 kinase without ATP.

Cellular response to norepinephrine: Cells ($3x10^{-5}$cells/35-mm dish) were incubated at 37℃ for 2 min with NE and 1mM $CaCl_2$ in the presence of 1μM of Metprolol. The reactions were terminated and extracted with $CHCl_3$/MeOH (1:2, v/v). IP_3 was separated above descrived method. The released DAG was determined by DAG assay sysem (Amersham, UK).(10)

RESULTS

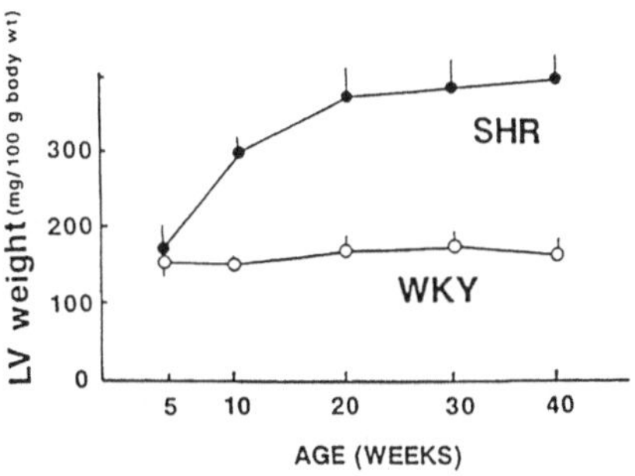

Fig.1 Left ventricular weight in SHR(●) was markedly increased compared to WKY(○) with age. (from ref. 1)

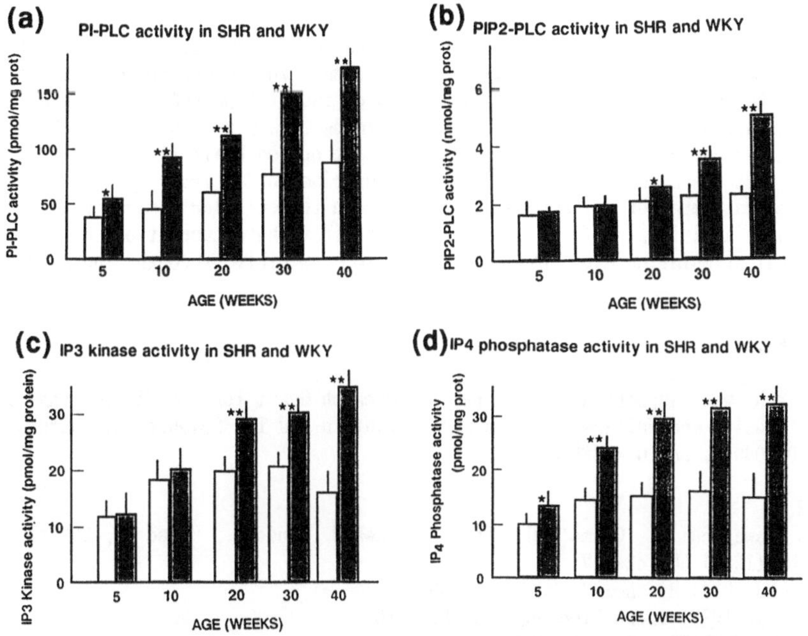

Fig.2

a:PI-PLC activity was significantly higher in SHR(■) compared with WKY(□)in all ages. Its activity of SHR at 40 weeks old was 3.3 fold higher compared with that of 5 weeks old.

b:In SHR(■) aged 20-40 weeks, PIP_2-PLC activity was increased compared with SHR aged 5-10 weeks and WKY(□) aged 20-40 weeks.

c:IP_3 kinase activity increased in SHR(■) with age compared with all ages except those between 20 and 30 weeks old. There were also significant increases in SHR aged 20-40 weeks compared with age-matched WKY(□)

d:IP_4 phosphatase activity was increased in SHR with age at 5-20 weeks. There were also significant differences between SHR (■) aged 5 weeks to 40 weeks and age-matched WKY(□). (from ref.1)

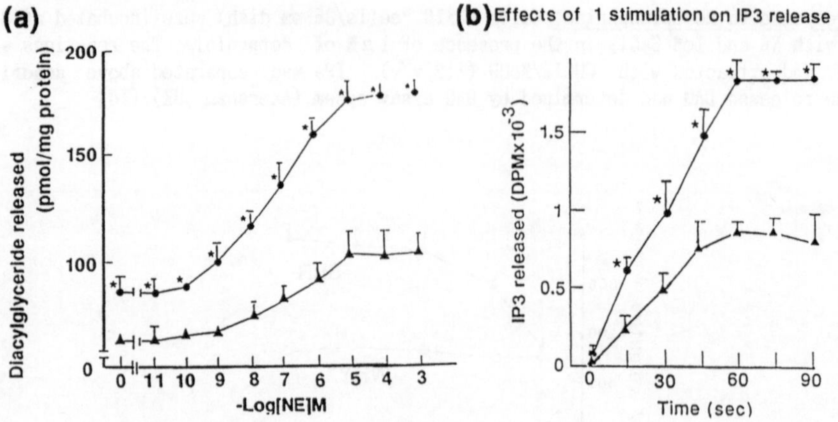

Fig.3
a:DAG release was markedly higher in SHR(●) than in WKY(▲) at the NE concentrations of 10^{-9} to 10^{-5} M in the presence of 1 μM of metoprolol. b:IP_3 release was markedly enhanced by 1 μM NE in SHR(●) compared with age-matched WKY(▲) in the presence of 1 μM of metprolol. (from ref.11)

DISCUSSION

In the present experiments in a cell free system, we demonstrated that basal levels of PLC, IP_3 kinase and IP_4 phosphatase activity increased in the cytosolic fraction of SHR compared to that of the WKY. But the accumulation of inositol polyphosphate under pathophys-iological conditions has not been studied. According to a previous study, the number of α_1-adrenergic receptors increases in SHR and hypertrophied heart (12). But there is a possibility that the stimulatoryeffect of norepinephrine in SHR myocytes is caused not only by the increased number of α_1-adrenergic receptor on the cellular membranebut also by the increased basal activity. These reports suggest that the accumulations of IP_3 and IP_4 after hormonal stimulation have physiological role, possibly through the alteration of Ca^{2+}levels.

ACKNOWLEDGMENT

This research was supported in part by a Research Grant for Cardiomyopathy from the Ministry of Health and Welfare of Japan and a Grant-in-Aid for Science and Culture of Japan, 01870041, 02404042, and 02454250.

REFERENCES

1. Shoki M. Kawaguchi H., Okamoto H., Sano H., Sawa H., Kudo T., Hirao N., Sakata Y., Yasuda H.,(1992) 56:142-147
2. Berridge MJ(1984) Biochem.J. 220: 345-360
3. Nishizuka Y.(1983) Trend Biochem. Sci. 8:13-16
4. Simpson P.(1986) Circ.Res. 56:884
5. Fujii S.,Kawaguchi H.,Okamoto H.,Saito H.,Togashi H.,Yasuda H.(1988) J.Mol.Cell Cardiol. 20:779
6. Renard D.,Poggioli J.(1987) FEBS lett. 217:117
7. Folch J.,Lee W., Sloane-Stanley GH.(1957) J.Biol.Chem. 226:497
8. Irvine RF.,Letcher AJ.,Heslop JP.,Berridge MJ.(1986) Nature 320:631
9. Dowmes CP.,Hawkins PT.,Irvin RF. (1986) Biochem. J. 238:501
10. Fukami K.,Takenawa T.(1989) J.Biol.Chem. 264: 14985-14989
11. Kawaguchi H., Shoki M., Sano H., Kudo T., Sawa H., Mochizuki N., Okamoto H., Endo Y., Kitabatake A. (1992) J. Mole. Cell Cardiol. in press.
12. Hanna MK., Khairallah PA.(1986) Arch.Int.Pharmacodyn.Ther. 283:80

Cardiovascular Effects of SK&F 64139, a PNMT Inhibitor, in Rats

TORU ENDO[1], HIROYUKI SATO[1], MASARU MINAMI[1] NAOYA HAMAUE[1], HIROKO TOGASHI[2], MITSUHIRO YOSHIOKA[2], and HIDEYA SAITO[2]

Department of Pharmacology, Faculty of Pharmaceutical Science, Higashi-Nippon-Gakuen University, Ishikari-Tobetsu, 061-02 Japan[1] and First Department of Pharmacology, Hokkaido University, Sapporo, 060 Japan[2]

KEYWORDS: SK&F 64139, PNMT inhibitor, cardiac nerve activity, catecholamine, vasodilating action

INTRODUCTION

PNMT catalyzes NE to Ep in the final steps of catecholamine synthesis. Pendleton et al. (1980) have reported that SK&F 64139 (SKF) is a potent and reversible inhibitor of PNMT (1). Because of the ability of SKF to cross the blood brain barrier (1), this compound lowers Ep levels both in the adrenal gland and in the CNS. The BP lowering effect of SKF was accompanied with a marked decrease in central PNMT activity. This further supports the interpretation that this is its main hypotensive mechanism (2). The present study was undertaken to elucidate the effects of SKF on BP, HR and adrenal catecholamine contents in rats. In order to elucidate the mechanism of cardiovascular effects induced by SKF, ICNA was also determined.

MATERIALS AND METHODS

General and ICNA recordings

Male Wistar rats (350-400g and 9-12 weeks old) were anesthetized with urethane (500mg/kg, i.p.) and α-chloralose (50mg/kg, i.p.). After immobilization was performed with gallamine triethiodide (10mg/kg, i.p.), respiration was maintained through a tracheal cannula connected to a rodent respirator (Harvard apparatus, Millis, MA, model 683). BP and HR were monitored continuously from the left femoral artery with a transducer (Nihon Koden, Tokyo, MPU-0.5A). Drugs were administered intravenously through a catheter inserted into the left vein. The inferior cardiac nerves were isolated from the right stellate ganglion and cut near the heart. ICNA was recorded from the central cut end of the nerve with bipolar platinum iridium wire electrodes as previously reported (3). ICNA was amplified, passed through a filter, displayed on an oscilloscope and quantified using a cumulative integrator (Nihon Koden, E1-601G). The amplified discharges were passed through a window discriminator (W-P Instruments, Hander, G, model 120). The discharge rates were counted by a real-time data analyzer (Nihon Koden, ATAC-450).

Catecholamine assay

Tissue NE, Ep and DA contents were measured using HPLC with an electrochemical detector (4). Protein was determined by the method of Lowry et al. (5).

Statistical analysis

Statistically significant differences were determined by Student's t-test. Values are expressed as mean ± SE.

---

[1]Abbreviation. PNMT, phenylethanolamine N-methyl-transferase; SK&F 64139 (SKF), 7-8-dichlorol, 2, 3, 4-tetrahydroisoquinoline; NE, norepinephrine; Ep, epinephrine; DA, dopamine; ICNA, inferior cardiac nerve activity; BP, blood pressure; HR, heart rate; CNS, central nervous system ; HPLC, high performance liquid chromatography.

RESULTS AND DISCUSSION

BP and HR

Maximal BP reduction was reached 15 min after SKF (5mg/kg and 10mg/kg, i.p.) administration and a significant hypotensive phase continued for up to 60 min. A dose-dependent reduction of HR was also observed after SKF was administered. Our data are in agreement with previous studies demonstrating the antihypertensive and bradycardic effects of SKF (1, 6). In present study, intracerebroventricular injection of SKF reduced the BP and the HR. SKF (5mg/kg, i.v.) increased the BP in spinalized rats. These results suggest that the central adrenergic mechanism may play a role in BP and HR regulation after SKF administration.

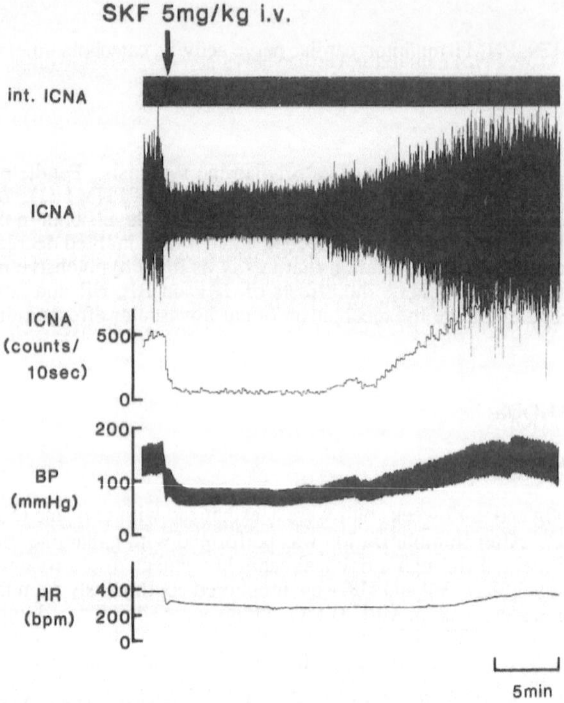

Fig.1. Effect of SKF on ICNA.

Effect on ICNA

A 5.0 mg/kg dose of SKF produced significant decreases in ICNA during the hypotensive phase (Fig. 1). SKF-induced ICNA changes coincided with changes in HR and BP after SKF injection. It has been reported that clonidine produced a decrease in HR and BP due to the reduction of central sympathetic outflow (7, 8). The negative chronotropic effect induced by SKF might be delivered mainly from the CNS.

Catecholamine contents

As shown in Fig.2, SKF-treated rats showed significant decreases in NE, Ep and DA levels of adrenal gland compared with those of vehicle-treated rats. This reduction may be due to sympathoinhibitory effect of SKF.

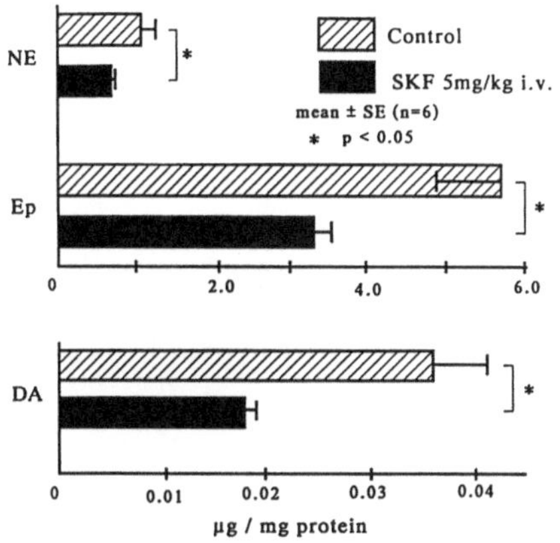

Fig.2 Effect of SKF on adrenal catecholamine content in rats.

In summary, SKF (i.v.) reduced BP, HR, adrenal catecholamine contents and ICNA in rats. In addition, central administration of SKF also decreased the BP and HR of rats. These findings suggest that the central sympathoinhibitory action of SKF may play an important role in SKF induced bradycardia. The bradycardic and vasodilatative actions induced by SKF may be useful in the treatment of the tachycardia and vasoconstriction of congestive heart failure.

REFERENCES

1.Pendleton, R. G., McCafferty, J. P., Roesler, J. M. (1980) The effect of PNMT inhibitors upon cardiovascular changes induced by hemorrhage in the rat. Eur. J. Pharmacol. 66, 1-10
2.Waeber, B., Gavras, H., Gavras, I., Chao, P., Kohlman, O., Bresnahan, M. R., Brunner, H. R., Vaughan, D. (1982) Evidence for a sodium-induced activation of central neurogenic mechanisms in one-kidney, one clip renal hypertensive rats. J. Pharmacol. Exp. Ther. 223, 510-515
3.Yoshioka, M., Matsumoto, M., Togashi, H., Minami, M., Saito. H. (1987) Central sympathoinhibitory action of katanserin in rats. J. Pharmacol. Exp. Ther. 243, 1174-1178.
4.Minami, M., Sano, M., Togashi, H., Sakurai, H., Saito, H. (1988) Stroke-related plasma norepinephrine, angiotensin II, arginine-vasopressin and serotonin concentrations in stroke-prone spontaneously hypertensive rats. In: Progress in hypertension, vol 1., H. Saito, H. Parvez, S. Parvez and Nagatsu (Eds), VSP, Vtrecht, pp89-114.
5.Lowry, O., Rosebrough, N., Farr, A. and Randall. R. (1951) Protein measurement with the folin phenol regent. J. Biol. Chem. 193, 265-275.
6.Biollaz, B., Biollaz, J., Kohlman, O., Jr., Bresnahan, M., Gavras, I. and Gavras, H. (1984) Acute cardiovascular effects of two central phenylethanolamine-N-methyl-transferase inhibitors in unanesthetized desoxycorticosterone-salt hypertensive rats. Eur. J. Pharmacol. 102, 515-519.
7.Isaac, L.(1980) Clonidine in the central nervous system: site of mechanism of hypotensive action. J. Cardiovasc. Pharmacol. 2(suppl 1), S5-S19.
8.Togashi, H.(1983) Central and peripheral effects of clonidine on the adrenal medullary function in spontaneously hypertensive rats. J.Pharmacol.Exp.Ther. 225, 191-197.

IX: Left Ventricular Hypertrophy and Myopathy

Expression of c-fos mRNA by Acute Pressure Overload in Perfused Rat Heart

JUNZO OSAKI, TAKASHI HANEDA, HIROTSUKA SAKAI, JUN FUKUZAWA, KIYOTAKA OKAMOTO, HIROKI TAKEDA, SETSUYA MIYATA, and SOKICHI ONODERA

First Department of Internal Medicine, Asahikawa Medical College, Asahikawa, 078 Japan

KEYWORDS : protooncogene c–fos, cAMP, protein synthesis, pressure overload

INTRODUCTION

It has been demonstrated that several mechanical or pharmacological overload to the heart induces immediate early gene expression such as protooncogenes and heat shock protein genes and accelerates the cardiac protein synthesis to lead to cardiac hypertrophy. Norepinephrine induces cardiac hypertrophy and specific gene expression in cultured rat cardiac myocytes via α_1–adrenergic receptor[1,2]. Mechanical stimuli (myocyte stretching) directly induce c–fos expression in cultured neonatal rat cardiac myocytes and this response was associated with protein kinase C activation[3,4]. In these experimental models the induction of specific protooncogene expression in response to several cardiac overload might be mediated by α_1–adrenergic receptor or protein kinase C–dependent signal transduction system. On the other hand, Morgan et al[5] have reported that increases in tissue cAMP content by acute pressure overload results in acceleration of protein synthesis rates in perfused adult rat hearts and that the effects of ventricular wall stretch by acute elevation of aortic pressure to accelerate synthesis may involve a cAMP–dependent protein synthesis mechanism. Our hypothesis was that protooncogene c–fos expression enhanced by acute pressure overload in adult rat hearts would play a transducing role in the cAMP–dependent protein synthesis mechanism in addition to protein kinase C–dependent mechanism. In the present study cAMP content, c–fos mRNA expression, and rates of protein synthesis were examined in adult rat hearts that were perfused at elevated aortic pressure or exposed to hormone receptor binding (glucagon) in order to determine whether c–fos expression by acute pressure overload coupled with an increase in cAMP content and continuously accelerated rates of protein synthesis.

MATERIALS AND METHODS

All animals used were male Sprague–Dawley rats, approximately 9–10 weeks old. Hearts were perfused as Langendorff preparations for 15 minutes with Krebs–Henseleit buffer containing normal plasma levels of 19 amino acids, 0.4 mM phenylalanine, and 15 mM glucose. The perfusate was maintained at 37°C and gassed with 95%O_2–5%CO_2. Following this preliminary perfusion, 20 ml of the same buffer containing 0.1% bovine serum albumin were recirculated at an aortic pressure of 60 mmHg. In experiments involving elevated perfusion pressure, aortic pressure was raised to 120 mmHg. Glucagon (1×10^{-6}M) was added to the perfusate at the beginning of recirculating perfusion. At the end of perfusion, hearts were rapidly frozen at the temperature of liquid nitrogen at time points indicated.

The cAMP content was measured by radioimmunoassay at 2 minutes of perfusion at aortic pressures of either 60 or 120 mmHg. Rates of protein synthesis were calculated by the incorporation of [^{14}C]phenylalanine (0.1 μCi/ml) into total heart protein during 2nd hour of perfusion using the specific radioactivity of phenylalanine in the perfusate.

Northern blot analyses were performed in hearts perfused for 2, 15, 30, 60, and 120 minutes. Total RNA was extracted using the acid guanidium–phenol–chloroform method. 15 μg of total RNA was electrophoretically fractionated through 1.2% agarose gels, and the quantity of RNA in each track was verified by ethidium bromide staining before transfer. The RNAs were blotted on the nylon membrane (Hybond–N+, Amersham). v–fos, 1.00 kb Pstl/Pvu2 fragment containing FBJ–MSV proviral DNA (TAKARA) was used as c–fos probe and labeled by random priming with [α-^{32}P]dCTP. Prehybridization and hybridization were carried out for 12 to 24 hours at 42°C in a solution containing 5×SSPE, 50% formamide, 5×Denhardt's solution, 0.5%SDS, and 20μg/ml sonicated salmon sperm DNA. After washing, membranes were exposed to X–Omat film for 2 or 3 days at –80°C and relative amounts of blots were determined by a densitometric scanner.

Comparisons were made initially using one–way analysis of variance (F–test). If the F–test was significant at $p<0.05$, the Dunnett method was used for subsequent comparisons between groups.

RESULTS

Both elevation of aortic pressure from 60 to 120 mmHg and exposure to glucagon at an aortic pressure of 60 mmHg in perfused rat hearts significantly increased tissue cAMP contents at 2 minutes of perfusion by 36% and 128%, respectively. Both elevated aortic pressure and glucagon significantly accelerated rates of protein synthesis during 2nd hour of perfusion by 43% and 46%, respectively (Table 1). In the next experiments, time course of c–fos mRNA expression was determined by Northern blot analysis (Fig.1 and Table 2). Basal levels of c–fos expression at an aortic pressure of 60mmHg could not be detected clearly at all time points. Elevation of aortic pressure from 60 to 120 mmHg rapidly increased c–fos transcript. Its expression was clearly detectable at 15, 30, and 60 minutes of perfusion, weakly at 120 minutes, and peaked at 15–30 minutes by 2.9–4.5–fold over control levels at the same time point. Exposure to glucagon at an aortic pressure of 60 mmHg also increased c–fos transcript. Its expression was clearly detectable at 15, 30, and 60 minutes of perfusion, weakly at 120 minutes, and peaked at 60 minutes by 2.3–fold over control levels at the same time point.

DISCUSSION

The molecular mechanism of signal transduction system to lead to cardiac hypertrophy by hemodynamic overload remains unknown. Several hemodynamic or pharmacological overload has been

Table 1 Effects of elevation of aortic pressure or exposure to glucagon on cAMP content and rates of protein synthesis.

Aortic pressure (mmHg)	Glucagon (10^{-6}M)	cAMP content (pmol/mg protein)	Rates of protein synthesis (nmol phenylalanine/g dry heart/hr)
60	–	4.49±0.54	673±83
120	–	6.09±0.91*	965±154*
60	+	10.23±1.37*	981±28*

cAMP contents were measured at 2 minutes of perfusion. Rates of protein synthesis were measured during 2nd hour of perfusion. Values represent means ± S.D. of 6–9 hearts.
* $p<0.05$ vs. at an aortic pressure of 60 mmHg without glucagon.

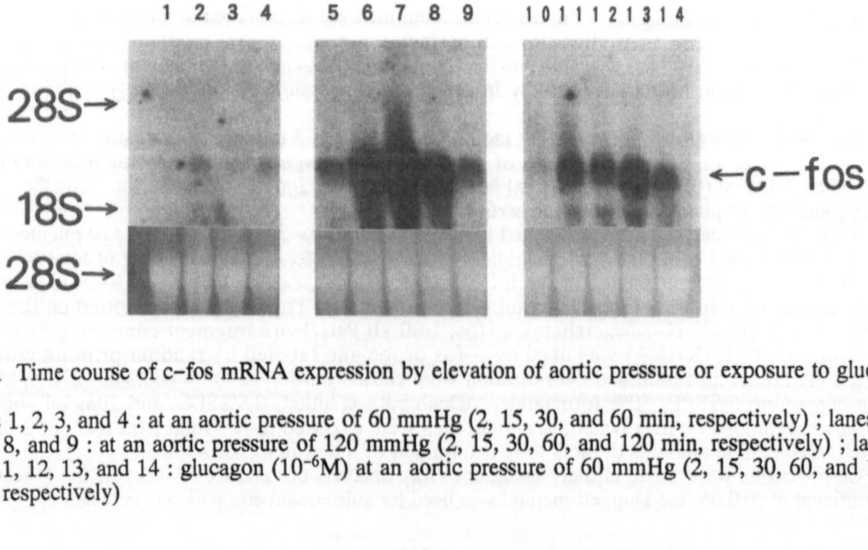

Fig.1 Time course of c–fos mRNA expression by elevation of aortic pressure or exposure to glucagon.
lanes 1, 2, 3, and 4 : at an aortic pressure of 60 mmHg (2, 15, 30, and 60 min, respectively) ; lanes 5, 6, 7, 8, and 9 : at an aortic pressure of 120 mmHg (2, 15, 30, 60, and 120 min, respectively) ; lanes 10, 11, 12, 13, and 14 : glucagon (10^{-6}M) at an aortic pressure of 60 mmHg (2, 15, 30, 60, and 120 min, respectively)

Table 2 The levels of c–fos mRNA expression at each time points by Northern blot analysis.

Aortic pressure (mmHg)	Glucagon (10^{-6}M)	Time of perfusion (min) 2	15	30	60	120
60	–	0.51±0.20	0.62±0.12	0.43±0.11	0.60±0.22	0.54±0.13
120	–	0.61±0.25	1.82±0.64*	1.95±0.62*	1.57±0.72*	1.02±0.25*
60	+	0.55±0.17	1.13±0.44	1.01±0.38	1.83±0.34*	0.81±0.24

The levels of mRNA expression are expressed as densitometry units.
Values represent means ± S.D. of 3–7 hearts.
*$p<0.05$ vs. at an aortic pressure of 60 mmHg without glucagon at the same time point.

reported to induce c–fos expression via α_1–adrenergic receptor or protein kinase C–dependent signal transduction system[1,2]. Recently, Komuro et al[3] have reported that exposure to protein kinase C stimulant (phorbol esters) intensely stimulates c–fos expression in cultured neonatal rat cardiac myocytes, but adenylate cyclase stimulant (forskolin) does it very slightly. Moreover, Komuro et al[4] suggest that mechanical stimuli (myocyte stretching) in cultured neonatal rat cardiac myocytes might directly induce cardiac hypertrophy and c–fos expression possibly via protein kinase C activation. These papers suggest that c–fos expression by hemodynamic overload may not be much associated by the cAMP–dependent mechanism.

Bauters et al[6] found that, in adult rat hearts, c–fos and c–myc protooncogenes expression was both sequentially and transitorily increased when the coronary flow was augmented. However, Kira et al[7] have reported that coronary flow could be dissociated from the stimulatory effect of higher aortic pressure on protein synthesis in adult rat hearts and that stretch of the ventricular wall, as a consequence of increased aortic pressure, could be the mechanical parameter most closely related to the increase in protein synthesis. In addition, Morgan et al[5] have reported that increases in tissue cAMP content by acute pressure overload or exposure to glucagon, forskolin, or IBMX accelerates rates of protein synthesis in perfused adult rat hearts. However, whether cAMP content regulates protooncogene c–fos mRNA expression and induces cardiac hypertrophy in adult rat hearts has not been investigated. The major findings of our experiments are that increased cAMP content at 2 minutes of perfusion by both elevated aortic pressure and exposure to glucagon in perfused adult rat hearts stimulates c–fos expression at 15, 30, and 60 minutes of perfusion and leads to acceleration of rates of protein synthesis during 2nd hour of perfusion. These results suggest that c–fos expression may couple with an increase in cAMP content and play a transducing role in the cAMP–dependent protein synthesis mechanism by acute pressure overload in adult rat hearts.

REFERENCES

1. Starksen NF, Simpson PC, Bishopric N, Coughlin SR, Lee WMF, Escobedo JA, Williams LT (1986) Cardiac myocyte hypertrophy is associated with c–myc protooncogene expression. Proc Natl Acad Sci USA 83 : 8348–8350
2. Ikeda U, Tsuruya Y, Yaginuma T (1991) α_1–Adrenergic stimulation is coupled to cardiac myocyte hypertrophy. Am J Physiol 260 : H953–H956
3. Komuro I, Katoh Y, Hoh E, Takaku F, Yazaki Y (1991) Mechanism of cardiac hypertrophy and injury —Possible role of protein kinase C activation— Jap Circ J 55 : 1149–1157
4. Komuro I, Katoh Y, Kaida T, Shibazaki Y, Kurabayashi M, Hoh E, Takaku F, Yazaki Y (1991) Mechanical loading stimulates cell hypertrophy and specific gene expression in cultured rat cardiac myocytes. J Biol Chem 266 : 1265–1268
5. Xenophontos XP, Watson PA, Chua BHL, Haneda T, Morgan HE (1989) Increased cyclic AMP content accelerates protein synthesis in rat heart. Circ Res 65 : 647–656
6. Bauters C, Moalic JM, Bercovici J, Mouas C, Emanoil–Ravier R, Schiaffino S, Swynghedauw B (1988) Coronary flow as a determinant of c–myc and c–fos proto–oncogene expression in an isolated adult rat heart. J Mol Cell Cardiol 20 : 97–101
7. Kira Y, Kochel PJ, Gordon EE, Morgan HE (1984) Aortic perfusion pressure as a determinant of cardiac protein synthesis. Am J Physiol 246 : C247–C258

Spontaneous Arrhythmias and Heart Rate Variability in Several Models of Cardiac Hypertrophy in Rat: a Holter Monitoring Study

FRANÇOIS CARRÉ, PHILIPPE COUMEL, RENÉ VICUNA, YVON LESSARD, SOPHIE BESSE, and BERNARD SWYNGHEDAUW
U 127-INSERM, Hopital Lariboisiére, Paris, France

KEY WORDS: experimental arrhythmias, supraventricular premature beats, aortic stenosis, cardiac hypertrophy, cardiothyrotoxicosis, heart rate variability, autonomous system, Holter.

Arrhythmias is a major risk factor in left ventricular hypertrophy (LVH) [6-9] and this is independent of the etiology and may occur whether coronary artery were normal or not. There are few animal models of arrhythmias [3, 10] and the capability of various models of cardiac hypertrophy to produce arrhythmias has been explored for the first time in our laboratory [3].

Spontaneous heart rate fluctuations, the so-called Heart Rate Variability (HRV), as others hemodynamics variables depends on the interaction of vagal and sympathetic nervous activity on the sinus node and studies of HRV constitute non invasives methods of investigation of the autonomic control of the cardio-vascular system [1, 4]. Recently clinical investigators have shown that HRV has a potential pharmacological interest [4] and could predict sudden death. Few studies were dealing with animals and more specially in the rat and none of them tried to correlate HRV to some biologicals parameters which better characterizes the autonomic nervous system [1, 2, 3].

The goal of the study was to summarize our recent findings concerning Holter monitoring in the rat and to show how it is possible to quantitate arrhythmias in unanesthetized animals in experimental models of cardiac hypertrophy [3]. In addition we would like topresent in a preliminary form our data concerning the analysis of HRV in the same animal species.

Methodology.

Thyrotoxicosis was produced in 2 month-old male Wistar rats by a daily intraperitoneal injection of L-thyroxine (0. 4 mg/kg body weight) for seven days. Abdominal aortic stenosis was performed by banding the suprarenal abdominal aorta [10, 11]. Senescent rats consists of 22 month-old animals. At that age they started to die spontaneously, the mortality rate being around 35-40 %.

Holter monitoring. The details of the technique have been previously published [3]. Electrodes were implanted under anesthesia in the back of the rat and attached on the inner part of the skin. They were connected through a swivel-tethering system to an amplifier and a Holter monitor running at 2 mm/s. The rats were placed into special cage and after 1-2 hours they began their normal day-time sleeping.

Data analysis. Recordings were printed and the total number of ventricular premature beats (VPB), supraventricular beats (SVPB), and atrio-ventricular block (AVB) were counted by visual analysis on comprimed printing report.

HRV analysis was performed_using a non spectral method previously described and validated in humans [4]. Briefly the programme is an ATREC II programme and consists in (i) digitazition and constitution of R-R intervals files, (ii) detection of short and long oscillations in the accelerations and deccelerations of heart rate. (iii) Results are displayed by the computer in terms of number of oscillations per time unit and mean amplitude in msec.The product amplitude times number of oscillations is expressed in msec. min^{-1}. It reflects the spectral power in frequency domain [Kauffman et al 1988; Coumel et al 1991]. (iv) For each rat we selected 3 samples of 5 minutes duration each according to the HR trends (low, medium and high).

Results.

Cardiac hypertrophy. Both thyrotoxicosis and banding aorta resulted in cardiac hypertrophy. Aortic stenosis also augmented atria and right ventricular weights. Senescence was associated with an increase in heart weight in mg, but the LVW/BW ratio was also augmented indicating a certain degree of mechanical overload in this model in spite of a normal blood pressure.

Arrhythmias. In normal young rats the mean 24h heart rate was 310 beats per min and premature beats were nearly absent. Cardiothyrotoxicosis resulted in a sinusal tachycardia and frequent (5/6) auriculo-ventricular block (AVB). No premature beats were seen. After banding abdominal aorta the incidence of supraventricular premature beats (SVPB) was increased [0.70 ± 0.3 SVPB per 24h in C *vs* 99 ± 61 in AS, $p<0.05$] while ventricular premature beats remained rare. During senescence all types of spontaneous arrhythmias, but specially supraventricular tachyarrhythmias, SVPB and AVB were frequent, most of the hearts had a permanent irregular activity [3].

HRV (preliminary data). As described above we made first a screening of differents central sequence in normal adult Wistar rats in order to select two groups of oscillations: Short Oscillations (SO) with a central sequence of 8-12 R-R intervals and border zones over 5 beats and Long Oscillations (L O) with a central sequence 15-30 R-R intervals and 5 beats border zone. SO were nearly abolished by atropine and insensitive to propranolol and are likely to be respiratory oscillations of the heart rate. In contrast LO were attenuated both by atropine and propranolol and seems to correspond to the sympathetic oscillations previously reported in human [1, 4].

The product amplitude times number of SO and LO are both negatively correlated with heart rate. Since isolated rat heart spontaneously beats at 2OO beats per min such a correlation is a clear indication that in vivo the heart rate of a rat is under a sympathetic control.

Preliminary data showed that the products amplitude times number remain unchanged by the process of hypertrophy. Nevertheless the situation in terms of heart rate fluctuations is not completely normal since for both SO and LO the product amplitude times number does not correlate with the heart rate as it normally does.

Discussion and conclusions.

Senescence and aortic stenosis in the rats represent valid experimental models of spontaneous arrhythmias occuring in the absence of ischemia or toxic agression. Spontaneous arrhythmias in rats has mainly a supraventricular origin. In the rat cardiothyrotoxicosis is a model of auriculoventricular block probably related to the tachycardia. Holter monitoring in rats may have several potential pathophysiological and pharmacological applications. In addition this technique allows the measurement of heart variability by a non spectral method of analysis.

The most striking feature of this study was the high incidence of arrhythmias during senescence. Old rats had almost no sinusal rate and the most frequent abnormalities were supraventricular arrhythmias. All senescent animals exhibited this type of electrical abnormalities. . Auriculo-ventricular blocks were also frequent and some typical examples of Luciani-Wenckebach periods were found. Whether the high lethality observed in this age group was due to arrhythmia has not been documented yet. With respect to arrhythmias, senescent rats resemble human [5, 6].

The high incidence of arrhythmias in pressure overloaded hearts is well-documented [4, 6, 7, 8, 9, 10]. In rats banding aorta results mostly in an increasing incidence of SVPB. Similar data have been reported in man [7, 8, 9]. The scarceness of ventricular premature beats in rats was unexpected and may be related either to the particularities of the calcium metabolism in this species, or only to the fact that abdominal aortic stenosis in the rat results in a well-compensated cardiac hypertrophy without failure even after several months, resembling to a hypertensive cardiopathy in man before the NYH stade I.

HRV was quantitated by non-spectral analysis [4], a method which allows to see the oscillations and to visually review the ECG recording.

This method was able to detect in the rat two heart rate oscillations as in human. One (SO) is vagally mediated and the other (LO) is mediated by both the vagus and the sympathetic systems. The control of the autonomous system on these two types of oscillations is confirmed by the correlation observed between heart rate and oscillations.

In this preliminary study HRV was not really affected by pressure overload since the amplitude times number product was unmodified for both SO and LO. Nevetheless we were able to show the limits of the process of adaptation since in hypertrophied hearts the two oscillations no more correlate with heart rate. no correlation between oscillations products and heart rate.

REFERENCES.

1. Akselrod S. Spectral analysis of fluctuations in cardiovascular parameters: a quantitative tool for the investigation of autonomous system. TIPS, 91: 6-9, 1988.

2. Benessiano J, Levy B, Samuel JL, Leclercq JF, Safar M, Saumont R. Circadian changes in heart rate in unasthetized normotensive and spontaneously hypertensive rats. Pflügers Arch 1983; 397: 70-72.

3. Carré F, Lessard Y, Coumel P, Ollivier L, Besse S, Lecarpentier Y, Swynghedauw B. Spontaneous arrhythmias in various models of cardiac hypertrophy and senescence in rats. A Holter monitoring study. Cardiovasc. Res. in press.

4. Coumel P, Hemida J, Wennerblöm B, Leenhardt A, Maisonblanche P, Cauchemez B. Heart rate variability in left ventricular hypertrophy and failure, and the effects of beta-blockade. A non-spectral analysis of heart rate variability in the frequency and the time domain. Eur. Heart J. 1991; 12: 412-422.

5. Fleg JL, Kennedy HL. Cardiac arrhythmias in a healthy elderly population. Chest 1982; 81: 302-307.

6. Levy D, Anderson K, Savage DD, Balkus SA, Kannel WB, CastelliWP. Risk of ventricular arrhythmias in left ventricular hypertrophy: The Framingham Heart Study. Am J Cardiol 1987; 60: 560-65.

7. Loaldi A, Pepi M, Gagostoni PG, Fiorentini C, Grazi S, Della-Bella P, Guazzi M. Cardiac rythm in hypertension assessed through 24 hours ambulatory electrocardiographic monitoring. Br Heart J 1983; 50: 118-126.

8. Mc Lenachan JM, Dargie HJ. A review of rythm disorders in cardiac hypertrophy. Am J Cardiol 1990; 65: 426-46.

9. Messerli FH, Ventura HO, Elilardi DJ, Dunn FG, Frohlich ED. Hypertension and sudden death. Increased ventricular ectopic activity in left ventricular hypertrophy. Am J Med 1984; 18-22.

10. Swynghedauw B. *Cardiac hypertrophy and failure.* Paris/London. INSERM/ J. Libbey pub.1990; 753 pp.

11. Swynghedauw B. *Experimentation animale en cardiologie.* Paris: INSERM-Flammarion 1987; 178 pp.

Does Angiotensin II Accelerate Protein Synthesis in Adult Rat Hearts?

TAKASHI HANEDA, JUN FUKUZAWA, SETSUYA MIYATA, JUNZO OSAKI,
YASUHIRO NAKAMURA, HIROTSUKA SAKAI, KIYOTAKA OKAMOTO,
HIROKI TAKEDA, and SOKICHI ONODERA
First Department of Internal Medicine, Asahikawa Medical College, Asahikawa, 078 Japan

KEYWORDS: angiotensin II, protein synthesis, adult rat heart, pressure overload

INTRODUCTION

Cardiac hypertrophy in regulated by a number of different processes such as hemodynamic load and circulating neurohumoral factors [1]. Angiotensin effects on cardiac hypertrophy are potentially of major importance and inhibitors of the renin–angiotensin system are effective therapeautic agents [2,3,4]. However, the effects of angiotensin II to stimulate cardiac hypertrophy could have been mediated by direct and indirect actions of the peptide on cardiac tissue. We have reported that elevation of aortic pressure in perfused adult rat hearts increases cAMP content and accelerates ribosomal formation and protein synthesis [5,6]. This model was used to examine the direct effects of angiotensin II on cardiac hypertrophy. The purpose of these expriments were to : 1) determine if angiotensin II accelerated rates of protein synthesis ; and 2) evaluate if angiotensin coverting enzyme (ACE) inhibitors prevented the effects of elevated aortic pressure on protein synthesis.

MATERIALS and METHODS

Hearts excised from male Sprague–Dawley rat (9–10 weeks–old) were perfused by Langendorff technique [5,6] with bicarbonate buffer gassed with 95%O2–5%CO2 and containing normal plasma levels of 19 amino acids, 0.4mM phenylanine and 15mM glucose. Following this preliminary perfusion, 20ml of perfusate were recirculated through hearts at an aortic pressure of 60 mmHg. In experiments involving elevated perfusion pressure, aortic pressure was raised to 120mmHg. Glucagon (1 X 10^{-6}M), angiotensin II (1 X 10^{-6}M) and ACE inhibitor, captopril (3.5 X 10^{-6}M), were added to the perfusate at the beginning of recirculating perfusion. At 2 min or 2 h of perfusion, hearts were frozen at the temperature of liquid nitrogen for measurements of cAMP content and rates of protein synthesis. cAMP contents at 2 min of perfusion were measured by RIA. Rates of total protein synthesis during 2nd h of perfusion were calculated from incorporation of [^{14}C] phenylalanine (0.1μCi/ml) into total heart protein using perfusate–specific radioactivity [6]. Myocardial contents in high energy phosphates were enzymatically determined in the same hearts used for measurements of protein synthesis rates.

RESULTS

Elevation of aortic pressure from 60mmHg to 120mmHg in perfused rat hearts increased cAMP content 27% and raised rates of protein synthesis 37% (Table 1). Glucagon, which increased cAMP content, also mimicked the effects of elevated aortic pressure on rates of protein synthesis (Table 1).

In the next series of experiments, angiotensin II and captopril were used to determine whether the renin–angiotensin system was involved in cardiac hypertrophy in adult rat hearts. Angiotensin II had no effect on cAMP content and protein synthesis in the hearts perfused at aortic pressures of 60 and 120 mmHg or with exposure to glucagon (Table 1). Captopril did not affect on cAMP content and protein synthesis in the hearts perfused at an aortic pressure of 60mmHg and failed to block the effects of elevated aortic pressure and glucagon on these parameters (Table 1).

Elevated aortic pressure, angiotensin II and captopril did not affect the levels of ATP, CrP, total adenine nucleotide and energy change potential (Table 2). Glucagon singnificantly increased CrP levels 23–42% in every group and did not change the levels of ATP, total adenine nucleotide and energy change potential (Table 2).

Table 1. Effects of elevated aortic pressure, glucagon, angiotensin II and captopril on cAMP content and total protein synthesis in perfused rat hearts

Additions	Aortic pressure (mmHg)	cAMP content (pmol·mg protein^{-1})	Protein synthesis (nmol phe·g dry heart^{-1}·h^{-1})
–	60	4.89±0.48	704± 90
–	120	6.21±1.02*	964±139*
glucagon	60	10.56±1.05*	981± 26*
angiotensin II	60	5.07±0.78	679±117
angiotensin II	120	6.57±0.63*	922± 99*
angiotensin II, glucagon	60	11.97±1.26*	941± 52*
captopril	60	5.49±0.33	720±109
captopril	120	7.17±0.96*	980±100*
captopril, glucagon	60	11.76±1.35*	985±107*

The levels of cAMP content or rates of protein synthesis were measured in 6–8 or 6–11 hearts, respectively, in each group. Values are mean±S.D.
*P<0.05 vs comparable parameter in hearts perfused at 60 mmHg in the absence of glucagon within the same group.

Table 2. Effects of elevated aortic pressure, glucagon and captopril on energy metabolism in perfused rat hearts

Additions	Aortic pressure (mmHg)	ATP	CrP	TAN	ECP
		(μmol·g dry weight^{-1})			
–	60	13.1±2.1	15.3±2.4	17.4±2.5	0.848±0.037
–	120	13.5±2.6	15.6±2.2	17.5±2.5	0.843±0.040
glucagon	60	13.4±1.6	21.7±2.7*	17.5±1.5	0.861±0.042
angiotensin II	60	13.6±2.2	16.2±3.0	17.6±2.6	0.853±0.025
angiotensin II	120	13.9±1.7	16.2±2.3	17.2±2.3	0.856±0.067
angiotensin II, glucagon	60	15.0±1.7	21.0±1.7*	18.7±2.0	0.868±0.038
captopril	60	13.7±2.0	16.0±1.9	17.0±2.6	0.876±0.027
captopril	120	13.6±2.4	15.6±2.4	17.0±3.1	0.878±0.020
captopril, glucagon	60	13.9±2.2	19.7±2.3*	18.1±2.2	0.861±0.026

TAN or ECP represents total adenine nucleotide or energy charge potential, respectively.
Values are mean±S.D. of 6–11 hearts.
*P<0.05 vs comparable parameter in hearts perfused at 60 mmHg in the absence of glucagon within the same group.

DISCUSSION

The renin–angiotensin system has emerged as a serious candidate in mediating cardiac myocyte growth. Kromer and Riegger [2] found that ACE inhibition reduced myocardial hypertrophy in experimental aortic stenosis in rats. Aceto and Baker [3] demonstrated that angiotensin II stimulated protein synthesis in cultured embryonic chick myocytes. Moreover, Baker et al reported that the pressure–overload cardiac hypertrophy in abdominal aorta–constricted rats was completely prevented by ACE inhibitor. These reports suggest that angiotensin II seems to play an important role in the regulation of cell growth and protein synthesis. On the other hand, Moalic et al [7] have reported that the expression of oncogenes coding for nuclear protein are not enhanced by angiotensin II in perfused adult rat hearts. Zierhut et al [8] showed that ACE inhibition did not reduce the development of cardiac hypertrophy in aortic constricted rats which were similar to experimental models used in the study made by Kromer and Riegger [2].

Since ACE inhibitors reduce total peripheral resistance and blood pressure, it is difficult or impossible to decide whether regression of cardiac hypertrophy is the result of the decreased afterload or a direct effect on the myocardium mediated by growth control. In our experiments of isolated perfused adult rat hearts, angiotensin II did not increase cAMP content and rates of protein synthesis and captopril failed to prevent the effects of elevated aortic pressure to increase cAMP content and rates of protein synthesis. These data strongly suggest that the renin–angiotensin system was not involved in the process of cardiac hypertrophy through mechanisms related to increased cardiac afterload and that as if angiotensin II could stimulate cardiac hypertrophy, its effects may have been mediated by indirect actions of the peptides on cardiac tissue. It has been demonstrated that adult rat ventricles have nearly no angiotensin II receptors in contrast to embryoric rat, rabbit and calf [9]. However, the reasons why angiotensin II has no effect on protein synthesis in our experimental model remain to be defined. Studies are in progress to evaluate whether and how the renin–angiotensin system involves in mediating cardiac hypertrophy.

REFERENCES

1. Morgan HE, Baker KM (1991) Cardiac hypertrophy–mechanical, neural, and endocrine dependnce–. Circulation 83: 13–25
2. Kromer EP, Riegger GAJ (1988) Effects of long–term angiotensin coverting enzyme inhibition on myocadial hypertrophy in experimental aortic stenosis in the rat. Am J Cardiol 62 : 161–163.
3. Aceto JF, Baker KM (1990) [Sar^1] angiotensin II receptor–mediated stimulation of protein synthesis in check heart cells. Am J Physiol 258 : H806–H813.
4. Baker KM, Cherinin MI, Wixson SK, Aceto JF (1990) Renin–angiotensin system involvement in pressure–overload cardiac hypertrophy in rats. Am J Physiol 259 : H324–H332.
5. Watson PA, Haneda T, Morgan HE (1989) Effect of higher aortic pressure on ribosome formation and cAMP content in rat heart. Am J Physiol 256:C1257–C1261.
6. Haneda T, Watson PA, Morgan HE (1989) Elevated aortic pressure, calcium uptake, and protein synthesis in rat heart. J Mol Cell Cardiol 21 (Suppl. I) : 131–138.
7. Moalic JM, Bauters C, Himbert D, Bercovici J, Mouas C, Guicheney P, Baudoin–Legros M, Rappaport L, Emanoil–Ravier R, Mezger V, Swynghedraw B (1989) Phenylephrine, vasopressin and angiotensin II as determinants of proto–oncogene and heat–shock protein gene expression in adult rat heart and aorta. J Hypertens 7 : 195–201.
8. Zierhut W, Zimmer HG, Gerdes AM (1991) Effect of angiotensin converting enzyme inhibition on pressure–induced left ventricular hypertrophy in rats. Circ Res 69 : 609–617.
9. Saito K, Gutkind JS, Saavedra JM (1987) Angiotensin II binding sites in the conduction system of rat hearts. Am J Physiol 253 : H1618–H1622.

Stretch Induces Hypertrophic Growth Through Renin-Angiotensin System in Cultured Neonatal Rat Myocytes

SETSUYA MIYATA, TAKASHI HANEDA, JUN FUKUZAWA, KIYOTAKA OKAMOTO, HIROKI TAKEDA, JUNZO OSAKI, HIROTSUKA SAKAI, and SOKICHI ONODERA
First Department of Internal Medicine, Asahikawa Medical College, Asahikawa, 078 Japan

KEYWORDS: angiotensin, cardiac hypertrophy, mechanical loading

INTRODUCTION

Cardiac hypertrophy occurs in response to various mechanical or hormonal stimuli [1]. Recentry, Baker et al [2] and Schunkert et al [3] reported that angiotensin-converting enzyme (ACE) activity, ACE mRNA expression, angiotensinogen mRNA expression and rate of angiotensin II production in heart were increased by pressure overload. Angiotensin II (A II) has two different receptors, such as type 1 angiotensin II receptor (AT_1) and type 2 angiotensin II receptor (AT_2) in heart [4].

In this study, we investigated whether stretch would increase RNA content and stimulate cell growth in neonatal cell cultures and whether renin-angiotensin system would be involved in stretch-induced cardiac hypertrophy in vitro.

MATERIALS and METHODS

Cell Culture

Primary cell cultures of cardiac myocytes were prepared from minced ventricular myocardium of 1-2 day old neonatal rats as described previously [5]. The myocytes were plated at a concentration of $4.1x10^5$ cells/2cm x 4cm x 1cm silicon dish which Yazaki's group originally created [6]. After an overnight incubation in MEM containing 10% newborn calf serum and 0.1mM BrdU at 37 °C in an atmosphere of 5% CO_2/95% room air, the attached cells were maintained in serum-free medium. The media were changed every 48 h over the time course of the experiments. The culture dishes were stretched by 15% from culture day 3 and passive stretch was maintained through the experiment. In some experiments, ACE inhibitor, captopril (10^{-6}M), or AT_1 antagonist, DuP753 (10^{-6}M) (gifted from Banyu C.O.), was added to media just before stretch stimulation. At the termination of the experiment, the cells layer were scraped with 0.5 ml volumes of 1x standard sodium citrate (SSC) containing 0.25% sodium dodecyl sulfate (SDS) and cell extracts were prepared from two dishes.

Total Protein, DNA and RNA Content

Protein content (μg/dish) in each culture dish was assayed by the method of Lowry. DNA content (μg/dish) in each culture dish was determined fluorometrically at an excitation wavelength of 360 nm and emission wavelength of 450 nm using 33258 Hoechst dye and calf thymus DNA as a standard. RNA content (μg/dish) in each culture dish was calculated by the absorbance at 260 and 232 nm as described by Munro and Fleck.

Rates of Protein Synthesis

In culture day 5, rates of protein synthesis was determined by assessing the incorporation of L-[U-^{14}C]phenylalanine (1 μCi/ml) for 2 h as described by McKee et al [7]. The cells were rapidly rinsed 3 times with ice-cold phosphate-buffered saline, incubated for 1 h on ice with 2 ml of 10% trichloroacetic acid, and dissolved in 0.5 ml of 1 N NaOH. Radioactivity was determined by liquid scintillation counting.

RESULTS

Stretch significantly increased RNA/DNA ratio by 14–16% at culture day 3 and 4 and Protein/DNA ratio by 21–22% at culture day 6 and 7 (Fig. 1 and 2). Rates of protein synthesis were determined to assess their contribution to protein contents during myocyte growth. Stretch significantly increased rates of protein synthesis by 15% (Table 1).

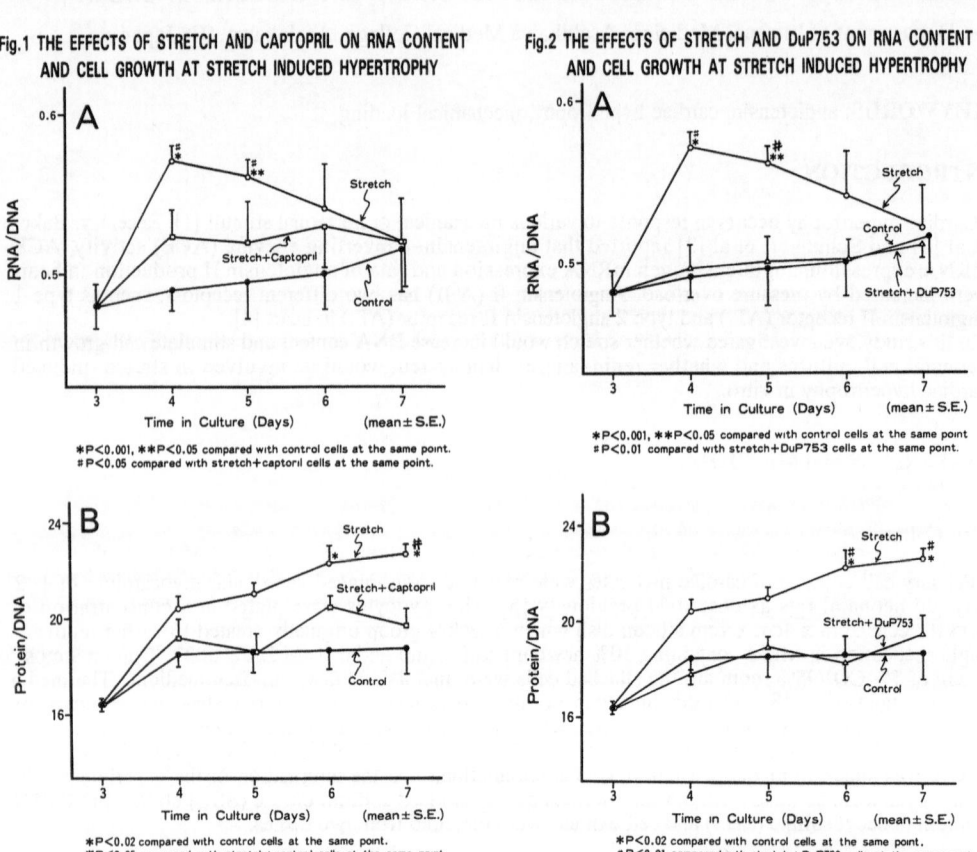

Fig.1 THE EFFECTS OF STRETCH AND CAPTOPRIL ON RNA CONTENT AND CELL GROWTH AT STRETCH INDUCED HYPERTROPHY

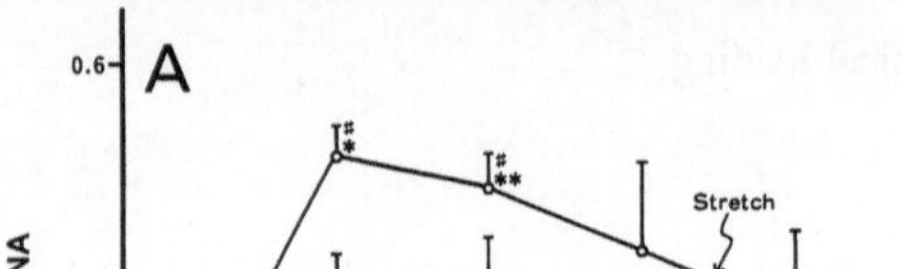

*P<0.001, **P<0.05 compared with control cells at the same point.
#P<0.05 compared with stretch+captopril cells at the same point.

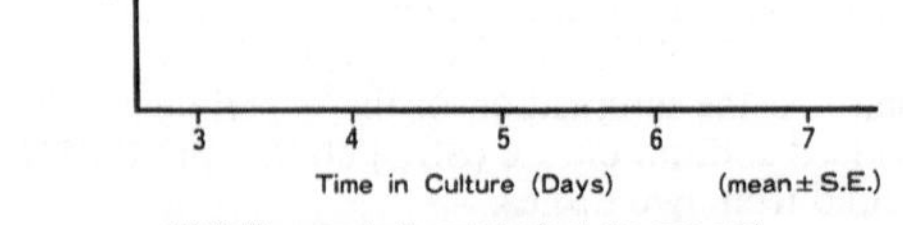

*P<0.02 compared with control cells at the same point.
#P<0.05 compared with stretch+captopril cells at the same point.

Fig.2 THE EFFECTS OF STRETCH AND DuP753 ON RNA CONTENT AND CELL GROWTH AT STRETCH INDUCED HYPERTROPHY

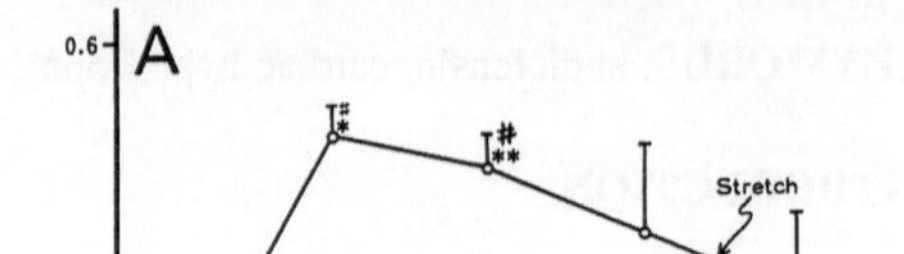

*P<0.001, **P<0.05 compared with control cells at the same point
#P<0.01 compared with stretch+DuP753 cells at the same point.

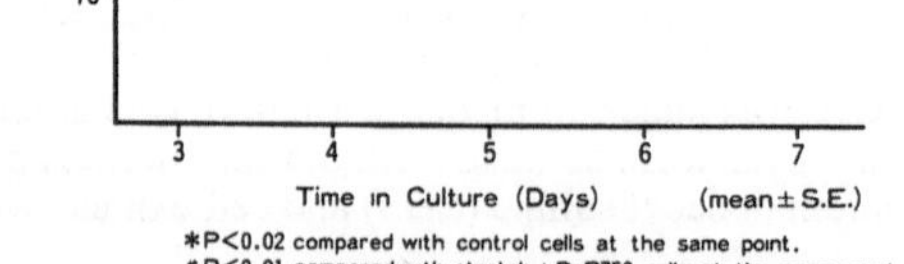

*P<0.02 compared with control cells at the same point.
#P<0.01 compared with stretch+DuP753 cells at the same point.

Fig. 1: Cardiocytes were stretched by 15% and captopril was added to a final concentration of 1x10⁻⁶M at culture day 3. Values at each point are mean±S.E. of 10 dishes in 5 different preparations.

Fig. 2: Cardiocytes were stretched by 15% and DuP753 was added to a final concentration of 1x10⁻⁶M at culture day 3. Values at each point are mean±S.E. of 10 dishes in 5 different preparations.

In the next experiments, whether ACE inhibitor or AT_1 antagonist prevented the effect of stretch on hypertrophic growth was studied. As shown in Fig. 1 and Table 1, captopril inhibited the increases in RNA/DNA ratio at culture day 4 and 5, and protein/DNA ratio at culture day 7 and the acceleration of protein synthesis rates induced by stretch. DuP753 also inhibited the increases in RNA/DNA ratio at culture day 4 and 5, and protein/DNA ratio at culture day 6 and 7 and the acceleration of protein synthesis rates induced by stretch as shown in Fig 2. and Table 1. Both captopril and DuP753 did not change RNA/DNA ratio, protein/DNA ratio and protein synthesis rates in non-stretched cells (data not shown).

Table 1. The effects of stretch and the inhibitory effects of captopril and DuP753 on [^{14}C] Phe incorporation.

	[^{14}C] Phe incorporation dpm/μg protein
Control	67.1±1.6
Stretch	73.9±1.7$^{*\,\$\,\#}$
Stretch+Captopril	66.0±2.1
Stretch+DuP753	65.5±1.1

Values are mean±S.E. of 6–10 dishes in 5 different preparations. $^{*}p<0.01$ vs. control, $^{\$}p<0.01$ vs. stretch+captopril, $^{\#}p<0.001$ vs. stretch+DuP753

DISCUSSION

Aceto and Baker [8] have reported that angiotensin II directly stimulates protein synthesis in cultured embrionic chick myocytes. Moreover, they have found that the renin–angiotensin system is a significant contributing factor to the cardiac hypertrophy that develops following abdominal aortic constriction in rats, suggesting that a localized cardiac renin–angiotensin system may have a paracrine or autocrine function in perpetuating the cell growth. On the other hand, Komuro et al [6] reported that passive stretching of neonatal cultured myocytes stimulated protein synthesis and induced the experession of c-fos protooncogene.

In the present study, we used the same experimental model that Komuro et al used and studied the relationship between passive stretch and the cardiac renin–angiotensin system. We found that stretching of myocytes increased RNA content and stimulated cell growth and that both ACE inhibitor and AT_1 antagonist prevented the increases of RNA content and the acceleration of cell growth by stretch. These results strongly suggest that activation of a localized cardiac renin–angiotensin system may be raised by stretch and that this activated system may have a autocrine or paracrine function in maintaining the cell growth process in this experimental model.

REFERENCES

1. Morgan HE, Baker KM (1991) Cardiac hypertrophy. Circulation 83: 13–25
2. Baker KM, Chernin MI, Wixson SK, Aceto JF (1990) Renin–angiotensin system in volvement in pressure-overload cardiac hypertrophy in rats. Am. J. Physiol. 259: H324–H332
3. Schunkert H, Dzau VJ, Tang SS, Hirsch AT, Apstein CS, Lorell BH (1990) Increased rat cardiac angiotensin converting enzyme activity and mRNA expression in pressure overload left ventricular hypertrophy. J. Clin. Invest. 86: 1913–1920
4. Rogers TB, Gaa ST and Allen IS (1986) Identification and characterization of functional angiotensin II receptors on cultured heart myocytes. J. Pharmacol. Exp. Ther. 236: 438–444
5. Haneda T, McDermott PJ (1991) Stimulation of ribosomal RNA synthesis during hypertrophic growth of cultured heart cell by phorbol ester. Mol. Cell. Biochem. 104: 169–177
6. Komuro I, Kaida T, Shibazaki Y, Kurabayashi M, Katoh Y, Hoh E, Takaku F, Yazaki Y(1990) Stretching cardiac myocytes stimulates protooncogene expression. J. Biol. Chem. 265: 3595–3598
7. McKee EE, Cheung JY, Rannels DE, Morgan HE (1978) Measurements of the rate of protein synthesis and compartmentation of heart phenylalanine. J. Biol. Chem. 253: 1030–1040
8. Aceto JF, Baker KM (1990) [Sar[1]] angiotensin II receptor-mediated stimulation of protein synthesis in chick heart cells. Am. J. Phisiol. 258: H806–H813

Does Hypertrophic Cardiomyopathy Change into Dilated Cardiomyopathy-Like Features?

MAREOMI HAMADA, MAKOTO SUZUKI, TAKASHI OHTANI, HIDEO KAWAKAMI, TAKAMASA KOBAYASHI, HIDEKI OKAYAMA, MITSUNORI ABE, HIROSHI MATSUOKA, TAKUMI SUMIMOTO, and KUNIO HIWADA

Second Department of Internal Medicine, Ehime University School of Medicine, Ehime, 791-02 Japan

KEYWORDS: hypertrophic cardiomyopathy, dilated cardiomyopathy, creatine kinase, MM isoforms, lactate dehydrogenase

INTRODUCTION

Hypertrophic cardiomyopathy sometimes progresses to dilated cardiomyopathy-like features [1-5]. The etiology of the progression remains to be determined. Recently, we reported a patient with hypertrophic cardiomyopathy who showed a persistent elevation of serum creatine kinase (CK)-MB and lactate dehydrogenase 1 (LDH1) activities for several years and developed dilated cardiomyopathy-like features [6]. Thus, the persistent elevation of cardiac enzymes might be closely related to the progression from a typical hypertrophic cardiomyopathy to a dilated left ventricle in the patient. To elucidate the prognosis of hypertrophic cardiomyopathy it is very important to know whether the cardiac enzymes elevation occurs usually in patients with hypertrophic cardiomyopathy or only in the specific type. The total CK activity of myocardial origin is composed of three different components, CK-MM, CK-MB and a lesser amount of CK-BB. CK-MM itself is also composed of three main isoforms, MMa, MMb and MMc. CK activity in the myocardium is primarily MMa, and in acute myocardial infarction a rapid and transient rise in MMa activity in the serum is observed. The serum MMa/MMc activity ratio is useful to estimate the process of myocardial injury due to myocardial infarction [7,8]. We recently reported that the measurement of MMa/MMc ratio was also useful to estimate the myocardial condition in patients with hypertrophic cardiomyopathy [9].

MATERIALS AND METHODS

Subjects

Twenty-two patients with hypertrophic cardiomyopathy (6 women and 16 men) and 14 normal controls (4 women and 10 men) participated in this study. The mean (±SD) systolic and diastolic blood pressures in patients with hypertrophic cardiomyopathy were 129±11 and 80±6 mmHg, respectively. The mean value of serum creatinine was 0.96±0.22 mg/dl. These values showed no significant differences between hypertrophic cardiomyopathy and normal controls. The mean ages of patients with hypertrophic cardiomyopathy and normal controls were 50±14 and 46±16 years, respectively.

Biochemical Procedures

<u>Measurement of total CK activity and CK-MB activity</u>
Venous blood was taken in the morning after overnight fasting, and the serum was stored at -70 °C until assayed. Total CK activity was assayed with the Merchauto CK (MERCK, Darmstadt, Germany) by a method based on the recommendations of the German Society for Clinical Chemistry [10]. Serum CK-MB activity was measured by cellulose acetate electrophoresis and fluorescence scanning using the modified of Wong& Swallen [11].

<u>Determination of CK-MM isoforms</u>
CK-MM isoform activity was assayed by a recently developed quantitative system in which the sample is subjected to high-voltage electrophoresis on dynamically cooled agarose gels (rapid electrophoresis: REP system, Helena Laboratories, Beaumont, TX, U.S.A) [9].

RESULTS

The total serum CK activity was 98.4±43.2 i.u./l in normal controls and 111.0±27.2 i.u./l in patients with hypertrophic cardiomyopathy. Serum CK-MB activity was significantly higher in patients with hypertrophic cardiomyopathy (7.8±3.8 i.u./l) than in normal controls (0.4±0.8 i.u./l, $p<0.01$). The MMa, MMb and MMc isoforms in normal controls comprised 11.3±3.0%, 21.5±4.4% and 40.7±11.5% of total CK-MM activity, and these values were significantly different from those in patients with hypertrophic cardiomyopathy (19.4±4.1%, 26.7±2.5% and 33.5±7.0%). As shown in Fig.1, the MMa/MMc activity ratio in patients with hypertrophic cardiomyopathy was significantly higher than that in normal controls. Fig.2 shows 201-thallium myocardial scintigrams in a patient progressed from typical hypertrophic cardiomyopathy into dilated cardiomyopathy-like features. On myocardial scintigram in 1988, hypoperfusion areas, as indicated by arrows, markedly extended. In this patient, persistent elevations of serum CK-MB between 3.0% and 8.5%, and LDH1 between 58.0% and 66.0% were observed for several years. The MMa/MMc activity ratio in this patient was 0.79.

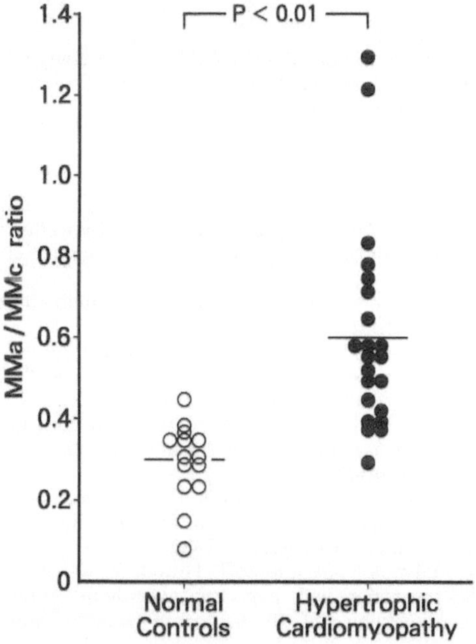

Fig. 1 Comparison of the MMa/MMc activity ratio in normal controls and patients with hypertrophic cardiomyopathy (Modified from ref. 9, with permission)

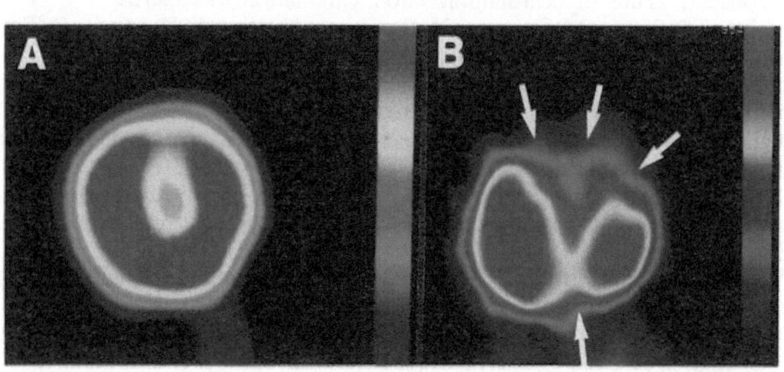

Fig. 2 Short axial tomograms in 201-thallium SPECT (A:1985, B:1988; from ref.6, with permission)

DISCUSSION

The results in this study show that a small amount of the myocardial tissue isoform of CK-MM (MMa) was constantly released in many patients with hypertrophic cardiomyopathy. This finding supports our previous observation of a persistent elevation of CK-MB and LDH1 activities in many patients with hypertrophic cardiomyopathy [12]. Several mechanisms for the release of MMa into the circulation in hypertrophic cardiomyopathy are possible. Myocardial ischemia seems to be one of the important factors. An inappropriate myocardial mass in relation to coronary arterial size [1], an abnormality of the intramural coronary arteries [13] and a decreased vasodilator reserve of coronary arteries [14] may contribute to myocardial ischemia in patients with hypertrophic cardiomyopathy. As shown in our presented patient [6], biochemical changes which suggest the evolution of hypertrophic cardiomyopathy into dilated cardiomyopathy-like features occur long before the echocardiographic method can detect any morphological changes. Therefore, to clarify the clinical course of hypertrophic cardiomyopathy, it is very important to check the serial changes of isoforms of CK and isoenzymes of CK and LDH.

CONCLUSION

A small amount of myocardial tissue isoform of CK-MM (MMa) is constantly released in many patients with hypertrophic cardiomyopathy. This finding points to a mechanism for hypertrophic cardiomyopathy to change, over time, to dilated cardiomyopathy-like features.

REFERENCES

1. Maron BJ, Epstein SE, Roberts WC (1979) Hypertrophic cardiomyopathy and transmural myocardial infarction without significant atherosclerosis of the extramural coronary arteries. Am J Cardiol 43:1086-1102
2. Ten Cate FJ, Roelandt J (1979) Progression to left ventricular dilatation in patients with hypertrophic obstructive cardiomyopathy. Am Heart J 97:762-765
3. Fujiwara H, Onodera T, Tanaka M, Shirane H, Kato H, Yoshikawa J, Osakada G, Sasayama S, Kawai C (1984) Progression from hypertrophic obstructive cardiomyopathy to dilated cardiomyopathy-like features in the end stage. Jpn Circ J 48:1210-1214
4. Yutani C, Imakita M, Ishibashi-Ueda H, Hatanaka K, Nagata S, Sakakibara H, Nimura Y (1985) Three autopsy cases of progression to left ventricular dilatation in patients with hypertrophic cardiomyopathy. Am Heart J 109:545-553
5. Nagata S, Park YD, Minamikawa T, Yutani C, Kamiya T, Nishimura T, Kozuka T, Sakakibara H, Nimura Y (1985) Thallium perfusion and cardiac enzyme abnormalities in patients with familial hypertrophic cardiomyopathy. Am Heart J 109:1317-1322
6. Hamada M, Shigematsu Y, Fujiwara Y, Sumimoto T, Hiwada K, Kokubu T (1990) Persistent elevation of cardiac enzymes in a patient with hypertrophic cardiomyopathy. With special reference to electrocardiographic, echocardiographic and 201-thallium myocardial scintigraphic findings. Jpn Circ J 54:354-360
7. Morelli RL, Carlson CJ, Emilson B, Abendschein DR, Rapaport E (1983) Serum creatine kinase MM isoenzyme subbands after acute myocardial infarction in man. Circulation 67:1283-1289
8. Jaffe AS, Serota H, Grace A, Sobel BE (1986) Diagnostic changes in plasma creatine kinase isoforms early after the onset of acute myocardial infarction. Circulation 74:105-109
9. Hamada M, Ohtani T, Sekiya M, Fujiwara Y, Sumimoto T, Hiwada K, Morita S, Tsukada H (1991) Serum creatine kinase MM isoforms in hypertrophic cardiomyopathy. Clin Sci 81:723-726
10. Recommendations of the German Society for Clinical Chemistry. Standardization of methods for the estimation of enzyme activities in biological fluids. (1977) J Clin Chem Clin Biochem 15:255-260
11. Wong R, Swallen TO (1975) Cellulose acetate electrophoresis of creatine phosphokinase isoenzymes in the diagnosis of myocardial infarction. Am J Clin Pathol 64:209-216
12. Hamada M, Ohtani T, Shigematsu Y, Fujiwara Y, Sumimoto T, Hiwada K (1990) Persistent elevations of serum cardiac enzymes in patients with hypertrophic cardiomyopathy [Abstract]. Jpn Circ J 54:786
13. Maron BJ, Wolfson JK, Epstein SE, Roberts WC (1986) Intramural (" small vessel ") coronary artery disease in hypertrophic cardiomyopathy. J Am Coll Cardiol 8:545-557
14. Cannon RO, Rosing DR, Maron BJ, Leon MB, Bonow RO, Watson RM, Epstein SE (1985) Myocardial ischemia in patients with hypertrophic cardiomyopathy: contribution of inadequate vasodilator reserve and elevated left ventricular filling pressures. Circulation 71;234-243

Likage Analyses of Familial Hypertrophic Cardiomyopathy

NUNECHIKA NOGUCHI, HIROKI SATO, HISAO ONOZUKA, TAISEI MIKAMI, MASAYUKI HASHIMOTO, HISAKAZU YASUDA, and AKIRA KITABATAKE

Departments of Cardiovascular Medicine, Hokkaido University, Sapporo, 060 Japan

keywords: linkage analyses, familial HCM, cardiac myosin heavy chain, PALB, missense mutation

INTRODUCTION

Hypertrophic cardiomyopathy (HCM) is a clinically and genetically heterogeneous disease. Nearly half of HCM shows familial occurrence wit hautosomal dominant inheritance. To investigate the causative genes of familial HCM, we performed linkage analyses by using RFLP (Restriction Fragment Length Polymorphism) method. In addition, we used SSCP(Single-strand Conformation Polymorphism) method to detect missense mutations within the beta cardiac myosin heavy chain(βMHC)which is known to be one of the causative genes for familial HCM.

CLINICAL ANALYSES

To identify a DNA marker linked to the gene responsible for HCM, family members with familial HCM were evaluated clinically. The diagnosis of HCM was based on the two-dimensional echo-cardiographic demonstration of unexplained left ventricular hypertrophy[1]and was made without knowledge of DNA patterns. None of the familiy members evaluated had a history of systemic hypertension or a·resting blood pressure greater than 140/90 mm Hg.

GENE-MAPPING STUDIES

Lymphoblastoid cell lines which were established by Epstein-Barr virus transformation or peripheral nuclear cells, were obtained from each family members. The samples of DNA were digested with a restriction enzyme, fractionated on 1% agarose gels, and transferred to transfer membrane. DNA probes were labeled and hybridized to transfer membrane. Filters were washed under conditions of high stringency and subjected to autoradiography for 24 to 72 hours with intensifying screens at -70°C[2].

RESULTS AND DISCUSSION

Seidman,C.E. has previously reported that maximum lod score of D14S26 which is located near βMHC is more than 9[3],and that different missense mutations in the βMHC can be identified in approximately 50 percents of families with HCM[4,5,6]. Therefore, we began our analyses with D14S26. But, we found crossing-overs between the causative genes and D14S26 in at least 3 Japanese familial HCM families. In addition, crossing-overs between βMHC and the causative genes have been confirmed by PCR-RFLP method ,and no missense mutation of MHC detected by SSCP method. These results demonstrated that familial HCM is a genetically heterogeneous disease.

Then we performed linkage analyses by using the other DNA markers. Only PALB which is located on chromosome 18q11.2-12.1[7,8] was co-inherited with the locus for familial HCM.

CONCLUSIONS

The causative loci for familial HCM are closely linked with PALB and missense mutation of βMHC appears uncommon in our family members with familial HCM.

REFERENCES

1. Maron BJ,Nichols PF,Pickle LD,Wesley YE,Mulvihill JJ (1984) Patterns of inheritance in hypertrophic cardiomyopathy assessment by M-mode and two-dimensional echocardiography. Am J Cardiol 53: 1087-1094.
2. Southern EN (1975) Detection of specific sequence among DNA fragments separated by gel electrophoresis. J Mol Biol 18:503-515.
3. Jarcho JA,McKenna W,Pare JAP,Solomon SD,Holcombe RF,Dickie S,Levi T, Donis-Keller H,Seidman JG,Seidman CE (1989) Mapping a gene for familial hypertrophic cardiomyopathy to chromosome 14q1. N Engl J Med 321: 1372-1378.
4. Tanigawa G,Jarcho JA,Kass S,Solomon SD,Vosberg HP,Seidman JG,Seidman CE (1990) A molecular basis for familial hypertrophic cardiomyopathy: α/β cardiac myosin heavy chain hybrid gene. Cell 62:991-998.
5. Geisterfer-Lowrence AA,Kass S,Tanigawa G,Vosberg HP,McKenna W,Seidman CE,Seidman JG (1990) A molecular basis for familial hypertrophic cardiomyopathy: A β cardiac myosin heavy chain gene missense mutation. Cell 62: 999-1006.
6. Watkins H,Rosenzweig A,Hwang DS,Levi T,McKenna W,Seidman CE,Seidman JG (1992) Characteristics and prognostic implications of myosin missen mutations in familial hypertrophic cardiomyopathy. N Engl J Med 326: 1108-1114.
7. Yoshikawa K,Yoshikawa N,Nakabeppu K,Sakaki Y.(1986) Two RFLPs associated with the human prealbumin gene(PALB). Nucl Acids Res 14: 3147.
8. Nishi H,Kimura A,Sasaki M,Wakisaka A,Matsuyama K,Koga Y,Toshima H, Sasazuki T (1989) Localization of the gene for hypertrophic cardiomyopathy to chromosome 18q. Circulation 80 (Suppl.II):II-457.

Presence of Angiotensinogen and Renin mRNAs and Angiotensinogen Protein in the Human Heart

YUKA ENDO[1], NAOKI MOCHIZUKI[1], HIROFUMI SAWA[1], FUMIO TOKUCHI[2], TOSHIYA SHINOHARA[2], YASUSHI FURUTA[2], HIDEAKI KAWAGUCHI[1], HISAKAZU YASUDA[1], AKIRA KITABATAKE[1], and KAZUO NAGASHIMA[2]

Departments of Cardiovascular Medicine[1] and Pathology[2], Hokkaido University School of Medicine, Sapporo, 060 Japan

KEY WORDS: renin, angiotensinogen, mRNA, immunohistochemistry, human heart

INTRODUCTION

The renin-angiotensin system acts to constrict vessels and enhance renal retention of sodium and water to raise the blood pressure. Angiotensinogen (ang-n) is synthesized in the liver and released into the blood. It is cut by renin, which is produced by the kidneys, and becomes angiotensin I. Angiotensin I is cleaved by angiotensin converting enzyme (ACE) into angiotensin II, which is an active pressor substance. Recently, the presence of cardiac renin-angiotensin system has been reported in some animals [1,2,3] but it has not been investigated fully in the human heart. Angiotensin II appears to be a stimulus for cardiac hypertrophy [4]. In clinical studies, ACE inhibitor has been reported to cause regression of cardiac hypertrophy [5]. Bearing these findings in mind, we studied the presence of ang-n, renin mRNAs and ang-n protein in human autopsy hearts and discussed its relation to cardiac hypertrophy.

MATERIALS AND METHODS

For ribonuclease protection assay (RPA) and reverse transcription (RT)-PCR analysis, RNAs from various organs obtained within 3 hours of death at autopsy were extracted using RNAzol followed by the acid guanidinium thiocyanate-phenol-chloroform method [6]. The expression of ang-n mRNA was examined using RPA, and renin mRNA was studied by RT-PCR, as renin mRNA had been not detected using RPA previously. For RPA of ang-n, human ang-n cDNA (sequence no. 395 to. 1805) [7] was inserted into the vector pAM 19 bidirectionally, then RPA was performed on several parts of the left ventricle (papillary muscle, endocardial layer, midcardial layer, epicardial layer, and conduction system), atrium and liver, using an RPA Kit (Ambion, Inc., Austin Texas). For RT-PCR analysis of renin, first we designed an upstream primer included in exon 8 and a downstream primer in exon 9 [8], composing of 20 bases respectively. cDNAs synthesized from RNAs of various organs using MuLV transcriptase mixed with random hexamer and RNase inhibitor were amplified by 20 cycles of PCR after the addition of both primers. The amplified products were electrophoresed and transferred to nitrocellulose membrane, then detected with digoxigenin-labeled renin cDNA using a chemiluminescence reaction. Immunohistochemical study on ang-n was carried out on nondiseased hearts and on a hypertrophic cardiomyopathic heart with a monoclonal antibody to human ang-n (a synthetic peptide, composed of 13 amino acids) developed newly using the *in vitro* immunization method, followed by the avidin-biotin peroxidase complex method.

RESULTS

RPA of Angiotensinogen in the Human Heart

An antisense cRNA probe used in this study was derived from the RNA vector (pAM 19) cleaved with Bst EII. RPA demonstrated that a single band of 407 nucleotides in length was protected in the liver, three layers of left ventricle, conduction system which contains His and major branching bundles and right atrium. In addition, the amount of ang-n mRNA from the epicardial layer was less than that from the endocardial layer in two cases of nondiseased hearts. The sense cRNA probe used as a negative control did not hybridize with RNAs from liver and heart. These results indicated that ang-n mRNA was present in human hearts and was expressed with a distributional difference.

RT-PCR of Renin in the Human Heart

RT-PCR of RNAs from human organs showed that target renin mRNA from the left ventricle, right atrium and kidney were amplified successfully, recognized on 1% agarose gels. The length of amplified complementary DNA fragments (241 bp) was quite different from that of the genomic DNA (441 bp) used as a positive control, which was confirmed using Southern blot analysis with human renin DNA labeled with digoxigenin. These results indicated that renin mRNA existed in the human heart.

Immunohistochemical Studies of Nondiseased and Hypertrophic Cardiomyopathic Hearts

Immunohistochemical analysis of ang-n was performed on the tissues fixed with 4% paraformaldehyde at 4℃ over night and embedded in paraffin. A positive immunoreaction was observed in the right atrium of both diseased and non-diseased hearts. However, the immunoreactivity in the left ventricles of nondiseased and hypertrophic cardiomyopathic heart was different. Positive immunoreactivity was found only in the subendocardium and conduction system in nondiseased hearts (Fig.1). On the other hand, intense and wide spread immunoreactivity was observed in the hypertrophic cardiomyopathic heart (Fig. 2). In control sections, no immunoreaction was found with pre-immune serum or pre-absorbed antiserum. These results revealed that ang-n protein which was present in specific areas of the nondiseased hearts seemed to become widely distributed and over expressed in the hypertrophic cardiomyopathic heart.

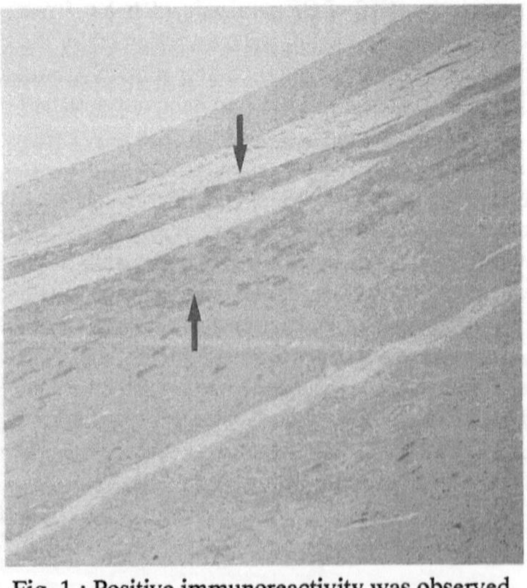

Fig. 1 : Positive immunoreactivity was observed in the subendocardial layer of the left ventricle in normal heart (arrow).

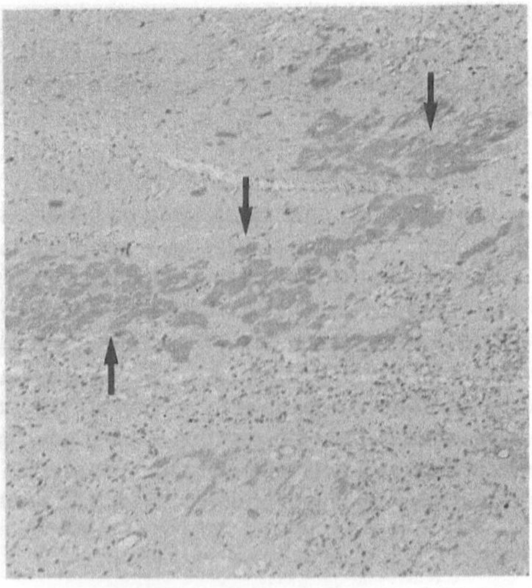

Fig. 2 : Wide spread immunoreactivity was found in the left ventricle of hypertrophic-cardiomyopathicheart(arrow).

DISCUSSION

In the present studies, we could demonstrate the presence of ang-n mRNA [9] and renin mRNA, suggesting the existence of the tissue renin-angiotensin system in the human heart. Before this study, we tried to examine the presence of renin mRNA using RPA. However, we could not detect the renin mRNA in human heart probably due to small amount of its message. When we applied RT-PCR method, we could show the presence of renin mRNA in human hearts. To confirme whether renin mRNA is translated into protein in the human heart, further immunohistochemical and/or biochemical studies will be required. In the present studies, we could point out that the localization and expression of angiotensinogen were different between the hearts without diseases and in the heart with HCM. Competitive RT-PCR and immunohistochemical study on renin are needed to examine the difference between those states. Tissue renin-angiotensin system in human heart may affect hypertrophic change of myocardium, though in the present we could not rule out the influence of the circulating renin-angiotensin system. The examination of the other element of the tissue renin-angiotensin system especially the presence of ACE in human heart will be further necessitated.

CONCLUSIONS

Angiotensinogen mRNA was detected in the human heart by RPA. Renin mRNA was also detected in the human heart by RT-PCR. Immunohistochemical studies showed that protein of ang-n was more abundant in the endocardial layer than in the epicardial layer of the hearts without diseases. This specific localization was consistent with that of ang-n mRNA. In the hypertrophied heart, ang-n was found to be widespread with intense immunoreactivity being observed in the ventricle, suggesting some role of tissue renin-angiotensin system in the human cardiac disorders.

REFERENCES

1.Kunapuli SP, Kumar A (1987) Molecular cloning of human angiotensinogen cDNA and evidence for the presence of its mRNA in rat heart. Circ Res 60: 786-790

2.Dzau VJ, Ellison KE, Brody T, Ingelfinger J, Pratt RE (1987) A comparative study of the distribution of renin and angiotensinogen messenger ribonucleic acid in rat and mouse tissues. Endocrinology 120: 2334-2338

3.Campbell DJ, Habener JF (1989) Hybridization in situ studies of angiotensinogen gene expression in rat adrenal and lung. Endocrinology 124 : 218-222

4.Khairallah PA, Robertson AL, Davila D (1972) Effect of angiotensin II on DNA, RNA and protein synthesis. In : Genest J, Koiw E (eds) Hypertension'72. New York, Springer-Verlag:212-220

5.Dzau VJ (1987) Evolution of the clinical management of hypertension. Am J Med 82 (suppl 1A):36-43

6.Chomczynski P, Sacchi N (1987) Single-step method of RNA isolation by acid guanidinium thiocyanate-phenol- chloroform extraction. Anal Biochem 162:156-159

7.Kageyama R, Ohkubo H, Nakanishi S (1984) Primary structure of human preangiotensinogen deduced from cloned cDNA sequence. Biochemistry 23:3603-3609

8.Imai T, Miyazaki H, Hirose S, Hori H, Hayashi T, Kageyama R, Ohkubo H, Nakanishi S, Murakami K (1983) Cloning and sequence analysis of cDNA for human renin precursor. Proc Natl Acad Sci USA 80:7405-7409

9.Sawa H, Tokuchi F, Mochizuki N, Endo Y, Furuta Y, Shinohara T, Takada A, Kawaguchi H, Yasuda H, Nagashima K (1992) Expression of the angiotensinogen gene and localization of its protein in the human heart. Circulation 86 (in press)

Alteration in Cardiac Renin-Angiotensin System in Spontaneously Hypertensive Rats (SHR)

TOSHIYUKI KUDO, HIROSHI OKAMOTO, NAOKI MOCHIZUKI, YUKA ENDO, HITOSHI SANO, KENJI IIZUKA, MIKAKO SHOKI, HIDEAKI KAWAGUCHI, AKIRA KITABATAKE, and HISAKAZU YASUDA

Department of Cardiovascular Medicine, Hokkaido University, Sapporo, 060 Japan

KEYWORDS: Angiotensinogen m-RNA, Angiotensin-converting enzyme (ACE), Spontaneously Hypertensive Rats (SHR)

INTRODUCTION

It has been demonstrated that components of the renin-angiotensin system such as renin, angiotensinogen (ATN), angiotensin-converting enzyme (ACE) and angiotensin II receptor exist within the heart and function independently from circulating renin-angiotensin system [1-4]. The potent myotropic actions of angiotensin II, as well as its effects on positive inotropism and chronotropism, make it likely that the heart is the site of a locally active renin-angiotensin system. It is suggested that angiotensin II is one of the contributing factors to regulation of cell growth, moreover, ACE inhibitors regress left ventricular hypertrophy. The purpose of this study is to determine whether intrinsic renin-angiotensin system play a role for the development and the regression of left ventricular hypertrophy in spontaneously hypertensive rats (SHR).

MATERIALS AND METHODS

Male SHR aged 11 weeks were divided into 6 groups and were assigned to administration of atenolol (A), bunazosin (B), captopril (C), nifedipine (N), trichlormethiazide (T) for 4 weeks and compared with a group without treatment (CONT) and age-, sex-matched Wistar Kyoto rats (WKY). After measurement of blood pressure, left ventricle (LV) was removed and membrane fraction was prepared. Total RNA was extracted and angiotensinogen (ATN) m-RNA was identified by ribonuclease protection assay. Angiotensin-converting enzyme (ACE) activity was determined in membrane fraction using radioassay by the method of Tess et al [5].

RESULTS

Systolic Blood Pressure

SHRs without treatment (15 weeks of age) had significantly higher systolic blood pressure compared with that in age- and sexmatched WKY rats ($p<0.001$). Antihypertensive treatment lowered systolic blood pressure in each group compared with that of SHRs without treatment. In groups treated with Ca antagonist and ACE inhibitor, systolic blood pressure showed decreases to the level of WKY rats (Figure 1).

Left ventricular weight-to-body weight ratio (LV/BW)

Figure 2 shows the left ventricular weight-to-body weight ratio (LV/BW). The LV/BW was significantly higher in SHRs compared with WKY rats. Antihypertensive treatment significantly decreased this ratio in each group.

Figure 1 Systolic Blood Pressure

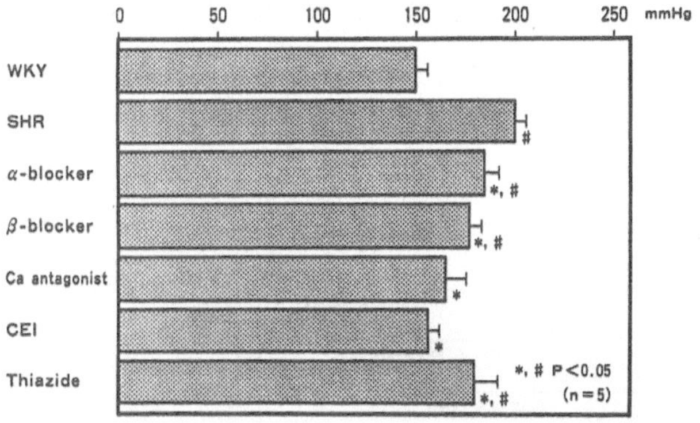

WKY, Wistar-Kyoto rats; SHR, spontaneously hypertensive rats;
α-blocker, SHRs treated with bunazosin (10 mg/Kg/day);
β-blocker, SHRs treated with atenolol (20 mg/Kg/day);
Ca antagonist, SHRs treated with nifedipine (20 mg/Kg/day);
CEI, SHRs treated with captopril (30 mg/Kg/day);
Thiazide, SHRs treated with trichlormethiazide (5 mg/Kg/day)
* $p<0.05$ v.s. control SHRs
# $p<0.05$ v.s. WKY rats without treatment

Figure 2 Left Ventricular Weight-to-Body Weight Ratio

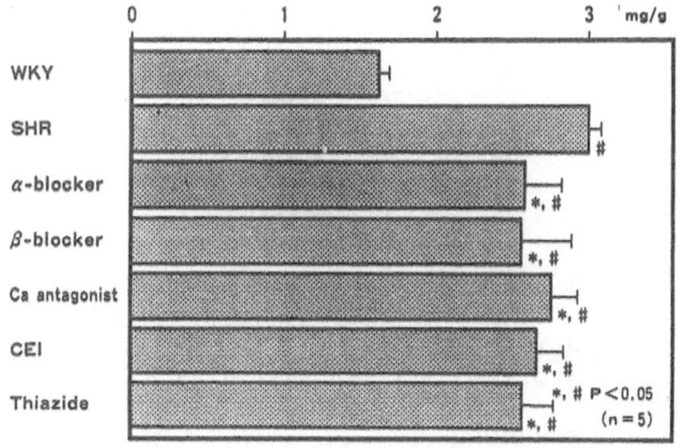

Angiotensin-Converting Enzyme (ACE) Activity

SHRs without treatment had a twofold higher ACE activity in left ventricular membrane fraction (0.127 nmol/mg protein) compared with WKY rats (0.067 nmol/mg protein). In each group treated with anti-hypertensive drugs, ACE activity was decreased [(C): 0.074, (N): 0.103, (T): 0.086, (B): 0.107, (A): 0.093 nmol/mg protein]. In SHRs treated with captopril and trichlormethiazide, ACE activity showed decreases to the level of WKR rats.(Figure 3)

Angiotensinogen (ATN) m-RNA Expression

Ribonuclease protection assay demonstrated angiotensinogen (ATN) m-RNA expression in the left ventricles. The electropholeic migration of cardiac ATN m-RNA was identical with rat hepatic angiotensinogen m-RNA, which used as a positive control (Lane 8). In left ventricular tissue from SHRs without treatment (Lane 2), cardiac ATN m-RNA showed two-fold higher signals than in WKY rats (Lane 1). The signal density for ATN m-RNA was determined by densitometry. In each group treated with antihypertensive drugs, the signals for ATN m-RNA were decreased to the level in WKY rats without treatment.(Figure 4)

Figure 3 ACE Activity in Membrane Fraction

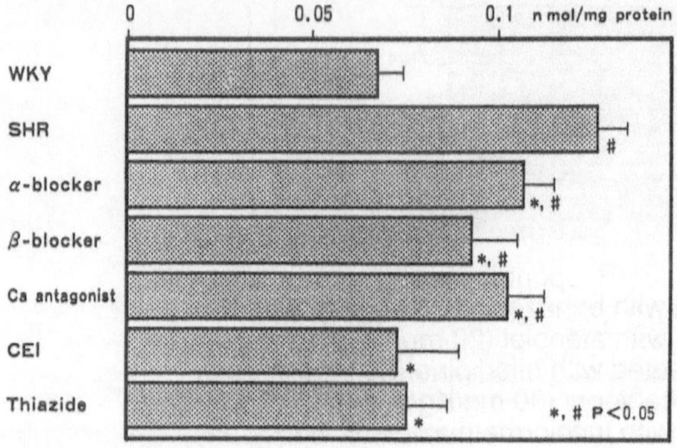

Figure 4 Angiotensinogen (ATN) m-RNA Expression

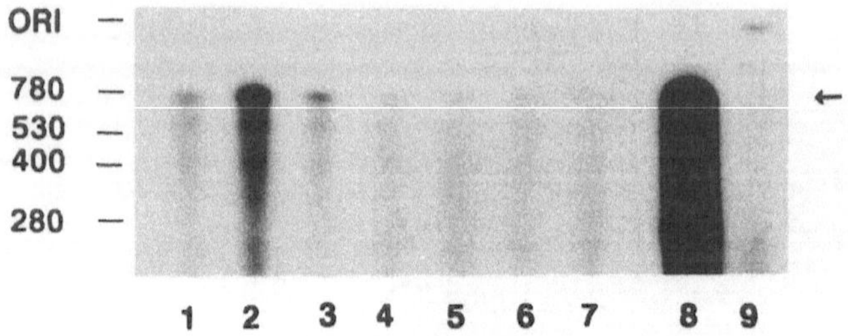

ORI indicates the origin of the applied samples.
The arrow indicates the position of RNA probe for ATN (712 base).
Lane 1, WKY rats;
Lane 2, SHRs without treatment;
Lane 3, SHRs treated with bunazosin;
Lane 4, SHRs treated with atenolol;
Lane 5, SHRs treated with nifedipine;
Lane 6, SHRs treated with captopril;
Lane 7, SHRs treated with trichlormethiazide;
Lane 8, Positive control for ATN m-RNA.

DISCUSSION

It is suggested that angiotensin II is a potent factor that regulate cell growth. It has been also demonstrated that components of renin-angiotensin system (RAS) exist within the heart. Thus, local production of angiotensin II may be responsible for the development of left ventricular hypertrophy (LVH). The present study was undertaken to determine whether intrinsic RAS is involved in the LVH and whether any alterations in cardiac RAS associated with the antihypertensive action can be demonstrated. The results showed a increased expression of angiotensinogen m-RNA and a higher ACE activity in hypertrophied heart of SHR. Antihypertensive treatment might have reversed the enhanced intrinsic RAS despite those different actions on blood pressure, which may lead to the regression of LVH. It has been found that angiotensin II stimulate protein synthesis in cultured cardiomyocytes [6]. This phenomenon was prevented by the Angiotensin II receptor antagonists. These direct effects of angiotensin II may be due to the activation of phospholipase C, which results in increases in inositol-1,4,5-triphosphate, diacylglycerol and proteinkinase C (PKC) activation [7]. Thus, cardiac RAS may play an significant role for the development of LVH. However, it is not known whether the other components such as renin and angiotensin II receptor can alter with pressure overload and other stimulations. Further studies are needed to elucidate the role of local renin-angiotensin system within the heart.

REFERENCES

1. Ohkubo H, Nakayama K, Tanaka T, Nakanishi S (1986) Tissue distribution of rat angiotensinogen mRNA and structural analysis of its heterogeneity. J Biol Chem 261:319-323

2. Lindpaintner K, Wilhelm MJ, Jin M, Unger T, Lang RE, Schoelkens BA, Ganten D (1987) Tissue renin-angiotensin systems: Focus on the heart. J Hypertens 5(suppl 2): S33-S38

3. Murphy TJ, Alexander RW, Griendling KK, Runge MS, Bernstein KE (1991) Isolation of a cDNA encoding the vasculat type-1 angiotensin II receptor. Nature 351: 233-236

4. Hirsch AT, Talsness CE, Schunkert H, Paul M, Dzau VJ (1991) Tissue-specific activation of cardiac angiotensin converting enzyme in experimental heart failure. Circ Res 69: 475-482

5. Stewart TA, Weare JA, Erdos EG (1981) Human peptidyl dipeptidase (converting enzyme, kininase II). Methods in Enzymology 80; 450

6. Baker KM, Aceto JF (1990) Angiotensin II stimulation of protein synthesis and cell growth in chick heart cells. Am J Physiol 259: H324-H332

7. Simpson P (1983) Norepinephrine-stimulated hypertrophy of cultured rat myocardial cells through an alpha1-adrenergic response. J Clin Invest 72: 732-738

Keywords Index